*A Mother's Work*

MEGAN VANGORDER

## *A Mother's Work*
Mary Bickerdyke, Civil War–Era Nurse

The University of North Carolina Press  *Chapel Hill*

*This book was published with the assistance of the Greensboro Women's Fund of the University of North Carolina Press.*

© 2026 Megan VanGorder
All rights reserved
Set in Arno Pro by Westchester Publishing Services
Manufactured in the United States of America

Library of Congress Cataloging-in-Publication Data
Names: VanGorder, Megan author
Title: A mother's work : Mary Bickerdyke, Civil War–era nurse / Megan VanGorder.
Description: Chapel Hill : The University of North Carolina Press, 2026. | Includes bibliographical references and index.
Identifiers: LCCN 2025045118 | ISBN 9781469692319 cloth | ISBN 9781469692326 paperback | ISBN 9781469692333 epub | ISBN 9781469692340 pdf
Subjects: LCSH: Bickerdyke, Mary, 1817–1901 | Women—United States—Social conditions—19th century | Motherhood—Social aspects—United States | Nursing—United States—History | Women nurses—United States—History | United States—History—Civil War, 1861–1865—Medical care | BISAC: MEDICAL / History | HISTORY / United States / State & Local / Midwest (IA, IL, IN, KS, MI, MN, MO, ND, NE, OH, SD, WI) | LCGFT: Biographies
Classification: LCC E467.1.B54 V36 2026 | DDC 973.7/75092 [B]—dc23/eng/20251114
LC record available at https://lccn.loc.gov/2025045118

Cover art: *Mary (Mother) Bickerdyke in Ohio,* 1898. Special Collections and Archives, Knox College Library, Galesburg, Illinois.

Parts of chapter 6 were published as "Special Acts of Justice: Mary Bickerdyke and the Extension of Civil War Veteran Care," *Indiana Magazine of History* 125, no. 2 (June 2025): 69–102. DOI: 10.2979/imh.0070. Reprinted with permission. No part of it may be reproduced, stored in a retrieval system, transmitted, or distributed in any form, by any means, electronic, mechanical, photographic, or otherwise, without the prior permission of Indiana University Press. For educational reuse, please contact the Copyright Clearance Center (https://www.copyright.com/). For all other permissions, contact IU Press at (http://iupress.org/meet/rights-and-permissions//).

For product safety concerns under the European Union's General Product Safety Regulation (EU GPSR), please contact gpsr@mare-nostrum.co.uk or write to the University of North Carolina Press and Mare Nostrum Group B.V., Mauritskade 21D, 1091 GC Amsterdam, The Netherlands.

*For "my boys"—David, Asa, Harrison, and Simon.*

## Contents

*List of Illustrations* ix
*Preface* xi
*Acknowledgments* xvii

Introduction 1

CHAPTER ONE
Mother, Before the War 14

CHAPTER TWO
Becoming Mother: The Civil War and the Development of Bickerdyke's Public Motherhood (1861–1863) 39

CHAPTER THREE
She Ranks Me: Asserting Motherhood in the Civil War (1863–1865) 68

CHAPTER FOUR
Mother-Guardian: Negotiating Institutional Care after the Civil War 94

CHAPTER FIVE
Mother-Nurse: Care-Switching Between Private and Public Motherhood 112

CHAPTER SIX
Special Acts of Justice: Mary Bickerdyke and Pension Claims 135

CHAPTER SEVEN
The Passing of the Mother: Mary Bickerdyke and Constructed Remembrance 155

Epilogue: What Did Mother Mean? 183

*Notes* 189
*Bibliography* 219
*Index* 235

## Illustrations

FIGURES

0.1  Mother Bickerdyke statue (illustration)  xii
0.2  Mother Bickerdyke statue at the Knox County Courthouse in Galesburg, Illinois  xiv
1.1  Dr. Benjamin Woodward and his wife Amanda, 1863  26
1.2  James Bickerdyke, age 16  35
1.3  Hiram Bickerdyke, age 5  36
2.1  Mary Jane Safford, "Angel of Cairo," 1867 engraving  44
2.2  Mary Ann Bickerdyke, "Mother" Bickerdyke, 1866 engraving  45
2.3  Florence Nightingale, "Lady with a Lamp"  61
2.4  "Midnight on the Battlefield"  61
2.5  Letter written by Mrs. Abbott  65
2.6  Sherman Abbott's gravesite  66
4.1  Illinois Soldiers' Orphans' Building in Normal, Illinois  99
4.2  Bickerdyke Hotel in Salina, Kansas  106
5.1  Organizers of the United States Sanitary Commission  115
5.2  Swift's Specific advertisement, 1886  127
5.3  Receipt for Mrs. J. H. Temmen, MD  128
5.4  Receipt for doctor providing Mollie Bickerdyke's cancer care  133
5.5  Dr. Brumbaugh's breast cancer treatment receipt  133
6.1  Mother Bickerdyke's memorial hymn card  137
E.1  Hiram's hieroglyphs  187

TABLES

3.1  1860 US Census data comparison of Chicago Sanitary Commission workers  82
7.1  Comparative Black literacy in Russell County, Kansas, 1880  160

## Preface

"Mother" Mary Bickerdyke's profound impact on the Civil War generation deserved a permanent and distinguished marker. And so, in the years after her death in 1901, the Mother Bickerdyke Memorial Association was formed in Galesburg, Illinois, to properly honor her life, which was dedicated to the care of the town's soldiers who had become aging veterans.[1] As the fiftieth anniversary of the Civil War approached, public interest in remembering Mother Bickerdyke after her death mirrored the memorial trends of the time.[2] In the early 1900s, monument fever captivated Civil War memorialists, and the Mother Bickerdyke Memorial Association set out to raise funds for a large public statue in her honor.

In 1904, the association commissioned Theo Alice Ruggles Kitson, a decorated Boston sculptor, to create a massive fourteen-ton bronze statue depicting Bickerdyke's compassionate care on the Civil War battlefield. The monument was set to be prominently displayed in front of the Knox County Courthouse in the heart of Galesburg, Illinois, Bickerdyke's hometown during the Civil War.[3] Before this commission, Kitson had completed a series of sculptures and relief portraits for the Vicksburg Memorial Park, where Mary Bickerdyke served as an agent and nurse for the United States Sanitary Commission in the aftermath of the 1863 siege.

This was to be the first major monument erected to celebrate a woman's Civil War service, and the American public took note. The press announced and recorded the ceremony, advertising the "Mother" Bickerdyke Monument. Hundreds of newspapers across the United States and Australia ran articles with titles such as "Mother Bickerdyke, War Nurse, Has a Monument Now," "Monument to Mother Bickerdyke Unveiled at Illinois Encampment with Ceremonies," and "'Mother' Bickerdyke Monument Will be Erected at Galesburg, Ill" (see figure 0.1).[4] Each was consistently attached with the message that "the name of Mother Bickerdyke stands preeminent."[5]

The ubiquity of this title was not an inevitable reflection of prevailing maternalist norms. While female Civil War nurses were often framed as caregivers to soldiers and were frequently described as tending to "their boys," not all prominent Civil War nurses were bestowed with the honorific of Mother. Clara Barton, Mary Livermore, Dorothea Dix, and Louisa May Alcott were recognized

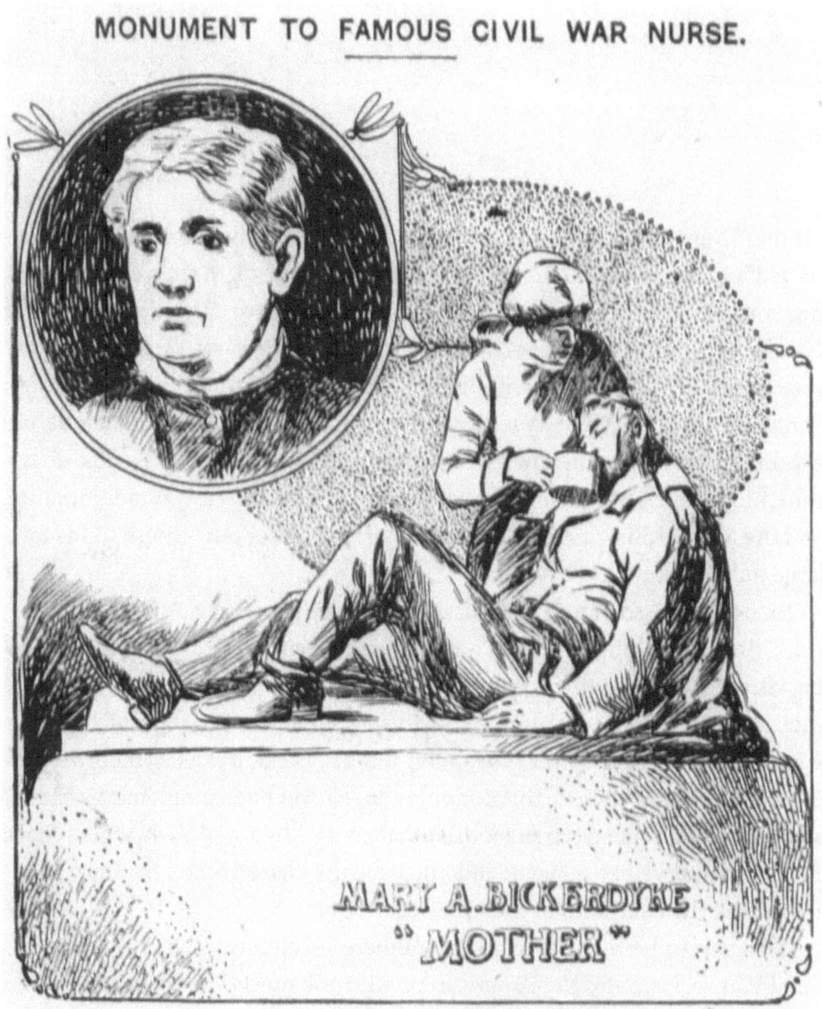

FIGURE 0.1 This illustration of the Mother Bickerdyke statue accompanied many articles featuring the news of the unveiling of Bickerdyke's monument. "Mother" is proudly attached to Mary Bickerdyke's legacy in the text of all the articles across the Midwest. Public domain.

for their wartime service, but none were popularly known in this explicitly maternal way. Bickerdyke stood apart from her peers as one thoroughly identified as Mother, indicating that this title did not simply emerge from cultural expectations but resulted from a deliberate construction. The press played a role in cementing this identity, but it was also one that Bickerdyke herself, her supporters, and veteran communities actively shaped, sometimes in ways that complicated or even challenged conventional gender norms.

The monument was unveiled on May 22, 1906, to commence the fortieth annual encampment of Illinois's chapter of the Grand Army of the Republic. By the time that the Bickerdyke statue was crafted, built, and ready for dedication in Galesburg, Bickerdyke's oldest son, James, who had long championed efforts to honor his mother, had died. The Mother Bickerdyke Memorial Association forged ahead and assembled a thoughtful program that demonstrated a deep knowledge and appreciation of Bickerdyke's local efforts and now immortalized legacy. It drew upon speakers who knew her, played the songs that once stirred her, and ended with "taps" played by residents of the Soldiers' Orphans' Home that she helped establish fifty years prior. An estimated crowd of 8,000 people filled the courthouse square to celebrate its unveiling.[6]

Richard Yates, the former governor of Illinois, gave a speech that underscored the deep impact Bickerdyke's care impressed upon soldiers. He echoed the sentiments of veterans, remembering her tender ministrations as she "sang songs of home and heaven to dying men while shot and shell fell in the midst of her field hospital."[7] In his speech, Yates recognized that Bickerdyke's contributions were invaluable and that "her insistence made every army commander realize the importance of her work."[8] Her unyielding insistence and refusal to be dismissed or delayed in her important work transformed compassion into action, and earned her the recognition and affection of both soldiers and officers alike.

The statue still stands proudly in the courthouse square in Galesburg (see figure 0.2). For eternity, Mother Bickerdyke kneels and props up a fallen soldier, tenderly bringing a bottle of liquid relief to his lips. Her appearance is generous and strong, and her countenance is concentrated on the task at hand: she is prepared to do whatever she can within her ability to guide this son on a dignified path to life or death, whatever may come.

Since the monument's dedication in 1906, Mary Bickerdyke's relative fame as a Civil War nurse has waned to distinctly local recognition. Some keen observers might recognize her from a short feature in Ken Burns's now-iconic 1990 PBS documentary series *The Civil War*. In the documentary, a warm baritone voice narrated an abbreviated version of her story over the pensive rhythms of a folksy fiddle and piano unmistakably derived from a simpler musical era while black-and-white images fade in and out of focus: "Mary Ann Bickerdyke, a Quaker widow and Sanitary Commission agent, traveled with the Union army through four years and nineteen battles, assisting at amputations, brewing barrels of coffee, rounding up cattle and chickens and eggs to feed the grateful men who called her Mother Bickerdyke. By the end of the

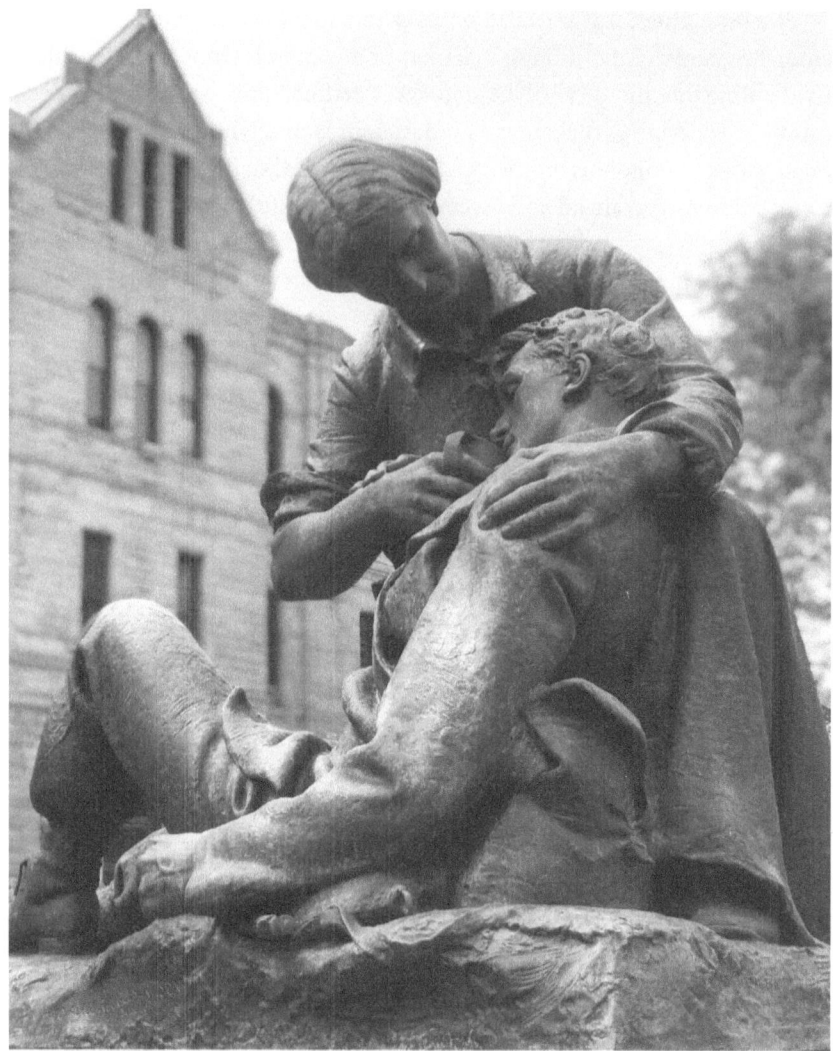

FIGURE 0.2 Mother Bickerdyke statue at the Knox County Courthouse in Galesburg, Illinois. The inscription on the statue reads, "Mother Bickerdyke; 1861—Army Nurse—1865; 'She outranks me' General Sherman." Photo taken by the author.

war, General Sherman said simply, 'She ranks me.'"[9] Soothed by the reassuring yet authoritative tones of documentary narration, viewers have practically no choice but to internalize the humble yet heroic summary of this woman known to posterity as Mother.

Even Ken Burns, in his massive data-collecting process to tell the story of the Civil War, revealed the constant redesign and revision of Bickerdyke's story in historical memory. Burns's research teams, perhaps unconsciously, copied and pasted the seemingly minute mistakes that have transformed Bickerdyke's story into a tidy myth, adding some texture to the otherwise simplified narrative of women who served in the Civil War. Burns is far from the only commentator, past or present, to inflate and morph Bickerdyke's story, affiliation, and impact. Such revision in this single instance reflects larger issues of historical construction and the craft of historical writing.

By the time that the Mary Ann Bickerdyke Papers were released to the public in 1977, repeated anecdotes about what her Civil War work and motherhood meant had become accepted fact, with little reason to look beyond the corroborated lore. In fact, there has been no major historical investigation of her life that utilizes the breadth of the available materials.[10] This book is an attempt to use the available archival materials to assemble and determine the value and meaning of "Mother's" work, both in her time and in ours.

## *Acknowledgments*

The publication of a book is an achievement that has only been possible because of the contributions of so many who helped me develop as a student, teacher, historian, and human. I want to begin by thanking my teachers at Oakdale Elementary, Parkside Junior High, and Normal West High School. Laura O'Donnell, Rexie Lanier, Lisa Preston, Jason Klokkenga, April Miller Fitzgerald, April Schermann, and many others: each modeled what it looks like to embrace lifelong learning. I have continued to learn, grow, and dream because teachers like you encouraged me to do so.

I am indebted to the academic community and generous teachers at Northern Illinois University who nurtured my ideas in their early stages. Jim Schmidt provided thoughtful feedback and urged me to trust my intuition as I pursued various leads in the research. Anne Hanley taught me to write clearly and compellingly, and I have done my best to follow her guidance. Beatrix Hoffman introduced me to the history of medicine and opened new ways of thinking about the past. The influence of these three teachers is present throughout this book.

Bringing this book to publication has been a team effort. My research benefited from the assistance of archivists and librarians. Michelle Krowl and Elizabeth Novara at the Library of Congress went above and beyond and sent scans of additional Bickerdyke materials. I am deeply grateful to María García at the University of North Carolina Press, who championed this project and guided it through publication. Erin Granville and Thomas Bedenbaugh, thank you for your keen editorial eye that helped shape the final revision. I also want to extend my gratitude to the two anonymous peer reviewers for their constructive critiques and astute suggestions, which strengthened the work. I acknowledge support from Indiana University Press and their attention to my sixth chapter, which was published as an article in the *Indiana Magazine of History*. Special thanks go to David Nichols and Dawn Bakken for their encouragement and time during that article's revision. Additionally, I would like to thank the Office of Research and Graduate Studies at Illinois State University for its support in completing this work.

My colleagues and friends have been supportive as I balanced teaching and research as an early career academic. I spent the first three years of my higher education teaching career at Governors State University. Eliot Fackler,

Lisa Pennington, and Cynthia Rousseau helped me to find my "professor voice" and proved to be incredibly supportive of each ambitious endeavor, including this book. My former teachers, many of whom are now my colleagues in the Department of History at Illinois State University, warmly welcomed me to the team and continue to guide my professional journey. Thanks especially to Andrew Hartman, Richard Hughes, and Christina Varga-Harris. I am also grateful for my students over the years, whose curiosity and enthusiasm remind me why historical work matters.

I've been fortunate to have cultivated friendships that have influenced my understanding of the history profession and helped me articulate the meaning of this book. Shae Smith Cox and Jonathon Jones provided collaborative opportunities and were exemplary models of productivity and ambition for early career faculty. Alex Lundberg and Thom Brown read early drafts when I first started studying Mary Bickerdyke and offered helpful comments over post-seminar hot wings.

I am indebted to dear friends who cheered me on and helped me maintain healthy life and work boundaries as I revised (and re-revised) this manuscript. Danielle Corple, you are such a good friend; you are a beautiful, talented, brilliant, powerful musk ox. I'll never be able to thank you enough for your friendship, wise insights, and attentive feedback. Laura Colee, thank you for always asking questions and for being my New York City research partner. I would be stuck in Grand Central Station without you. And Denise Ludwig, thanks for always hyping me up and reminding me that I am capable. I am beyond fortunate to have friends like each of you invested in my success.

Above all, I am profoundly grateful to my family. My parents, Bill and Sally Cummins, encouraged me to pursue my dreams and instilled in me the confidence to take up space wherever I go. From a young age, they nurtured my love of history and travel by taking me to historical sites across the United States—experiences for which I remain profoundly thankful. My husband and sons have been my greatest source of love, strength, and perspective throughout this journey. David has been my steadfast partner, offering unwavering support as I conducted research and wrote. He has always believed in this project, but he believes in me more; it has made all the difference (insert David chanting "Book tour!" here). My sons have provided joyful distractions, growing alongside this book's development. As the project has aged, so have they, and with that passage of time has come an endless cycle of "mom guilt" as I stepped away to work on the book. Yet, in their own ways, they have reassured me that my work matters. Their love, patience, and presence have shaped me as much as anything in these pages. This book and the insights within it would not exist without them.

*A Mother's Work*

# Introduction

"Mother knows best." A simple three-word phrase that is meant to disarm all who might question the authority that comes from a mother's command. If someone finds themselves on the receiving end of this irrefutable zinger, attempting a comeback is risky. This phrase is more than a retort, it is an instruction to defer, a signal to cut one's losses, and a reassurance that unparalleled wisdom has been imparted. But what does it mean, and what has it ever meant?[1] What mothers know and have known is an essential investigation into the fundamental process of society-building. Becoming and being a mother in the United States is an integral societal role, but its complexities and evolutions over time have eluded current understandings of historical motherhood in America.

Cultural demands on mothers have expected them to perform the duties assigned to their gender while raising their children to be healthy, productive citizens and members of society. Before the twentieth century, women performed maternal and household duties despite the significant risks of child and maternal mortality that threatened growing families. After becoming a mother, a woman needed to make daily decisions about how to aid in the preservation and maintenance of the household. For most American women, this meant arduous household management in addition to supporting their spouse's earned income with their own productive labor. Practically, women had to work both inside and outside the home to ensure the family's financial stability, all while raising children full-time.

Historically, women have been pushed into these demanding emotional and physical labor arrangements for a variety of reasons. Many women were forced to work without supportive childcare, so they strapped their children to their bodies, brought older children to their workplaces, and necessarily carried on with their labor. Slowly, over centuries, support systems and alternative arrangements for mothers became more commonplace as women demonstrated the necessity of earning income outside the home. Such systems were not always ideal, unlike today's curbside enrichment daycare services, which boast trained and compassionate teachers to provide temporary care during a mother's workday. Instead, a mother's work outside the home sometimes required children to live in institutions or be placed with family or community members as half-orphans or in destitute conditions, a practice that became more common during the nineteenth century. These solutions were not undertaken lightly, as mothers understood the societal expectations to provide their children with moral instruction and health care. As workers, women were obviously still mothers, but the social and cultural acceptance of their labor away from the home was held in question, as domesticity continued to be the dominant norm in the United States.

The Civil War constituted a brief period when, for the first time on a large scale, close to 20,000 women left their homes to serve in the war effort in some capacity.[2] Of those women, 3,000 were officially employed as nurses while others worked as sanitary agents; yet others served in various commissions or were camp followers.[3] In the service of national preservation or independence, women became essential agents in the wartime economy. Childcare institutions were tested as the adult population in both the North and South committed their professional efforts to the conflict. After the war was over, many mothers returned to lives of domesticity. Others, like Mary Bickerdyke, found clarity in a new professional calling amid the chaos of war.

Mary Ann Bickerdyke was a poor, widowed mother from Galesburg, Illinois, who was recruited to care for sick and wounded Union soldiers across the Western theater during the American Civil War. Once she decided to enter wartime service, she left her young sons in the care of others and became a surrogate mother to Union army soldiers on the front lines. She left behind a life of lower-class struggle and obscurity, only to find a professional calling that valued the skills she had developed through maternal medical training. The war provided an opportunity to refine those medical skills while also yielding a measure of authority as a mother-figure among soldiers who preferred homestyle therapeutics for their various ailments rather than the institutional solutions offered by Civil War doctors and hospitals.

Bickerdyke's professional decisions both during and after the war caused her to grapple with the multiple meanings of motherhood as she found ways to be a mother while operating outside the contemporary norms of domesticity as a worker. During the war, Bickerdyke became nationally known for her ability to marshal aid resources, organize massive makeshift hospitals, and provide individualized, compassionate care for young men away from home. She was a deputy mother for men who had only known illness or hardship under the loving supervision of their own mothers, and in this way, she endeared herself to thousands of men who embraced her willingness to stand up for their care and protection. From the early days of the conflict, soldiers were drawn to her pragmatic and assertive yet familiar style of medical care. As a result, she became widely known as "Mother" Bickerdyke among the rank-and-file soldiers. At the same time, Bickerdyke's assumption of her professional role distanced her from her biological sons and introduced a significant contradiction in her maternal identity.

She attended nineteen battles on the Western Front, became acquainted with a veritable "Who's Who" of Civil War influence, and never relented in her commitment to transform American medical institutions after the war's conclusion. In some ways, Bickerdyke represents a nineteenth-century Forrest Gump, bumping up against war heroes and highlighting her efforts as a diligent worker in the background of regional and national events that demonstrated the growing reach and influence of national systems during and after the Civil War. Her journeys from the beginning of the Civil War until her death took her across the United States, where she found herself involved in pivotal moments in the nation's institutional development.[4] As a professional "mother" who acted as a health care authority and as a mother to her own children, Bickerdyke was constantly wrestling with what it meant to be a mother in each role she embodied.

The complexities, ambiguities, and contradictions of Bickerdyke's various maternal roles throughout her life offer a valuable example for better understanding historical motherhood. Bickerdyke lived during a time in US history when society dramatically transformed to reflect an explosion of new scientific understanding as well as emergent political realities in the wake of the Civil War. The nation's population was devastated by the war's toll, and the Union victory over the Confederacy offered a "rebirth" to Americans. Women's work during the war demonstrated the need for a reevaluation of women's professionalism and their ability to productively contribute to roles that had previously been reserved for men. Bickerdyke's experience addresses how public performances of femininity and motherhood during the Civil War era influenced popular ideas and conversations about mothers for the rest of the century and into the present.

This work examines the transformation of one woman's mothering work as it evolved from strictly unpaid love-based labor within the realm of domesticity into a professional authority and ability that translated her mothering into tangible economic value. Specifically, Bickerdyke fostered and persistently applied palliative care procedures and hospice care protocols that met her individual patient's needs. This approach contributed to a generation of patients who came to expect an extraordinary level of care and became increasingly familiar with women's ability to provide it in a manner that reflected both the comfort measures of Victorian death expectations and the medical adeptness of a new scientific age. Mary Bickerdyke was a participant and agent in transitional historical processes that began during the Civil War and stretched into the Progressive Era. She took her household training to the front lines, where her style and effectiveness as a nurse created professional opportunities after the war's conclusion. She worked at a local level all over the United States in both private and public settings, providing aid and medical care to soldiers and their families until her death in 1901, effectively helping thousands of Americans in the process.

Bickerdyke was raised in a pre–Civil War culture that valued domestic permanence, so these dominant cultural beliefs were challenged by the realities of life for a poor widow. Her valuable professional skills demanded that she leave home and forced her to navigate the tension between tradition and necessity. Despite her esteemed competency as a community health care professional before the war, Bickerdyke spent her entire life encountering systems and institutions that were not designed for women's labor or the maternal competencies cultivated in domestic settings. Women were, for example, taught to care for the young and the dying within their homes, but they could not obtain professional medical training without social position and location.[5] Bickerdyke's attempt to extend her private maternal competencies and training into the public arena suggests an evolving public interpretation of women's impact on both the short- and long-term outcomes of the Civil War. Her incredible life journey unravels the traditional pre–Civil War understandings of patriotism, women's roles, and motherhood and transforms them into new expressions of health care, child welfare, and a broader cultural acceptance of women's professionalism through their persistent efforts to apply their skills in the professional world.

While her lifetime contributions seem clear, Bickerdyke's legacy and place within the national narrative have been reduced to her Civil War experience. There has been minimal scholarship that comprehensively examines her life. Bickerdyke has been the subject of several biographies, which gives the incorrect impression that an evaluation of her contribution has been told to its most fruitful extent. However, she has never been the subject of a serious historical biography and only receives passing mentions based on secondary material that circulated in repetitive form beginning in the late 1800s. The existing published material on Bickerdyke leaves the larger scope of her life and work untold and does not indicate the importance of her experiences for interpreting major shifts in women's history and the history of medicine in the second half of the nineteenth century.

Bickerdyke's story as "Mother" merits a much deeper examination that confronts the confusing complexities of her maternal identity and her negotiation with identities that fall outside maternal norms. Scholars who examine only her actions as "Mother Bickerdyke of the Western Front" or only her decisions as a biological mother miss the opportunity to understand the fundamental shifts in America's societal roles that occurred after the Civil War. To assume that Mary Bickerdyke was anything like most female agents in the United States Sanitary Commission (USSC) or that her motherhood was associated with the middle-class demonstration of moral authority belies the historical record for the sake of simplifying what is undeniably complex. Bickerdyke has served the purpose of historians; some of her actions and traits, which at times contradicted cultural conceptions of women's appropriate behavior, have been applied to scholarly arguments that situate her story neatly into place. Bickerdyke appears as a supporting character in historical scholarship on women of the Civil War era, consistent with the USSC memoirs that addressed Bickerdyke's wartime performance.[6] For example, Nina Silber's *Daughters of the Union* recognized Bickerdyke's maternal authority but suggested that she demonstrated an internalization of her subordinate position as a woman in the army.[7] However, a closer examination reveals that Bickerdyke's gendered position did not inhibit her from acting outside the typical norms of behavior in the domain where she had authority—as a mother. She, in fact, *insisted* on insubordinate actions to achieve various ends for her "boys," the soldiers, which led to her termination from the commission before the war's end.

The history of mothers and the experience of motherhood contribute to family and women's history, but they are also a part of economic, political, and intellectual history.[8] My study of Mary Bickerdyke's negotiation of working motherhood intervenes in the historiography of women, childhood, and Civil War literature that addresses the "alternate wartime geography" that directed women to make decisions based on the material conditions of war instead of the "ideological constraints of gender or the limitations of the middle-class imagination."[9] The emphasis on women from Eastern states in the bulk of historiography about the war and its effects on women's professional opportunities positions Bickerdyke as a different kind of Civil War nurse, one who was self-trained and appointed from a culturally and economically different background than women like Clara Barton and Dorothea Dix. Bickerdyke's social and economic context in Ohio, Illinois, and Kansas provides an example of how the Civil War permanently changed all American women's conception of their roles within the household, sensing their efficacy and autonomy to carry out traditionally male roles. Whether a poor

Northern mother or a wealthy Southern woman, redefinitions of working motherhood took place across geographic regions.[10]

Bickerdyke's mobility and application of medical skills challenge prevailing narratives about mid-nineteenth-century American motherhood, which were largely shaped by cultural ideals in the eastern part of the country. Scholars such as Emily Abel and Conevery Bolton Valenčius have argued that in the Midwest, maternal caregiving was both a response to environmental conditions and a means of professional advancement.[11] However, Bickerdyke's informal training and self-identification as a botanic physician complicate these findings, demonstrating that maternal styles of care also functioned as practical responses to public health crises, urbanization, migration, and rural medical scarcity. These insights add geographical context to Civil War–era medical histories, which tend to emphasize the indispensable role of women on the battlefield but often generalize their professional experiences based on the Eastern theater.[12] The intersection of Civil War medical histories and studies of settler and frontier women remains underexplored, leaving figures like Bickerdyke at the margins of both fields.

This study of "Mother" Mary Bickerdyke intersects with the robust historiography of nineteenth-century women and mothers. My episodic treatment of late nineteenth-century experiences through a feminine lens offers depth and nuance to the historical analyses of other well-known and prominent women of Bickerdyke's era.[13] Bickerdyke's intersection with social welfare institutions, constant displacements and migrations due to economic or political pressures, pension work, and class fluidity provide human-level insights into the experiences of women who fluctuated between the working and middle classes in the post–Civil War Midwest and West.[14] A story like Bickerdyke's promises a similar contribution to that of Martha Hodes's *The Sea Captain's Wife* in that Bickerdyke, like Hodes's Eunice, internalized appeals to universal womanhood from contemporary culture and was an "extraordinary women who led an extraordinary life by making momentous decisions within a world that offered her few choices."[15] As a result, Eunice and Mary Bickerdyke resigned themselves to working-class versions of domesticity, where the home and the extension of home activities were symbolic acts of dignity, reaching toward the security of the middle-class ideal while sacrificing the deeply embedded concepts of domestic home life. Indeed, Bickerdyke's documented individual experience as a real and representative mother demands a reexamination of scholarly ideas about the maternal image most often portrayed in the sentimental print culture of the mid to late nineteenth century.[16] Hardly a sentimental woman, Bickerdyke employed her rugged Midwestern practicality to propose a cultural shift in motherhood values and demonstrate the need for continued studies of women's experiences that occurred outside domestic spaces.

This book investigates the experience and worldview of a Midwestern, lower-class widow and wage earner during the Civil War and postwar period. An examination of a woman like Mary Bickerdyke answers a call made by Stephanie McCurry in *Women's War*. McCurry envisioned war histories from women's perspectives because their experiences "transform our vision of war" and break down the artificial constructs that exclude women from wars.[17] Bickerdyke proved that women belonged to the realm of the state and war, not just to family and peace. Her maternal responsibilities were intertwined with her activism, advocacy, and employment. Like McCurry's case studies, Bickerdyke's experiences demonstrate how the human-scale perspective pulls into the record the "allegedly 'private' but highly consequential matters of marriage and the family, revealing the way war disorders even these fundamental relations of social and political life."[18] Bickerdyke's biological children, James and Hiram, were often separated from their mother, moving between various social and educational institutions. Over time, both sons expressed distress at their early independence and the absence of maternal care, offering a perspective that complicates existing narratives of Civil War childhood.[19] Unlike the prevailing trends in mother-child relationships of the era, Bickerdyke's experience reflects the sacrifices and tensions that could accompany wartime caregiving.[20] Yet, despite this divergence, she remains memorialized as a quintessentially benevolent Civil War mother. This contrast underscores the need for a more nuanced approach to the mythologizing tendencies of early Civil War histories, which often simplify or idealize women's maternal roles during the conflict.

Bickerdyke's experience offers a more surgical view of women's transition as mothers from the private to public sphere during the nineteenth century. Her life and professional aspirations, grounded in traditional female motherwork, suggest that individual processes of professional work were complicated, insecure, and risky as women ventured outside the home into spaces that did not provide support for those who broke with culturally embedded notions of motherhood. Instead, Bickerdyke's example demonstrates that even professionally driven women—whether out of desire or necessity—struggled to find work that satisfied their needs as workers, their commitment to their field, and their motherhood. She did not fit into the broader molds that historians have since identified such as the Victorian "cult of domesticity" or the later phenomena of "scientific motherhood." As such, her example provides insight into the margins of historical trends and emphasizes the contingency that arises from human experience. The analysis of localized and immediate social connections uncovers collective meanings that quickly changed in the midst and aftermath of the American Civil War. The historical everyday serves to reveal the fracture lines of cultural demarcations within class and demographic categories, such as mothers and women.

This work employs a microhistorical approach to life writing. It examines how episodes in one woman's life reveal the changing meanings of motherhood and professional competencies for women in the second half of the nineteenth century. The specifics of this study interrogate Bickerdyke's life and maternal experience to uncover the multiple Mother Bickerdykes that together represent the complexities and contingencies of women's lives and work during this period. In a microhistory, an author takes a small unit of analysis and explores how the subject provides insight into subtle, everyday human experiences. Currently, there is no defined American school of microhistory.[21] As a result, American works of microhistory tend to rely on aspects of more developed international schools of thought from the Italian, French, and German historians who created more defined approaches.[22] These collective works established a consensus that microhistories take obscure events and people and seek to explore whether they are significant for constructing a deeper understanding of history. The approach looks deeply into the abyss to identify the "unknowable" and then explores those dimensions to add texture, meaning, and depth to our present knowledge of the past.

The text will adhere to several tenets of a self-determined American school of microhistory: a small unit of primary analysis; a micro-macro link or some indication of the wider implications of the analysis; transparency, in which the author acknowledges unanswered questions as they arise in the research process; and the use of an academic narrative style. Unlike a traditional biography, which often seeks a cohesive narrative arc and emphasizes the interplay between the personal and political, microhistory focuses on a small unit of analysis to uncover broader historical patterns, even when an individual's life does not conform to a singular, overarching narrative. This approach departs from the feminist biography's emphasis on the biographer's engagement with the subject and the subject's interiority, instead prioritizing the ways in which a life, or moments within it, illuminate deeper historical structures and contingencies.[23] This study uses key episodes in Bickerdyke's experience to explore shifting conceptions of motherhood and professional competency rather than constructing a cradle-to-grave account of her life.

A combination of national and local archives, contemporary newspapers, and census records has been used to bridge documentary gaps and expand the scope beyond personal papers to encompass the broader implications of Bickerdyke's maternal experience. The simplified redundancy of Bickerdyke biographies stands in contrast to her extensive 1,800-item digitized archive at the Library of Congress. Many rich stories and contexts in this archive remain unexplored by professional historians. This collection, spanning from 1845 to 1905, predominantly contains correspondence from Bickerdyke's long life. The items from the 1890s, including dated correspondence from box 2 and box 4, reveal Bickerdyke's extensive involvement in veteran pension cases. Constructing her maternal role from existing correspondence in the Library of Congress was aided by cross-referencing with regional archives holding smaller portions of her collection. This process, combined with the use of digital paleography, confirmed Lydia Foster's role as Bickerdyke's primary amanuensis, or ghostwriter, who recorded her pension work in the final decade of Bickerdyke's life and career.[24] These archival strategies have made it possible to reconstruct a more nuanced narrative of Bickerdyke's professional life and the careful construction of her motherhood.

The resulting narrative represents a type of disruption in the carefully preserved and celebrated image of Mary Bickerdyke. Bickerdyke biographies, which were consistently published from the mid-1880s through the 1970s, have taken on a mythic quality, transforming Bickerdyke into a legend rather than depicting her as a complex historical actor. Mary Bickerdyke's legacy was often mythologized in the image of a saintly mother, her care framed as the expression of patriotic and self-sacrificing womanhood. These narratives, born from soldiers' campfire reunions and biographers' flourishes, often reduce her work to tender acts of nurturing and moral cheer. Comparisons to Florence Nightingale further solidified this mythos, presenting Bickerdyke as an "American Nightingale" while stripping her of the pragmatism and authority she exercised on the front lines. Some biographers, like Jenkin Lloyd Jones, even fabricated familial ties to the Mayflower and Revolutionary War heroes to craft a lineage that elevated her cultural status and aligned her with idealized American values through heredity. Such simplifications obscure the more transgressive and complex realities of her professional work and identity.

The book challenges these mythologies by recovering the intentionality and contradictions of Bickerdyke's legacy. It highlights her active role in shaping her public image while also exposing the persistence of falsehoods in her constructed memory. It uncovers previously unexamined figures who were key to Bickerdyke's success, such as Lydia Foster, a young Black woman responsible for dictating Bickerdyke's pension correspondence. Bickerdyke's history can instruct on the types of occupations and resources that were available to working mothers, the ways in which relationships of power were formed and cultivated, and the strategies that mothers used to aid others. Additionally, Bickerdyke's papers direct careful readers to the discussions of race and womanhood. Bickerdyke, who claimed modestly progressive ideals regarding racial equality, was not an activist for racial equality in any sense of the word. Publicly, her venerable status as a mother was predicated on a White womanhood that held more cultural value in the nineteenth century and persists today. In fact, there were identifiable moments when Bickerdyke could have taken a more progressive stance on both gender and racial equality, but she deliberately chose not to use her growing influence among veterans and the American public to do so. As will be seen, Bickerdyke was acutely aware of how social and racial dynamics could be used to her advantage in life and in historical memory as she rose to fame toward the end of her life.

The book's analysis of her maternal journey should not be regarded as something normative, ideal, or laudatory, even in the nineteenth century. The major themes that emerge tell the story of how Bickerdyke took her experiences from the Civil War and revised them to fit into an expanding definition of what it meant to be known as a public mother defined by her labor. By reframing her maternal identity, I demonstrate how Bickerdyke strategically wielded the title of "Mother" as a form of professional and moral authority while navigating gendered limitations within Civil War medicine. Ultimately, I critique the sanitized heroism attributed to Bickerdyke and replace it with a nuanced analysis that acknowledges her agency, pragmatism, and the racial and class dynamics underpinning her legacy.

The first chapter is a detailed examination of Mary Bickerdyke's life before and during the Civil War, focusing on her role as a mother and caregiver. It situates Bickerdyke's story within the broader context of Midwestern settler life, the development of medical practices, and the social and political landscape of the Civil War. This provides a fuller understanding of how individual experiences both shaped and were shaped by larger historical processes. Bickerdyke's experiences of loss, displacement, and informal medical training shaped her and prepared her for wartime service. Her maternal relationship with her sons was deeply affected by her professional decisions. Historians have noted Bickerdyke's separation from her sons, but they often leave the analysis at that. Only Jane Schultz has noted Bickerdyke's "epistolary neglect" of her sons during the war, while others seem to chalk up Bickerdyke's absence during the war as patriotic domesticity; she was employing her medical skills to serve the country, as so many men were also doing.[25] Historians have yet to account for her postwar activities that continued to prevent Bickerdyke's direct domestic involvement in her children's lives. Chapter 1 dissects Bickerdyke's private motherhood and traces her transition toward a civic and public mother. Importantly, I introduce the concept of "care-switching," which describes how Bickerdyke adapted her maternal and caregiving skills to professional settings.

The second and third chapters explore different phases of Civil War involvement for Mary Bickerdyke and establish that maternal authority was respected as a form of medical competency during the Civil War. "Mother" Mary Bickerdyke used her private experiences and training as a mother in the public and professional sphere as an efficient USSC agent and eventual nurse for the United States Army. She attained and maintained a level of maternal moral authority; indeed, at times, she pulled moral rank and inverted the rigid and gendered structures of the Union army. Though women were hired as agents, they were not often given the tools to function outside of the prescribed roles within the male-dominated institution.[26] Additionally, Bickerdyke's medical authority was solidified throughout the Civil War as she provided surrogate motherhood, homestyle comfort measures, and palliative care to sick and dying soldiers. Her social position as a respected mother framed the practitioner-to-patient dynamic in a way that comforted soldiers, many of whom were experiencing medical care away from a familial setting for the first time. Chapters 2 and 3 present a broad overview of her personal and professional medical journey and offer a new perspective on the historiographical material that currently exists on the history of American medical authority. Predominately doctor-dominated narratives do not adequately address how Americans evolved from the ubiquitous cultural practices of home medical care at the beginning of the nineteenth century to a near-exclusive reliance on highly regimented institutions by the turn of the century.

Chapter 4 explores Bickerdyke's postwar activities, showing how her involvement with private, local, state, and national institutions extended her maternal commitment to veterans and their families. She believed it was a mother's responsibility to ensure that soldiers—the sons of the nation—and their families were properly attended. She envisioned herself in the role of civic motherhood, marshaling health resources to serve those populations. She primarily worked within institutions but always adhered to her own maternal procedures to ensure that increasingly impersonal medical organizations remained accountable to their end of the bargain when it came to providing health care.

Chapter 5 suggests that the pragmatic strategies developed by widows, such as migration and wage earning, mitigated the economic difficulties caused by the loss of a spouse. Bickerdyke employed a "motherhood of convenience" after the death of her spouse, accepting work that used the nursing skills she had cultivated during the Civil War. Motherhood of convenience refers to the strategic adoption or performance of maternal roles such as caregiving, nursing, or domestic care to secure economic survival or social legitimacy in the absence of traditional family structures. Mary Bickerdyke's nursing style and her commitment to preserving traditional, compassionate end-of-life care signaled her participation in pioneering palliative care practices that repudiated the developing norms and social order of institutionalized medicine in the postwar period. Her practices, which were not sanctioned by medical professionals of the late nineteenth century, reflected the generations-old desires of men and women to die at home or receive compassionate care that resembled familial therapeutics.

Chapter 6 surveys Bickerdyke's work as a pension attorney and guardian for individual veterans navigating the US Pension Bureau. Bickerdyke was one of a few women to occupy this type of role, and she was able to do so because of the overwhelming requests from veterans who desired a "mother's care." Mother Bickerdyke viewed guardianship, both official and unsanctioned, as an extension of her maternal duties, which began to be recognized as professionally valuable during her service as a Civil War nurse and agent at the USSC. The chapter situates her experience in a broader context of health activism and emerging maternalist policies and suggests that the pension advocacy leveraged by Civil War nurses set the stage for welfare reform that benefited women. Bickerdyke's ability to navigate formal institutions and informal networks of care after the Civil War underscores the complex and often contradictory ways in which gender shaped politics.

The final chapter interrogates the intentional construction of Mary Bickerdyke's legacy during the final years of her life and after her passing. The analysis uncovers the intersections of class and race by focusing on Mary Bickerdyke and her Black housekeeper and amanuensis, Lydia Foster. Only one of Bickerdyke's biographers mentioned Lydia Foster but did not provide any information about her role as Bickerdyke's live-in servant, secretary, and ghostwriter. The concealment of Lydia Foster's servitude behind the memory of Mother Bickerdyke's later-life accomplishments raises understudied questions about motherhood. Whether the decision to withhold credit from

Foster was deliberate or simply a consequence of historical context that habitually concealed Black contributions, the effect was that Lydia Foster was rendered invisible while Mother Bickerdyke's fame was bolstered in her final years and continues to be upheld in historical representations. The public saw an esteemed White mother hitting her professional stride in her later years while the labor, voice, and intellect of a Black woman was ultimately behind her success. Mother Bickerdyke's prominence as a "Mother" in historical memory was built on Lydia's intentional obscurity. Chapter 7 concludes with the efforts of her family and friends to preserve and maintain a carefully curated legacy that upheld a reputation for patriotic service and virtue after her death.

Mary Bickerdyke's conception and use of her maternal identity was an evolutionary process shaped by time and experience. She loved the name "Mother" in every iteration of its meaning: as a mother to her sons and to the sons of the Union army, as a nurse, and as a guardian. Knowing this, those around her continued to attempt to secure those honorable maternal images for the ages. Up until now, their efforts have been largely successful. At the same time, Mary Bickerdyke was merely human; she was a mother who made mistakes and entered into bargains that demonstrated her humanity. Re-examining her carefully preserved historical image throughout this book does not diminish her contributions to history or the cultivated legacy that surrounds her. Instead, it should encourage readers to question an all-or-nothing approach to historical heroes and heroines. "Mother" may have known best, but she gained that knowledge through the trial and error of her work.

CHAPTER ONE

# Mother, Before the War

The early 1800s were a time of significant change in the Old Northwest. European American settlers began establishing farms, clearing forests for timber, and building roads and canals in central Ohio. This period marked the beginning of a shift from a predominantly natural landscape to a more agricultural and settled one, laying the groundwork for the extensive agricultural development that would characterize central Ohio in the decades to come. Mary Ann Ball was born in 1817 in Knox County, located amid central Ohio's slowly developing dense forests. Growing up, she experienced both the perils of settler life and Ohio's rapid industrialization and urbanization. In Knox County, the population more than tripled, from 8,326 in 1820 to 28,872 by 1850. More dramatically, Cincinnati, where Mary lived as a young adult, skyrocketed from a population of 9,642 in 1820 to 161,044 in 1860.[1] The rural upbringing of her youth was transformed by a burgeoning Midwestern metropolis, fostering economic, social, and cultural values distinct from those of the cities of the eastern United States.

Regional histories depict the Midwest as the site of a republican good life and a symbol of American progress; however, these social developments were almost exclusively available to White citizens and, at that, mostly males.[2] Such a construction of the social order of the Midwest suggested a continued conservative public role for women as upholders of private virtue. For White women in the Midwest, the situation more resembled "the politicized domesticity of a Catharine Beecher," who endeavored to train female educators in the Old Northwest in the hopes that their intellectual and spiritual development might influence children, families, and thus the society around them.[3] The "cult of true womanhood" is a well-known historical analytic devised by Barbara Welter in her landmark 1966 article. She wrote, "The attributes of True Womanhood, by which a woman judged herself and was judged by her husband, her neighbors and society, could be divided into four cardinal virtues—piety, purity, submissiveness, and domesticity. Put them all together and they spelled mother, daughter, sister, wife—woman."[4]

Bickerdyke came of age in rural Ohio in the 1820s and 1830s, as the "cult of true womanhood" was at its height in American cultural consciousness. These normative formulations of gender and femininity provided the conventional wisdom that women's intrinsically superior morality needed to be cultivated and protected in the home.[5] This was especially true for women in middle-class to upper-class settings. Trials in women's higher education, primarily in seminary settings, coincided with the common school movement. A beneficiary of these education movements, Bickerdyke gained the ability to read and write, but those skills were limited to practical applications. In her youth and young adulthood, she was equipped with what she needed, but not much more. It was not until the Civil War that her lack of education became an issue.

While the diffusion and perpetuation of dominant cultural tropes was true to some extent, historian Kristin Hoganson has pointed out the danger of such assumptions: "Histories of the rural Midwest have emphasized the particular isolation of women, bound to home by male privilege, tied tighter by the unremitting burdens of childbearing, child care, and tasks such as cooking, cleaning, vegetable raising, poultry tending, dairying, sewing, and food preservation. . . . To write such stereotypes into the past creates further distortions, because rural communities have never been static."[6] Mary Bickerdyke's life serves as a valuable example of the dynamic roles that Midwestern women played during the transitional period prior to the Civil War. Her upbringing was dominated by a narrative of loss and displacement rather than any domestic training. This instability drove Bickerdyke to constantly move, seek living and working arrangements, and develop skills that would support her continued livelihood.

Mary Bickerdyke offers a compelling case study of how women in the nineteenth century navigated the complex terrain between traditional domestic roles and emerging opportunities for public service and work. This chapter argues that Bickerdyke's personal history of loss, displacement, and informal medical training prepared her to engage in a process of care-switching, adapting her maternal and caregiving skills to professional settings during the Civil War. A look into Bickerdyke's life before the war and during its initial stages, with particular attention to her relationships with her biological sons and the soldiers under her care, offers new insights into the tensions and transformations that shaped women's experiences of motherhood, work, and identity in the Civil War era. Bickerdyke's story challenges traditional narratives of women's wartime roles and illuminates the complex ways individual experiences reflected and reshaped broader social and historical processes. Through a close analysis of primary sources and engagement with relevant historiography, this chapter contributes to ongoing debates about the significance of gender, family, and caregiving in nineteenth-century

America while also introducing the concept of care-switching as a framework for understanding women's adaptive strategies in times of crisis and change.

When Mary was two years old, her mother died, leaving her father to transfer Mary's care to her grandparents. Widowed men in the nineteenth century typically either remarried quickly after a spouse's death to replace a mother and household manager or sent their dependent children to live with relatives.[7] Mary's father remarried quickly, and he began a new family with Mary's stepmother. Mary remained in her grandparents' household, but they died in quick succession when Mary was only twelve years old. After her grandparents passed in 1829, her father sent her to live with her uncle and chose not to make a place for Mary in his household with his second wife and Mary's half-siblings.[8] So, by the time she entered adulthood, Mary Ball had been displaced twice from her primary caretakers, first after her mother's death when she was two years old and then again before she was a teenager when her grandparents and guardians died.

A general lack of data sources has made it difficult to discern broad mortality trends in this region of the country; thus, family histories offer valuable information on life expectancies in these western localities.[9] Death was common enough in the Ohio country that cultural norms developed to ensure that normative gender roles could still be performed, as seen with Mary's father, who seemed unwilling to raise a child without a maternal substitute and chose to distance himself from any reminder of that previous familial arrangement. Though this was not reflective of any discernible pattern, her father's decision would not have been uncommon or seen as especially cruel. For her part, Mary Ball seemed to accept her father's decision without any outward or written display of bitterness or contempt, never mentioning any feelings of neglect.[10] It seems plausible to deduce that such arrangements were expected and reasonable solutions for caretaker mortality. Bickerdyke's family history can serve as a useful case study to fill in the gaps presented by regional variation in mortality during the nineteenth century.

From a young age, Mary took on the role of a lower-class domestic worker, employed in housework and nanny positions across Ohio, from Cleveland to Cincinnati.[11] Little reliable documentation exists to trace her late adolescence and early adult years. What is verifiably true is that as an unskilled domestic worker, Mary was exposed to some of Ohio's most powerful families, including when she nannied for Cleveland's mayor, Sam Starkweather, from 1845 to 1846.[12] In this role, Mary observed upper-middle-class domestic life. While living in the Starkweather household, she cared for their young son and maintained the house. Her observations and assigned duties for a powerful family in a growing city taught her middle-class household management.

Caregiving dominated women's lives as they worked within the household. Young girls from diverse social situations were expected to absorb informal medical training, not only to benefit their immediate family and to aid their own mothers in family medical practice, but also to prepare them for their future charge as household managers of health and wellness.[13] By and large, the underappreciated caretaking role was considered one of the baseline obligations of women's work in their household sphere rather than recognized as a skill that could be leveraged in the marketplace to secure a livelihood, as Mary Ball did in the Starkweather household.

In 1847, Mary Ball married widower Robert Bickerdyke, stepping into the role of mother to his four children from a previous marriage—a responsibility she had been denied in her own childhood. At the time of their marriage, Robert's children included Jane (age 17) and Joseph (age 19), as well as two younger siblings, Robert (age 9) and Mary (age 4).[14] Robert Bickerdyke was a locally renowned but seldom employed musician who reportedly excelled in the double bass and toured seasonally.[15] When not performing, he found contract work as a painter. The newlyweds faced immediate hardship: later that year, their first child together, John, died just days after birth. In 1848, a devastating flood forced the family to leave their Cincinnati home, destroying much of what they owned.[16] Despite these challenges, the Bickerdykes continued to grow their family, welcoming James in 1850 and Hiram in 1854. Through both triumphs and struggles, they remained locked in an ongoing battle against Robert's poor health and his lack of steady employment.[17]

The Bickerdykes moved farther west in 1856 to help with Robert's recovery and seek medical care.[18] With at least three small children in tow and very little to their name, the Bickerdykes trekked across the prairie to resettle their family. Their choice to seek remedies and therapeutics in the western climes of Keokuk, Iowa, and Galesburg, Illinois, suggests a values-based decision concerning medical matters. Rather than seeking treatment for Robert's chronic illness at the more advanced hospitals of the East Coast, they prioritized an environment where they could explore diverse therapies that aligned with their beliefs about chronic care. The Eastern United States experienced faster development of modern hospitals and training programs than states in the Midwest or West. This development did not reflect a lack of population growth in the middle and western regions throughout the nineteenth century. Instead, new medical norms experienced a slow westward diffusion as they encountered unique cultural characteristics. While doctors with orthodox medical training became more effective in curing patients, advancements in technology and health institutions often resulted in less holistic patient care. The Bickerdykes appear to be an example of that slow diffusion. As a family, they obviously preferred a holistic regimen for chronic ailments that plagued Robert.

During the nineteenth century, technological and scientific breakthroughs drastically changed medical practices and Americans' understanding of health. They also changed unevenly based on regional, social, and cultural forces. Orthodox medicine's adoption of European models of scientific empiricism, new technologies, and policies strengthened its professional authority by the twentieth century. The state and medical institutions became more compatible as scientific innovations proved to the American public that diseases could be effectively managed or eliminated through professional medicine and its practice. The social and scientific upheavals of the nineteenth century affected the scope of American medical care, from individual medical treatment to the implementation of federal public health measures. The Bickerdykes did not rely on these innovations; instead, they pursued forms of care that emphasized holistic, home-based, and experiential remedies over the treatments emerging in professional settings.

The Bickerdyke family settled into life in Galesburg, folding themselves into the community. Their move reflected a broader pattern of east-to-west migration, which fueled rapid population growth and the cultural transmission characteristic of such dramatic shifts. In the Old Northwest and the West, the region's "vaunted individualism" coexisted with an equally strong push for social organization.[19] Both impulses found expression in churches, seminaries, new political parties, clubs, and reform societies. As families established themselves in "hometown communities," the Midwest emerged as a social and political model for a "national American individualistic bourgeois society."[20] Amid their newly adopted community, Robert's health improved enough for him to resume playing the double bass, earning recognition as a "leading instrumental musician" with the Galesburg Academy of Music.[21] After settling in Galesburg, the Bickerdykes welcomed their final child together, Martha, in 1858.

Mary Bickerdyke continued to manage the household and oversee Robert's care, treating him at home when necessary. In April 1859, he was reported to be "full of vigor and life," but he was suddenly "taken with a fit" and became gravely ill.[22] If Mary sought the expertise of local doctors, she still retained primary responsibility for his care and made the crucial decisions as he lay waiting for the inevitable. Medical care was often a collaborative effort between trained doctors and home caregivers in small, close-knit communities like Galesburg. Physicians relied on the knowledge of household caretakers, recognizing their deep familiarity with the patient's condition and daily needs.[23] When intervention was possible, these care teams worked together to determine the most effective therapeutic approach. However, if a prognosis pointed toward death, attention shifted from treatment to ensuring a "good death." In the nineteenth century, women played a central role in orchestrating this transition, ensuring that the dying were physically comforted and spiritually prepared. As hope for Robert's recovery faded, Mary likely took on this role, tending to his body while providing the reassurance and presence expected of a devoted wife. Within just a few days, his condition worsened, and Robert Bickerdyke passed away. In his final moments, Mary's role was not only that of a caregiver but also a guide, ensuring that his passing aligned with the cultural expectations of a peaceful and dignified death.[24]

Robert Bickerdyke's death marked the loss of a husband and father, leaving Mary to navigate the practical and social realities of widowhood. In the wake of his passing, she faced the challenges of sustaining her household without the traditional economic and social security that a husband provided. Like many widows in her position, she turned to informal community care networks often reinforced by church congregations and professional associations. The Galesburg Academy of Music wrote to the family after Robert's death, providing their official condolences and sympathy for the "great affliction you have been called upon to suffer."[25] The music academy did not offer material assistance, but its acknowledgment of the family's hardship reflected the broader community's recognition of their suffering. In contrast, the Galesburg Congregational Church played a more direct role in providing tangible aid, reinforcing the vital role of religious institutions in supporting widowed households. The church was the foundation of Mary's community ties and involvement, and she continued to rely heavily on its help and Christian charity. Practically, her options were to remarry or to pursue work that engaged the skills she developed as a mother and as a former housekeeper. At the time of Robert's death, Bickerdyke was forty-two years old and at the end of her childbearing years. The outlook of another suitor to care for her and her children was logistically difficult and, more importantly, not a prospect that she desired.

Mary Bickerdyke's sorrow deepened only a year after losing her husband when tragedy struck the family again. On April 8, 1860, her two-year-old daughter Martha passed away.[26] The circumstances of her death remain unclear, but the weight of this second loss so soon after Robert's must have been devastating. Left to shoulder her grief while caring for her surviving children, Mary faced yet another painful reminder of the fragility of life and the limitations of her intention to provide care for her family. Mary did not have the luxury to grieve to the extent that cultural norms permitted.[27] Her circumstances, as was certainly the case for other poor frontier families, demanded that she continue her daily duties as a mother to her surviving children and, now, as the sole provider.

Over the decade of her biological motherhood before the Civil War, Bickerdyke developed a fortitude marked by the reality and risk of loss that was intimately connected to a love extending beyond the grave. From the early days of her marriage, Bickerdyke cultivated practical experience caring for her husband and adapting regularly to difficult circumstances with limited resources. Having lost her own mother at an early age, she lacked the traditional maternal training that many young women received during adolescence. Instead, she developed her medical aptitude through intense experiences that tested her competence and forced her to learn out of necessity rather than through formal instruction. The deeply personal work of home caregiving—especially in the wake of two family deaths in close succession—provided Mary Bickerdyke with a sense of purpose in her ability to offer comfort and care. Historian Emily Abel has noted that nineteenth-century caregiving both "exacted a terrible toll and conferred significant benefits" on those who took on the responsibility.[28] For Bickerdyke, these experiences not only honed her practical medical skills but also solidified a sense of purpose. Having endured the emotional and physical demands of caregiving within her own home, she was uniquely positioned to extend her expertise beyond it. The very skills she cultivated in the private sphere of family life soon propelled her into the public world of nursing, where she transformed personal loss into a professional calling.

Mary Bickerdyke's decision to work after her husband's death was not a choice. There was not yet a formalized federal system of support or welfare for widows and children. While most states and localities offered some form of poor relief, these highly regulated systems, such as asylums or orphanages, were generally a last resort and used only when community relationships could not meet immediate needs. Galesburg citizens understood that she was "fighting poverty for herself and four children" after her husband's death.[29] Bickerdyke's experience reflects the broader challenge women faced as they became mothers, raised families, and negotiated the economic demands of survival. Mary Bickerdyke was an ordinary woman whose life offers a view of the tension between traditional notions of female domesticity shaped by class privilege and the ways that some mothers had to operate outside the home in the workplace. Mary Bickerdyke lived in the space between these conflicting maternal and feminine models, and like most women who became mothers in the mid-nineteenth century, she adapted the deluge of social advice in a way that fit her own personal, practical applications.

She did have some agency in the type of work that she might pursue to provide for herself and her children. After Robert's death and before the war's outset, Bickerdyke hired herself out as a "botanic physician" to local Galesburg families in need, leaving her younger children in the care of their older half-sister while she worked.[30] The title of botanic physician signaled an extension of basic household skills expected of a mother and indicated a cultivation of specialized knowledge of medicine even to a small degree. While "botanics" did not constitute a formally recognized occupation with professional standards and training, practitioners distinguished themselves from homeopaths. By the mid-1840s, popular botanicism had outgrown its rugged beginnings and found renewed popularity in more "respectable" and professional schools of practice, like the Eclectic Medical Institute chartered in Cincinnati in 1845.[31]

There is no direct evidence of Mary Bickerdyke's training in botanic medicine or her awareness of the prevalence of this practice in the West, but her decision to brand her business as botanic suggests a philosophical underpinning to her medical practice. It indicates Bickerdyke's commitment to a holistic approach, free from systematic methodology, that considers the patient's overall health and then relies on both historical use and increasingly on modern scientific research to understand the efficacy and mechanisms of plant-based treatments.[32] Her decision to style her practice as botanic also demonstrated her desire for legitimacy, to be trusted by those who came to her for care. The botanics, led by Samuel Thomson and his system, emphasized education and science in an empirical embrace of nature's apothecary, using language that appealed to the common people. His book, *New Guide to Health; or Botanic Family Physician* (1822), provided homemade remedies for various illnesses and pointed to a general contempt for conventional medicine and orthodox medical practice. Thomsonians relied on a literate public to explain and disseminate their system of healing.[33] In a region where medical self-reliance was a cultural necessity and professional doctors were scarce or distrusted, Bickerdyke's embrace of botanic medicine would have bolstered her credibility, aligning her with a healing tradition that empowered ordinary people and made her care both familiar and trustworthy to those she served.

Household practitioners employed a wide range of techniques and bridged orthodox and unorthodox thought by consulting neighbors, relatives, and manuals to arrive at diagnostic decisions. By the beginning of the Civil War, those who identified as botanic physicians were descendants of Jacksonian-era developments in American medical practice, which were tied to westward expansion and a disdain for specialized knowledge. The role of non-elite and competing healers, such as Samuel Thomson, created a fractious medical environment. Western settlers relied on self-help books like John C. Gunn's *Domestic Medicine* and Thomson's *New Guide to Health*, as well as consultations with household members, to deal with sickness. This confluence of medical authority and dependence on household tradition reflected an approach to healing that "dovetailed with the boisterous political rhetoric of self-reliance in the Jacksonian period."[34] Home practitioners were predominantly women in the household who received medical training through familial tradition and published instructional tracts. Women were trusted to manage family or neighborhood care unless extreme medical circumstances prompted a call to a professional doctor. The struggle for medical authority and autonomy played out across America in the nineteenth century, with many household practitioners claiming sovereignty over family and community medical decisions.[35] By the time of the 1860 census, Bickerdyke's medical training consisted of her maternal confrontation with disease and death. As a botanic physician, Bickerdyke could effectively leverage that training to move her family out of poverty.

In the medical marketplace, Bickerdyke competed with trained physicians for paying patients. While some Americans acknowledged the gradual cultural diffusion of scientific knowledge and professional medical training, there was a viable contingent of ardent democratic Jacksonians who still preferred a mother's hand to a doctor's scalpel because of their convictions about the proper relationship between knowledge, authority, and deference.[36] Bickerdyke gained medical practice and training because there was an individualistic remnant within her community that trusted her abilities and hired her. She was part of what some considered the "medical counterculture," offering natural and traditional remedies. A reasonable argument can be made for such a claim, given that half of Ohio's population adhered to botanical programs when Thomson released his household medical guides.[37] Thomson believed that orthodox or university-trained physicians were endangering their patients with toxic minerals such as tartar emetic (antimony) and calomel (mercurous chloride). He became convinced that nature's apothecary was the source of health and healing, and he developed a system of herbal remedies.[38] This was the foundation of botanic medicine: using nature and common knowledge as methods of medical care. This approach appealed to female household practitioners across the country who lacked formal education but were eager to supplement their own medical knowledge for the benefit of their families.

Later biographers characterized Bickerdyke's Galesburg practice as "more nearly a Homeopathist . . . as she made use of any treatment or medicine which commended itself to her judgement."[39] This distinction is misleading and may more accurately reflect the author's gendered association with categories of medical philosophies that emerged in the mid-nineteenth century. Historian Anne Taylor Kirschmann asserts that homeopathy's popularity and appeal stemmed from the public's embrace of its gentle remedies as well as its association with women's reform movements.[40] Later in her life, Bickerdyke became involved with temperance movements, which may have contributed to the confusion. More likely, Bickerdyke's claim to medical knowledge as a botanic physician communicated her familiarity with natural remedies and her self-training in the principles of sanitation and household health, while also suggesting her openness to emerging natural therapeutics.[41] If anything, this designation represented the early development of what would become her signature style and bring her such adoration among Civil War soldiers: the deft balance between a mother's care and the efficacy of a medical professional.

Death, grief, and their processes were intertwined with family and community, and Mary Bickerdyke saw herself as a capable helper when life was in the balance. While there were some who broke from such therapeutic systems in favor of clinical observation and pathological anatomy, there were still contingents of patients who held to decades-old traditions of medical practice in Galesburg. These traditions would be tested in new ways when the Civil War displaced young men from their mother's expert care.

## The War Came to Galesburg

When the Civil War commenced in April 1861, President Abraham Lincoln's call for 75,000 troops awakened towns across the North to rally to defend the United States. In Galesburg, several companies were formed in May 1861, with many more to follow. By the war's end, Knox County took pride in its contributions, boasting that there were "only seven counties in the state that furnished a larger number of soldiers than Knox County, and none that filled their quotas more promptly."[42] This deep sense of duty and swift mobilization reflected how Galesburg residents saw themselves: committed, sacrificial, and unwavering in their support of the Union cause.

When the war broke out, Galesburg was firmly Republican, and there was little question of the town's stance on the war's purpose. Deeply rooted in the evangelical fervor of the second Great Awakening, Galesburg had gained a reputation as a "hot-bed for abolitionism" in Illinois.[43] Mary Bickerdyke never publicly proclaimed affiliation with the abolitionist movement, but the Bickerdykes would have been keenly aware of the positions on Black equality taken by their chosen congregation as well as the general impulses of the college town where they lived.

Galesburg was the fifth stop on the Lincoln-Douglas debate circuit that featured the rising Republican Party candidate. The candidates' speeches took place on October 7, 1858, and attracted over 15,000 observers from Galesburg and its surrounding towns. The founders of Knox College and Galesburg were profoundly antislavery and were shaped by the Oberlin College tradition. This refers to the antislavery, evangelical, and coeducational ethos of the college, which influenced Galesburg's founders and fostered its reputation as a hub of abolitionist activism. In the years after the passage of the Fugitive Slave Act of 1850, Galesburg became an enclave for freedom seekers who felt "as free from capture when within its limits as if in Canada."[44] As a result, the debate provided a fitting time and place for Lincoln to strongly attack Stephen A. Douglas's position on slavery.[45] There is no record that the Bickerdykes attended the day's festivities, but no Galesburg resident would have been able to escape the community fervor surrounding the event.

In Galesburg, Mary Bickerdyke immersed herself in religious and political circles that prepared her for patriotic action. Bickerdyke attended Galesburg's First Congregational Church, which was led by Rev. Dr. Edward Beecher. Beecher's influence extended far beyond the pulpit; he was part of a renowned family deeply embedded in the most pressing reform movements of the era. Born into the reform-minded Beecher dynasty—son of Rev. Lyman Beecher, brother to the famous preacher Henry Ward Beecher and *Uncle Tom's Cabin* author Harriet Beecher Stowe—Edward Beecher was no stranger to the nation's "firestorms of reform."[46] The Beechers collectively shaped religious thought, women's rights activism, and abolitionism, making their name synonymous with moral and social transformation. Beecher came to Illinois after his Yale education and a short tenure leading a Boston congregation. Upon being invited to lead Illinois College in Jacksonville as its first president, Beecher set out to implement "true systems of theology and right social organizations" in the young interior state, hoping to re-create the reform work that he had begun in the East.[47] Beecher was eventually called to lead his Galesburg church in 1855, arriving a few years before the Bickerdykes. He took up active abolitionist work in the town that used the convergence of several railroads to the advantage of freedom seekers traveling to Chicago.[48] This reformist energy surrounded Bickerdyke, shaping her worldview and preparing her for the work that lay ahead. The same commitment to justice and action that animated Galesburg's abolitionist movement would later propel her into service when the nation called on its citizens to act.

By the time the Civil War began, Galesburg's churches and organizations were well-practiced in mobilizing their community for a cause. They swiftly rallied around local families to support the newly formed military companies, soon confronting the stark realities of war firsthand. In May 1861, Beecher led the charge to clearly articulate the meaning and purpose of the unfolding conflict. With a committee of other Illinois Congregationalist ministers, Beecher asserted that "the Union instituted by our fathers fresh from the battles of liberty, was intended to preserve and favor freedom, and limit and discountenance slavery . . . that as the war is but the ripe and bitter fruit of slavery, we trust the American people will demand that it shall result in relieving our country entirely and forever of that sin and curse."[49] There was a clear moral, patriotic, and religious purpose for war, according to Beecher, and both God and the founders would vindicate their crusade to cleanse the country from the sins of slavery. Armed with this conviction, Galesburg's sons went to the front.

Dr. Benjamin Woodward, from Galesburg, was stationed in Cairo, Illinois, where he and other Union army surgeons promptly identified the conditions in the barracks as nothing short of a medical crisis (see figure 1.1). Woodward described the conditions as follows:

> I was ordered to the charge of the general hospital at Cairo, ILL., a large, three-story brick building, intended for a hotel. The walls were rough, unplastered, and the third story had only loose rough boards for a floor. Gathered into that place were about 300 sick men—camp diarrhoea, dysentery, typhoid fever, and measles. No ice to be had, the water just out of the foul Mississippi river; no nurses but men from the ranks, all unused to the care of the sick; no changes of underclothes; no convenience for bathing; no nice cooking for the sick. In the midst of such suffering and disorder nothing but the warm heart and willing hand of woman could bring order out of chaos.[50]

The situation was dire, and swift action was imperative. Amid the squalor and suffering, Woodward knew that Mary Bickerdyke was a person capable of imposing order and care in such conditions. His request for her assistance

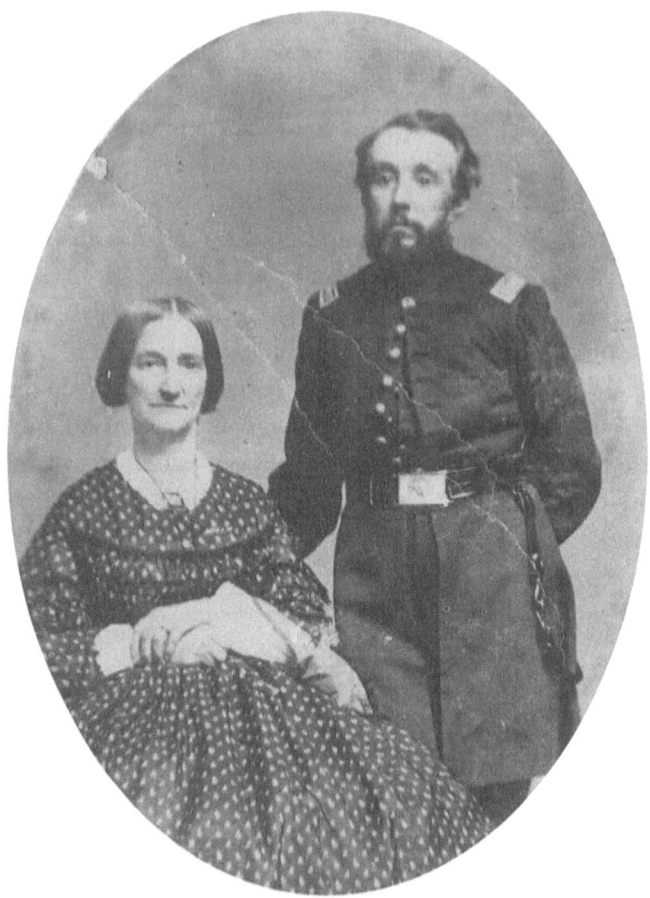

FIGURE 1.1 Dr. Benjamin Woodward and his wife Amanda. This photograph was "taken when father came home on his first furlough Galesburg, 1863." Woodward was Mary Bickerdyke's first point of contact during her Civil War service. Courtesy of the Abraham Lincoln Presidential Library.

moved swiftly through the ranks, reaching General Ulysses S. Grant, who approved Woodward's request. With that, Bickerdyke was summoned to the barracks at Cairo in the summer of 1861 as a force for transformation in the Union's fight against disease and neglect.

Before the war, Woodward's medical practice in western Illinois coexisted and perhaps even competed with Mary Bickerdyke's botanic practice. In the Western states, where trained physicians were scarce, settlers relied on a blend of orthodox medicine and practical, experience-based treatments to sustain their communities. Rather than viewing Bickerdyke's work as inferior,

Woodward recognized the value of diverse approaches to healing. In many cases, traditional medical practice and domestic caregiving worked in tandem, each filling critical gaps in patient care. This dynamic became painfully evident in Cairo, where Woodward quickly realized that the soldiers assigned to care for the sick lacked even the most basic medical knowledge. In civilian life, tending to the ill had largely fallen to female household members, neighbors, or relatives, with doctors stepping in only when specialized treatment was required, and was typically within the home.[51] Antebellum health care had long been the domain of women, who understood that a "comfortable sickroom" was as vital to recovery as any medical intervention.[52] Now, given the chaos of war, Bickerdyke was poised to bring that same logic of care to the overcrowded, unsanitary hospitals of the Union army.

The jarring change in this system came with the onset of the Civil War, when explicitly gendered lines were drawn between male and female practitioners in the ranks. Physicians faced complex questions during the Civil War and developed collaborative and professional responses to those challenges, making the war a critical period of development for nineteenth-century professionals.[53] Shauna Devine argues that many doctors took advantage of the collaborative opportunities presented by the Civil War and, as a result, redefined and reshaped American medicine. Female medical intervention contributed to the massive adaptations necessitated by the war.

While the historical record confirms Woodward's written request and Bickerdyke's arrival in Cairo between June and August 1861, the way this moment has been remembered reveals a more profound cultural significance.[54] Over time, authors have reimagined the circumstances of her recruitment, crafting narratives that elevate her call to service into something more mythological than a simple request for a medical professional's aid. These exaggerated accounts not only lack documentary evidence but also reflect the symbolic weight of Bickerdyke's wartime role. They reveal how Bickerdyke's story and legacy became intertwined with broader cultural ideals of duty, sacrifice, and feminine resilience.

In 1952, prolific young adult biographer Nina Brown Baker published *Cyclone in Calico: The Story of Mary Ann Bickerdyke*. From 1940 to her death in 1958, Baker produced over a dozen biographies of famous world figures. Her subjects spanned an impressive chronological and geographical range, from Peter the Great to Simón Bolívar, Amerigo Vespucci, *and* Nellie Bly. Baker's rapidly produced books integrated the available historical detail from the canon of past biographies into storybook prose that was both narratively captivating and still largely historically accurate. Baker's writing followed the conventions of the young adult genre, prioritizing accessibility and moral lessons over the emerging academic rigor of professional historians. As a result, her biography of Bickerdyke is more of an inspirational story than a strictly historical work. While Baker's vivid storytelling brings Bickerdyke's legacy to life, it also makes it difficult for readers, especially young ones, to distinguish between documented fact and her interpretive embellishments.

*Cyclone in Calico* presented a dramatized and heroic version of Bickerdyke's life, much like a Disney adaptation, bringing her story out of relative obscurity nearly five decades after her death. The book began with an imagined 1861 pulpit call as Edward Beecher implored his Galesburg congregation to send needed supplies to the illness-ridden army camp at Cairo, Illinois. The scene, theatrically fictionalized, was shaped around true historical details but infused with the conjured dramatization of Beecher and the congregation at Galesburg, Illinois.

Instead of his usual sermon, Beecher read the desperate letter from Dr. Benjamin Woodward to his congregation. The doctor's petition wrenched at the heart as it described neglected and untended young boys and men who had left their homes months prior and were now suffering from want of care. According to Baker, the preacher's words were a siren call to Bickerdyke, who sat dutifully in her pew and spang to service at the pastor's words. Bickerdyke was armed with maternal and medical competence that drove her to the self-assured resolution: "If the men had had proper care, the sort of care they would have had at home, they might not have died at all."[55] The citizens of Galesburg, according to Baker, knew that Bickerdyke was the one best suited for the job, and she was brought before the church. She accepted the congregation's nomination with a humble sense of duty and ability.

As Baker imagined it, Bickerdyke stood to speak to the congregation. "I'll go to Cairo," she said, "and I'll clean things up down there. You don't need to worry about that, neither. Them generals and all ain't going to stop me. This is the Lord's work you're calling me to do. And when I'm doing the Lord's work, they ain't nobody big enough to stop me."[56] Throughout the book, Baker injected dialogue that conveyed Bickerdyke's simplicity, typecasting her in a country-bumpkin role that contrasted with the distinguished and educated doctors and reformers with whom she interacted in the Union army and the USSC. Although Baker did not think her subject was altogether unintelligent, Bickerdyke's character in the book spoke with a twang, used contracted phrases, and often asked ignorant questions. She was depicted as unpretentious and culturally different, proving that she was the opposite of women like Mary Livermore who flaunted their education, refinement, and "Boston fussiness about grammar."[57]

In *Cyclone in Calico*, Baker's portrayal of Bickerdyke highlights the challenges she faced as a respected but unconventional female medical practitioner in the nineteenth century and emphasizes her struggle for recognition and the complex social dynamics that shaped her career. First, Bickerdyke's call to the front and the community's recognition of her abilities demonstrate the cultural importance of female medical practitioners. The overstated narrative of spiritual and community support affirmed Dr. Woodward's confidence in Mary Bickerdyke's ability to provide medical expertise to the Union's efforts. Second, Baker portrayed Bickerdyke as being simple. Even as a respected medical practitioner, Mary Bickerdyke was not formally educated. In fact, Bickerdyke spent her life and career fighting to prove her ability to perform medical interventions. Respectability was important in the nineteenth century, and Bickerdyke constantly navigated social and professional situations that dismissed her abilities or qualifications based on her pedigree and socioeconomic position. As she reflected on her youth, Bickerdyke collaborated with biographers toward the end of her life to address her perceived shortcomings—her lack of education, notable familial lineage, and direct maternal training—that might cause a critical American public to hesitate in wholeheartedly celebrating her designated role as a civic mother.

In late-life biographies and memoirs, false narratives persisted about her early life, pedigree, and preparation for her eventual success in the public sphere, as though her accomplishments during the Civil War needed to be legitimized by an idealized past rather than standing on their own merits. For example, many biographers have suggested that Bickerdyke received academic training under the teaching and preaching of Charles Grandison Finney, president of Oberlin College.[58] Bickerdyke had proximity to the coeducational experiments at Oberlin College, which have been viewed as an enlightened development in women's higher education. At the Ohio seminary, women were educated, but the equality of that education in the nineteenth century was questionable.[59] Women who attended the college came from middle- to upper-class families and were primarily trained for "intelligent motherhood and properly subservient wifehood."[60] Proximity was not the same as enrollment, and Bickerdyke never attended any institutions of higher learning, including Oberlin.[61] Instead, she was taught in the school of affliction, trained in her family as a caretaker. Another recorded but likely false bona fide recounted her training in emergency medicine under

Dr. Reuben D. Mussey of Cincinnati during one of the city's cholera outbreaks.[62] Mussey was a celebrated doctor and professor of surgery at the Medical College of Ohio at the time; however, no records suggest he personally trained Bickerdyke during the public health crisis in 1849.

Despite claims linking Bickerdyke to prominent Ohio figures, both instances have been thoroughly debunked, revealing the persistence of historical inaccuracies in the retelling of Bickerdyke's life. These false claims reflect a backward projection of status, which only makes sense when we consider what it meant to "earn" the honorific of a publicly venerated mother. The attempts to bolster her credentials were entirely unnecessary, as Bickerdyke became a revered "Mother" precisely because she did not conform to traditional markers of culturally sanctioned maternal success. Her boys, which included her biological sons and those she affectionately adopted through professional care, loved her not in spite of this distinction but because of it.[63] Baker's portrayal of Bickerdyke's simplicity in speech and demeanor aligns more closely with the historical record than these exaggerated tales.

Bickerdyke put in an extraordinary amount of work on behalf of others whom she designated as needing care and attention. Her benevolence was lateral; she served men whose station in life was similar to her own, unlike many reform-minded humanitarians of her era who took a top-down approach to care. From the beginning of her public career, she engaged in her work with her boots on the ground and understood the needs of her patients and care recipients through her shared experience as a fellow member of the working class. Her efforts to advocate for the common soldier were valiant, empathetic, and progressive for her time.

Mary Bickerdyke's historical legacy portrays her as a singular force of nature who asserted her pragmatic regimen of care throughout her life, despite her limited access to professional training or education.[64] Unsurprisingly, though, her success was never completely the result of her own merits or accomplishments. Her ability to care-switch between homegrown remedies and emerging medical techniques, her willingness to take risks, and her boldness in experimenting with a variety of ventures were predicated on a wide range of support. Mary Bickerdyke was propelled into public arenas largely because those around her recognized her capacity and competence for providing care that could effectively help people's lives. As she entered positions that typically required professional training, Bickerdyke relied heavily on those around her to perform tasks beyond her abilities. When she entered into service during the Civil War, she was determined not to let her lack of educational background deter her from pursuing larger goals and purposes.

She consistently enlisted the help of those around her to gain prominence, prestige, and position within her institutional arrangements.

When Bickerdyke received the request to join Dr. Woodward and assist in the Union army efforts, it presented a job opportunity that allowed her to support her family while serving a greater moral purpose. The immense suffering of the Civil War turned Mary Bickerdyke from a poor, middle-aged widow into an active and legendary nurse, agent, and organizer. She brought her informal training and personal experiences with death and dying into a professional and public setting.

Care-Switching: Leaving Her Boys to Care for "Her Boys"

As she transitioned out of her home context and into public professional practice, Mary Bickerdyke was seen as "a woman rough, uncultivated, even ignorant but a diamond in the rough," refined by her situational inheritance of "hardihood" that made her "by nature fitted for the work in which she became noted."[65] Women become "fitted" for work in Civil War field hospitals by demonstrating their ability to care-switch—that is, their capacity to transfer and translate their domestic medical training into a professional environment. This skill allowed women to extract the caregiving expertise cultivated in the home and apply it to compensated labor. For Bickerdyke, this shift profoundly shaped her relationship with her sons, as her professional decisions redefined the nature of her maternal role. At the same time, her ability to deploy maternal care in professional settings was instrumental in her rise to fame as "Mother" Bickerdyke.

"Mother" Mary Bickerdyke has been the subject of historical discussions about women's roles in the Civil War, but little attention has been given to how her public persona intersected with her private life as the mother of two sons and a step-mother. The Civil War forced her to adapt traditional maternal care, reshaping both the meaning and practice of motherhood in her life. For widowed women like Bickerdyke, motherhood was culturally rigid but practically malleable—able to accommodate economic necessity and in this case, civic action. Bickerdyke's case is particularly noteworthy because she leveraged her fame as a civic "mother" to secure employment far from her biological sons, raising the question of whether she ultimately belonged more to the nation's community of veterans than to her own family circle.

Historians have pointed out that Bickerdyke left her sons; however, their analysis often stops there.[66] Apart from Jane Schultz, who noted Bickerdyke's "epistolary neglect" of her sons during the war, most historians seem to chalk up Bickerdyke's absence to patriotic domesticity. She chose to employ her medical skills to serve the country, as so many men were doing.[67] Most accounts of Bickerdyke's story overlook her postwar activities, which continued to limit her direct domestic involvement in her children's lives.

Widowhood compelled Bickerdyke to depart from the traditional domestic economy, and the need to provide for her children also opened an opportunity to assert her professional independence, placing her on a path that diverged from most women in the USSC. The Civil War thrust Bickerdyke into a new phase of her maternal development, and the opportunities prompted by her employment forever altered her relationship with her sons. The narrative of Civil War sacrifice is well documented, but it also rests on the assumption that women largely returned to the status quo of the domestic economy after their wartime duties were over. This was untrue of Mary Bickerdyke, who continued to distance herself from the cultural constraints of domesticity by leaving her sons in the care of others while she was popularly lauded as "Mother" to soldiers. Her experience differed dramatically from that of her female colleagues in the USSC because of her economic and marital status.

Importantly, Bickerdyke adapted her ideas of culturally acceptable motherhood in the private sphere and carved out spaces for herself as a public mother through the process of care-switching. The term refers to the process by which women adapt and apply their domestic caregiving skills to professional and public settings, particularly during times of crisis or social change. This terminology is derived from the concept of "code-switching," wherein behavior or language is adapted from informal to formal settings to gain social acceptance. In Bickerdyke's case, care-switching was a behavioral adjustment involving therapeutics, language, and a general willingness to play by the rules of the game when it resulted in personal advantage or benefited patients under her care. The necessity to activate care-switching was rooted in the social, economic, and cultural conditions of nineteenth-century America, which included the gendered ideology of separate spheres, the professionalization of medicine, and the impact of the Civil War on family life and women's roles.

Engaging in professions that relied on care-switching offered professionalizing women in caring professions with new opportunities for empowerment and autonomy. Women who chose to pursue caring professions in the mid-nineteenth century often did so because these occupations fit into the cultural expectations of women's labor.[68] After overcoming that gendered barrier to entry, women could enter professional spaces where their knowledge and instincts were affirmed and respected. Through care-switching, women like

Mary Bickerdyke were able to exercise greater control over their lives and make decisions that challenged traditional gender roles and expectations. Women who successfully adapted their caregiving skills to professional settings often gained public recognition and respect for their contributions, which could enhance their social status and influence. For Bickerdyke, care-switching provided a sense of purpose and fulfillment, allowing her to make a meaningful impact through her work.

Mother Bickerdyke made decisions that reflected both the economic pressures she faced as a widow and her evolving professional ambitions. Her engagement in care-switching in Union camps, hospitals, and battlefields was not only a necessity for employment but also a means of asserting authority over medical practices that aligned with her values. At times, she embraced this shift willingly; at other times, she did so begrudgingly, recognizing that leveraging her maternal expertise was often the only way to secure influence in male-dominated medical spaces. Through this fluid navigation of roles, she advanced her career while also shaping battlefield and hospital care through a maternal lens.

Bickerdyke's professional ambitions did not exist in isolation from her personal commitments. She remained invested in the well-being of her biological children, even as she extended her maternal care to wounded soldiers who came to see her as their own. In every role she assumed—nurse, administrator, advocate, and surrogate mother—she wrestled with the emotional weight of her choices. The pull of fulfillment and heartache accompanied each move, as she sought to balance her devotion to her family, her professional aspirations, and her commitment to the countless soldiers who relied on her care. Through this complex negotiation of identities, Bickerdyke redefined the boundaries of maternal labor, proving that care was not just a private duty but a powerful public force.

Most likely, the seemingly drastic decision to leave her children was predicated on some combination of elements that were both practical and patriotic, both maternal and extra-maternal. A sense of loyalty to the Galesburg community's call for help at the Cairo army camp, her personal recruitment, and a national crisis prompted her to work both inside and outside the maternal instincts and boundaries that shaped the rest of her professional life. Some early biographers preferred to attribute her decision to a feminized patriotism, a version of the same impulse that drove men to enlist and leave their families for the perils of war. They conceived that Bickerdyke made the decision as part of a calling rife with religious undertones. She was compelled not by the prospect of economic survival; rather, "with a tender, patriotic heart, Mrs. B. felt called upon to go."[69] Of course, that patriotic justification was an attractive and admirable quality, but for women with household obligations—especially a woman with no means to compensate a governess or family member—the notion of leaving young dependents and struggling to provide for their basic care undercut the core tenets of domesticity.

From 1861 until at least 1868, the Bickerdyke boys did not live with their mother. When Bickerdyke left Galesburg for the war, she made a controversial decision to break the security of the home circle and leave her young children without a parent present. Her children were charged to the ladies of Galesburg and Bickerdyke's home church, who took over as community mothers, aiding Mary E. "Mollie" Bickerdyke, James and Hiram's stepsister, who was sixteen years old when Bickerdyke left for the war.[70] Their wartime correspondence is sparse, but James's letters to his mother throughout 1868 reveal some of the hardships that the Bickerdyke boys endured because of their mother's remote employment. It is evident from the course of his life that James Bickerdyke, Mary's elder biological son, bore the brunt of the emotional trauma that his mother's absence inflicted. He spent the entirety of his mother's life vying for her attention and attempting to prove his worth through his professional success.

James Bickerdyke was consistently riddled with worry (see figure 1.2). As the elder brother in charge of himself and his younger brother, such a disposition made sense. When his mother left for the front in 1861, the eleven-year-old boy could not yet grasp what it meant to develop the emotional resilience needed to endure her sudden and indefinite absence. James took on the primary responsibility of reporting to his mother, requesting her assistance with various needs, and keeping her apprised of his own and Hiram's educational progress.[71] He yearned for his mother to come home and did not shy away from making the request. James wrestled with his own patriotism as he developed an awareness of the war efforts and his tangential participation in the Union cause. On the one hand, he wanted his mother for his own comfort, inserting requests like, "How long before you come back to see us? I would walk 5 miles to see you if you was [sic] so near." But only a few lines later, James recognized his mother's calling to the sons at war, telling her to "give my love to all the Soldiers."[72]

Hiram Bickerdyke, Mary's younger son, was six years old at the war's start when she left for Cairo (see figure 1.3). Affectionately called "Sugar," Hiram's personality contrasted with his older brother's.[73] Much less serious and far more adventurous, Hiram often frustrated James, causing their mother to occasionally have to intervene. She advised James, "Don't let friend nor foe stir up your mind about Hiram for you can no more carry Hiram on your shoulders than you can carry the United States. You are constitutionly [sic] differ-

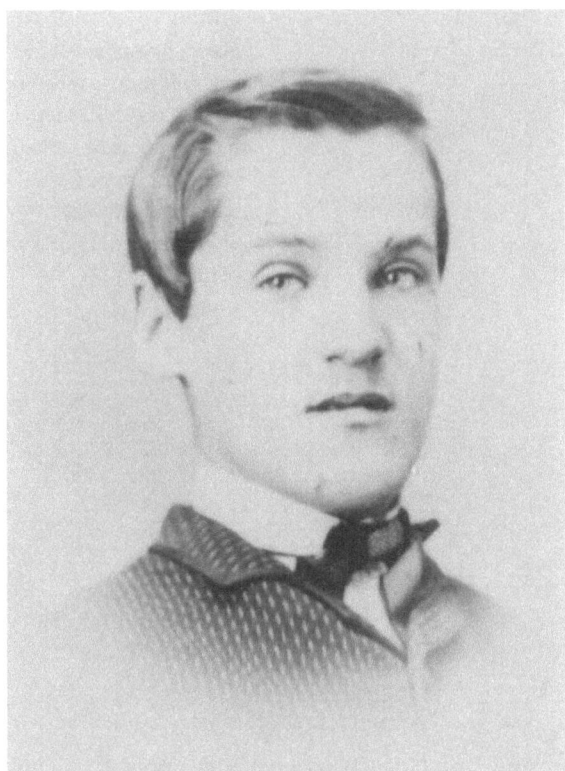

FIGURE 1.2
James Bickerdyke, while a student at Beloit College, age 16. Courtesy of the Library of Congress.

ent, but you are to [sic] dear brothers."[74] While constitutionally different, the two brothers were intimately bonded, and throughout their youth, James was Hiram's keeper.

After leaving in July 1861, Bickerdyke returned home on furlough only twice during the war.[75] While their mother served during the war, Hiram suffered from chronic auditory illness and experienced hearing loss, which required continuous medical attention.[76] Hiram's caretakers, James included, struggled to reconcile Mother Bickerdyke's attentive care to soldiers with Hiram's relative motherless suffering. Hiram never mentioned that his mother's distance during his dangerous illness affected him, perhaps being too young and accustomed to other surrogate mothers to feel the ache for his own mother's presence like his older brother did. Mary Bickerdyke's decision to remain on the battlefield through the end of the conflict deprived her sons of care as well as the money needed for prescriptions. While Bickerdyke worked to maintain her legacy as a revered middling mother, her biological sons suffered from her absence while entrenched in working-class struggles.

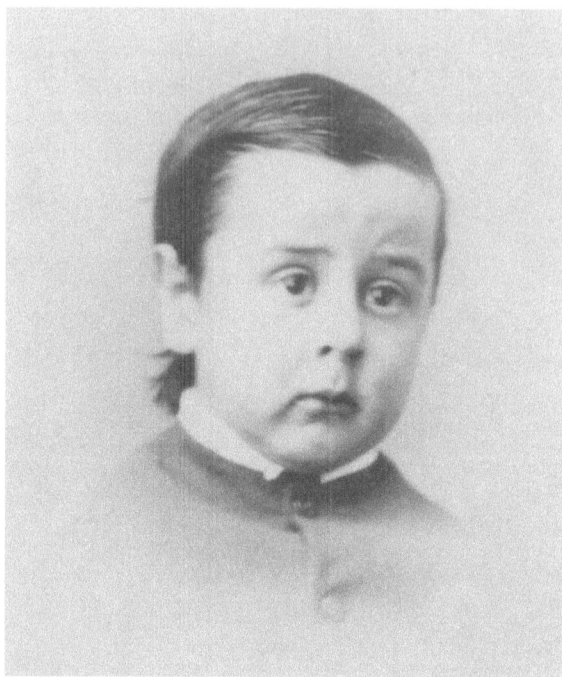

FIGURE 1.3
Hiram Bickerdyke at five years old, one year before Mary Bickerdyke left for her service to the Union army. The image was taken by a Chicago photographer. Courtesy of the Library of Congress.

Unlike Mary Livermore and Jane Hoge, who were both upper-class Chicago women who worked for the USSC and could afford to hire help while managing their duties from local offices, Bickerdyke spent the war years constantly relocating her sons among friends, teachers, and boarding houses.[77] During the war, Hiram and James alternated between working-class and middle-class living arrangements, between rural and urban lives, subject to their mother's wishes, wages, and developing social networks. By the time the guise of a settled home environment manifested for the Bickerdyke boys, they were eighteen and fourteen years old.

Bickerdyke's absence from home and her decision to abandon domestic maternity for the role of battlefield "Mother" have garnered varied interpretations. In response to the anticipated judgment about her choice of patriotic duty over domestic responsibility, postwar biographers L. P. Brockett and Mary Vaughan praised Bickerdyke's patriotic zeal, characterizing it as "even stronger than her love for her children," framing potential maternal neglect as situationally appropriate or merely another sacrifice demanded by the war.[78] Another, more candid evaluation came from her initial recruiter Dr. Benjamin Woodward. In 1888, he reflected that women who chose to leave their homes, even for such a national duty, were "often maligned and despised . . .

as one who debased herself."[79] He acknowledged that the patriotic narrative served as a fragile shield, crafted to protect a woman's dignity and reputation in the face of criticism for leaving home. Martin Litvin, a more recent Bickerdyke biographer, defended his "patron saint" against such attacks and described how Bickerdyke's initial arrangements were perfectly acceptable.[80] Both defenders and detractors miss some crucial points in Bickerdyke's decisions, tending to focus more on individual character than on economic pressures or expanded opportunities for women's employment.

During the Civil War, motherhood and childhood changed, alongside every other aspect of civilian and family life. Historians have written about the evolving concepts of motherhood in the nineteenth century, noting the varied childrearing practices across regions and social classes.[81] While some historians note the diversity of childhood experiences across these categories, scholars of historical childhood depict types of mothers broadly, leaving little room for women like Bickerdyke, who did not fit neatly into a category.[82] James Marten argued that wartime home front experiences "politicized" children. The Bickerdyke children were acutely aware of the war from their mother's letters, but the extent of their war-related politicization was naming a pet bird "Lincoln."[83] In *Huck's Raft*, Steven Mintz argued that while the Civil War disrupted families and exposed children to "adult realities," it caused parents to become more protective of their children, suggesting that "postwar parents strengthened and intensified family bonds."[84] This was certainly not the case for the Bickerdykes.

The Bickerdyke family, like many others across the nation, experienced separation because of wartime circumstances. For some, the home served as a refuge from the daily humiliations of poverty and wage labor—a space where a mother could privately uphold the security and dignity associated with the American middle-class ideal of domesticity.[85] But the home, with all that it symbolized to Bickerdyke and others, could not substitute for the necessity of work for provision. As a result, poorer families or homes with single mothers were sometimes forced to place their children in orphanages, another growing institution that emerged from the Civil War's carnage. The isolated conditions of Western life often left greater distance between familial support and resulted in less stable temporary arrangements, like those experienced by James and Hiram throughout the war.

By the mid-nineteenth century, puritanical views on childhood had evolved as an emphasis on childhood innocence and parental warmth gained cultural acceptance.[86] By this period, a child's "age of innocence" extended to roughly fifteen, though it varied by class, region, and race.[87] The Civil War, as several historians have argued, unsettled these norms, exposing children to the anxieties and responsibilities of wartime life.[88] Mary Bickerdyke's long absence, for example, left her children to navigate this vulnerable development stage without her daily care. Each son was undoubtedly affected by the combination of these arrangements, and their individual trajectories underscored the need for a more precise historical inspection of the effects of shifting motherhoods and Bickerdyke's care-switching.

Mary Bickerdyke made a consequential decision when she left her sons to serve in the Civil War. She knew her course was unusual, but that did not deter her from continuing to choose remote working arrangements after the war's conclusion. Her wartime employment introduced a constant tension in Bickerdyke's motherhood: a lifelong attempt to balance her biological motherhood with a newfound civic motherhood, operating within a care-switching dynamic. During the war, she began to frame her absence in terms of a combined patriotic and maternal duty. When her boys, just eight and twelve years old, begged her to come home, she turned their plea into a lesson in self-sacrifice: "Now my dear children would you have me leave these wounded men and come home to you today and take you away to find our pleasure together? Or would my little boys exercise their patriotism and self-denial and wait until this terrible campaign is ended? I shall leave the question with you dear and you must write and tell what you wish me to do."[89] Dutifully, the boys expressed whatever sense of patriotism they could muster, echoing the soldier-sons their mother had chosen to serve. After the war was over, Bickerdyke reflected on her decisions, using her Christian faith to attempt to make peace with herself and her children: "Now my darlings I have laid you on the *Alter* [sic] of the Lord as all these years of separation his spirit has been with my spirit that he might watch over you and guide you when the cold storms beat."[90] Still, the tension was present. Even as she pronounced her assurance, she admitted that her "mother's heart yearns for her two darlings on the Western Prairie," a poignant reminder of the emotional cost of balancing private love and public duty.[91]

Mary Bickerdyke could have returned to her sons after the war as she had promised them in her letters. Instead, she abandoned the cultural expectations of domestic economy and engaged in a motherhood of her own design, shaped by professional opportunity and economic potential. Her domestic ideal, which was already marginal because of her socioeconomic and marital status, was altered by wartime duty that caused her to displace the hearth for the campfire.

CHAPTER TWO

# Becoming Mother
## *The Civil War and the Development of Bickerdyke's Public Motherhood (1861–1863)*

While soldiers and surgeons were familiar with the untimely loss of life in their prewar communities, nothing could have prepared them for the devastation that swept through army camps and battle lines. At the war's outset, modern medicine was notoriously inadequate, its implementation hindered by "inexperienced . . . arrogant, negligent" army doctors whose patient loads far exceeded their training. Jane Hoge, a prominent humanitarian and leader of the Chicago Sanitary Commission, later reflected that doctors seemed powerless against the relentless forces of disease and death, condemning soldiers to die before they had even reached their regimental assignments.[1] The collective despair was not entirely misplaced because by the end of the conflict, 63 percent of Union casualties were wrought by disease compared to only 19 percent of deaths by battle.[2]

Fortunately for the Union army, the indomitable Mary Bickerdyke, described as a force of nature akin to the "prairie-plough and thunderstorm," was there to confront the relentless "subsoil" of disease.[3] Equipped with the practical know-how and a maternal force of will, Bickerdyke did not singlehandedly stop gastrointestinal illness from ravaging General Ulysses S. Grant's forces. In contrast to army doctors, however, she brought comfort and a working understanding of hygiene and cleanliness. In her own household and the community where she had practiced botanic medicine, she had battled the same diseases and fought to prevent their spread. As expected of a female caretaker, she remained at the bedside when her remedies failed, offering solace to patients.

Mary Bickerdyke did not enter the war with the widely recognized title of "Mother." Rather, it was a reputation that grew over time during the Civil War. It is likely that the genesis of the honorific came from usage among the rank-and-file with whom Bickerdyke interacted; it then became part of United States Sanitary Commission (USSC) correspondence and was subsequently reprinted by the press during the war years. In 1863, a small newspaper in eastern Illinois admonished the community's young women to contribute to the war effort alongside the community's mothers. One young woman wrote: "Our mothers, breaking away from social duties, spend a day of each week cooking for the soldiers. Can we do less? . . . Can you turn a deaf ear to the eloquent appeals of Mrs. Colt? Can you look upon indifference upon the brave example of 'Mother Bickerdyke'? No indeed!"[4] From the front, fellow USSC workers praised her work and her popularity among the fighting force: "The soldiers fully appreciate 'Mother Bickerdyke,' as they call her, and her work."[5] By the end of the war, Bickerdyke's reputation even seeped into newspaper advertisements for washing machines. In Brooklyn, J. Ward and Co. sold "Union Washing Machines and Wringers," bragging that "Mrs. Bickerdyke, 'the mother' of the Fifteenth Army Corps, has one in her possession, and although it has washed over 200,000 articles of soldiers' and hospital clothing, yet it is as good to-day for all practical purposes as when it started on its journey."[6] Popular usage of "Mother" Bickerdyke, which separated her from other women in the USSC, proliferated after memorial literature became a popular genre. Her legacy was further cemented through postwar memorial literature, including Jane Hoge's *The Boys in Blue* (1867) and L. P. Brockett and Mary Vaughn's *Woman's Work in the War* (1867), which solidified her status as the enduring maternal figure of the Union army.

But how did she *become* "Mother?" A reexamination of Bickerdyke's Civil War record from contemporaneous accounts provides effective descriptors and reveals new insights into the changing role of motherhood because of the Civil War's familial displacement. The versatility of her labors within the USSC shows that her competencies as a domestically trained health provider were equal to the demands of ailing soldiers who constantly faced death from illness and injury. Bickerdyke's work to prevent death while providing comfort to the dying and their families during the Civil War signals an individual effort to offer professional palliative care and suggests that the origin of the twentieth-century subset of hospital specializations such as hospice care has a much longer history tied to female practitioners like Mother Bickerdyke.

Bickerdyke developed a pragmatic protocol for end-of-life care both before and during her association with the USSC. When she faced death and dying on the front lines, Bickerdyke acted as a liaison between dying soldiers and their home communities. In this way, she served as a maternal substitute at the bedside during a person's transition from life to death. She sought to fulfill the dying person's final wishes and communicate those final moments to anxious family members waiting for reassurances that their loved one was well cared for, demonstrated a fortitude of faith, and could be properly identified and buried. Her professional contributions have been overshadowed by her maternal identity and the nature of historical memory and its construction. Palliative care found its origins in the professional practice and hired work of mothers like Mary Bickerdyke and was largely influenced by the nineteenth-century understanding of a mother's role in the dying process.

Bickerdyke appears as a supporting character in historical scholarship on women of the Civil War era, consistent with the USSC memoirs that addressed Bickerdyke's wartime performance and contributions.[7] She has served the purpose of historians: some of her actions and traits, at times contradictory to cultural conceptions of women's appropriate behavior, are deftly applied to scholarly arguments that situate her story within the culturally acceptable roles of motherhood and domesticity. Most notably, Nina Silber's *Daughters of the Union* recognizes Bickerdyke's maternal authority but suggests that Bickerdyke demonstrated an internalization of her subordinate position as a woman in the army. Silber argues that Bickerdyke "epitomized the lesson that war imparted to the ranks of female nurses: the virtue of proper obedience."[8] Rather than seeing maternal authority as a space of mere compliance, Bickerdyke's example suggests that motherhood could serve as a vehicle for stretching, and sometimes defying, the behavioral expectations placed on women in military contexts. In the Civil War era, women like Mary Bickerdyke, those without the bona fides of formal medical training, gained repute and esteem for their ability to manipulate gendered archetypes to create a standard for end-of-life care in professional settings.

Bickerdyke maintained a level of maternal moral authority that was respected as a form of medical competency, and she became an efficient USSC agent and eventual nurse for the United States Army. At times, she pulled moral rank and inverted the rigid and gendered structures of the Union army. Though women were hired as agents, they were not often given the tools to function outside the constrained roles defined by the male-dominated institution.[9] Additionally, Bickerdyke's medical authority was solidified throughout the Civil War as she provided surrogate motherhood, homestyle comfort measures, and palliative care in a public environment for sick and dying soldiers.

## Entering the Province of Men: Gendered Authority in Civil War Medicine

The USSC had a complex bureaucratic structure that represented an emerging worldview. Specifically, this model valued order, science, structures of authority, and male leadership.[10] From the nationalist perspective, state relief and sanitary work were wasteful mechanisms prone to disorganization and favoritism. While many states eventually conceded local benevolent efforts to the efficiency of a national program, the USSC never successfully countered the impulse toward local control.[11] It was much more integrated into the eastern efforts of the war, where several institutions competed for access to soldiers' aid and well-being throughout the conflict.

When Bickerdyke first arrived in Cairo, Illinois, in 1861, she was unaffiliated with any institution and followed her instincts to work alongside surgeons while attending to sick and dying men. Dr. Benjamin Woodward was familiar with her skill set and felt that Bickerdyke would be an asset to assist medical professionals at the growing Union depot in Cairo, but he did not have any authority to formally grant her that position.[12] Like many Americans, Woodward and Bickerdyke did not anticipate a prolonged conflict when the war commenced. So, with the encouragement of her home community and a personal invitation from a reputable doctor to help as she was able, Bickerdyke went to Cairo unaffiliated and unpaid.

Bickerdyke was one of many women who, driven by patriotic fervor and confidence in their domestic medical skills, rushed to the front to serve as volunteer nurses. One Cairo doctor found himself inundated by women who sought to express their support for the war effort by volunteering as nurses.[13] As seasoned medical practitioners in their households, the women brought their expertise to the army. The war displaced men from the comforts of home, where they were accustomed to having meals prepared, clothes washed, and houses cleaned by women. As diseases crept into the camp, the men were away from their usual caregivers. The replacement care of the Union camp was strikingly bleak and often consisted of squalid and unsanitary conditions, particularly in the early days of the war before the USSC attempted to intervene.

While most female volunteers lacked professional medical training, Mary Bickerdyke arrived in Cairo with credentials. As a botanic physician, she possessed a "vigorous, brusque, and capable" constitution that equipped her to combat the dismal conditions in Cairo. Her training and disposition allowed her to assert her medical authority despite military restrictions on women's involvement in the conflict's early months. The trip to Cairo revealed the need for organization, and Mary Bickerdyke stayed on to help implement hygienic measures in the camp.[14] Bickerdyke, who was still unpaid, was accompanied by a local volunteer, Mary Jane Safford, who had been working in Cairo's regimental hospitals since late April or May 1861.[15] Safford was accustomed to caring for the sick; she often assisted her mother in treating family members and ill neighbors, and Cairo's army hub provided an opportunity for her to serve. She became known for reading Bible passages to sick soldiers and ministering to them, earning the moniker "the Cairo angel."[16]

The two women represented different approaches to the assertion of women's authority in medical care, despite the protests of military personnel who desired regulation, protocol, and ultimately, male professionalization of wartime medicine (see figures 2.1 and 2.2). On the one hand, Mary Safford, the "angel," was young, beautiful, untested in the field, and untrained in formal medicine. What she lacked in scientific training she compensated for with her attention to patient care, earning the adoration of her patients, who saw her presence as a "breath of spring borne into the bare, whitewashed rooms—like a burst of sunlight."[17] Safford's approach was appreciated by soldiers and colleagues, including Bickerdyke, but the arrangement was ultimately unsustainable. Upper-middle-class women like Safford had little exposure to death, suffering, and the physical demands of caregiving. In general, their families had greater access to medical interventions, more knowledge about medical advancements, or more money to hire home caregivers or servants to perform the grueling physical and emotional labor associated with health management. Eventually, Safford succumbed to the harsh conditions of wartime work as weeks of service began to take their toll. By April 1862, Safford would often collapse and become unable to attend to her duties, prompting a family physician to state that "nothing except removal from Cairo could save Mary from more relapses and the danger of possible death."[18] Ultimately, Safford withdrew from war work and spent the next four years convalescing in Paris.

On the other hand, Mary Bickerdyke became the quintessential depiction of female medical care in Cairo and on the Western theater. She resolved to work in hospital administration, despite facing many challenges from male organizers. She was practiced in making diagnoses and vested with the authority to make life-and-death decisions. Mary Bickerdyke and other Civil War mother-nurses understood how to take charge of a sickroom.[19] In a regimental hospital, Civil War soldiers keenly felt the literal distance from their own mothers and were reassured by the presence of a familiar medical authority. Mother Bickerdyke could withstand exposure to the environment, disease, and adversity because she, like other mothers, had been weathered and trained to do so. Both the "angel" and the "mother" were necessary categories in the war hospital, but the mother archetype, as demonstrated by Bickerdyke, proved to be more sustainable as an extension of prewar female medical care.

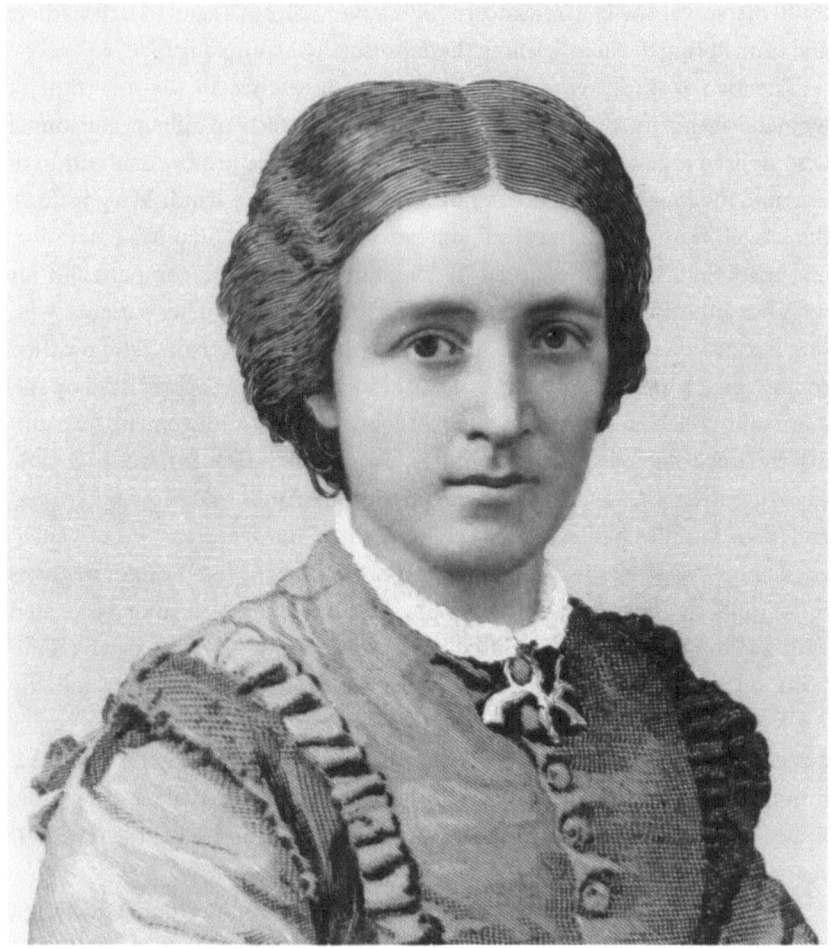

FIGURE 2.1 Mary Jane Safford, "Angel of Cairo." Born in 1834, Safford ministered to the sick and dying men in Cairo, Illinois. After the Battle at Fort Donelson, Safford was joined by Mary Bickerdyke, who directed Safford's work. Safford, who worked with great resolve, became ill as a result of her tireless work and the unpleasantness of Cairo's environs. She left her work at Cairo to convalesce in a healthier environment: Paris. This steel engraving was created after the war and first appeared in L. P. Brockett's *Woman's Work in the Civil War*, published in 1867. Note the difference in demeanor and expression between Safford and Bickerdyke's engraving, shown in figure 2.2. Courtesy of the Library of Congress.

In the opening days of the war, volunteers were confronted with the suffering and poor health conditions in the camps. Even before shots rang out, sickness assaulted young soldiers who encountered the precarious environment in Cairo.[20] Diseases ravaged newly enlisted troops as officers and doctors struggled to enforce hygienic practices. As soon as Bickerdyke arrived at

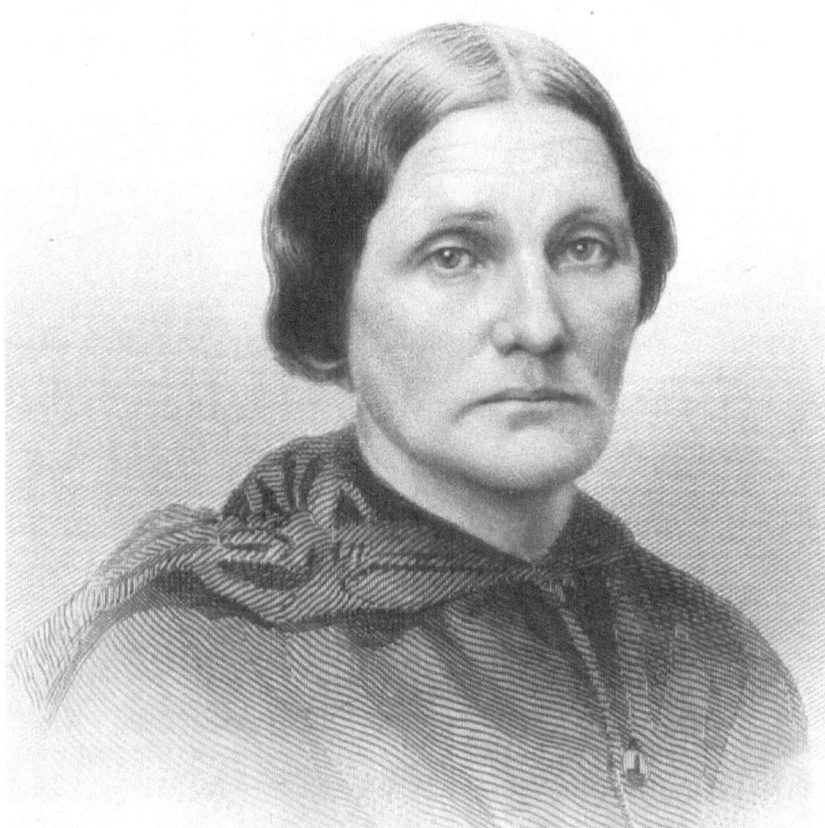

FIGURE 2.2 Mary Ann Bickerdyke, "Mother" Bickerdyke. Born in 1817, Bickerdyke embodied maturity and life experience—as a mother to young children and recent widow—that provided the authoritative "homestyle" medical care under the auspices of the United States Sanitary Commission in Cairo. This 1866 steel engraving by A. H. Ritchie demonstrates her seriousness of character; her face is marked with the lines of experience and a sturdiness of resolve, mentioned by those who observed her at work. This engraving was also published in *Woman's Work in the Civil War* and stands starkly in contrast to the softer features afforded to Safford. Bickerdyke remained in her position as field agent for the USSC throughout the war, engaging constantly in the battle against disease and trauma. Courtesy of the Library of Congress.

the campgrounds in southern Illinois, she encountered a young, enlisted man who was so sick with typhoid fever that he could not recognize anyone around him.[21] Finding the boy in such a dire state, Bickerdyke resolved to remain at his bedside, providing care and comfort until his family could arrive to be with him in his final moments. Reflecting on this experience, she recalled her role as a surrogate: "With the best care that could be given him by the surgeon and myself, we revived him till his father arrived—his family is among my best friends today."[22] Forging a connection with the dying and their surviving loved ones was not just an incidental duty but a defining aspect of Bickerdyke's approach to care. This deeply personal philosophy was shaped by her own familial experiences and an intrinsic understanding of maternal relationships. Because her work began voluntarily, her loyalty lay less with formal institutions than with the soldiers and families who depended on her in their most vulnerable moments.

As soon as it was practicable, the USSC extended its organizational reach to the western outposts of the war to support their efforts. In October 1861, leaders of the USSC toured the Western Department, which included Cairo. They expressed disapproval of its abysmal hygienic conditions and urged the Chicago branch to commence with more thorough inspections and recommendations for improvement.[23] Using the USSC's template for sanitary evaluation, the Chicago branch formed a committee to inspect the depots and hospitals in Cairo and the surrounding area and recommend improvements. The Chicago Sanitary Commission report highlighted the ineffectiveness of the current organization of health management under the supervision of the army.[24]

Bickerdyke and other women fought tirelessly for medical authority against male-dominated national organizations, determined to apply their skills and benevolence in efficient and practical ways while the slow machinery of a massive care system struggled to take shape. As the protocols for USSC operations began to develop on the Western theater, Mary Bickerdyke was expected to adhere to its evolving institutional principles and objectives. One of the main tenets of the sanitary mission was unity of purpose in systematic resource distribution.[25] In its official documentation, the USSC threatened that "no one can be allowed to work in the name of the Commission who does not work in subordination to this common purpose."[26] This was a struggle in the Western Department of the USSC because competition between local, state, and national aid organizations undermined the USSC's core nationalizing principles.[27] Mary Bickerdyke mirrored the sentiments of Illinois citizens and initially refused to rely on the promise of the USSC to deliver a system of organization. Like other women from the North, Bickerdyke recognized the need for hospital supplies, but instead of utilizing this new system, she depended on personal connections to obtain what was needed in what she deemed the most reliable manner. Bickerdyke noted that "finding the great necessity of clean clothing to change our patients with, I commenced to write all over the country for hospital clothing, and it was astonishing how readily the loyal women responded."²⁸ At least in the early part of the war, local communities and their soldiers' aid societies were far more motivated to send supplies to troops who were directly connected to the donors.²⁹

Bickerdyke's first battlefield action came when she cared for the wounded soldiers who were transported back to Cairo, Illinois, from the Battle of Belmont in Missouri on November 7, 1861. From that time forward, her care regimen became well known among the soldiers of the West. When Second Lieutenant Lemuel Adams returned to Cairo after being shot in the forearm and held as a prisoner for several weeks after the battle, he could not help but praise Bickerdyke's care. His inadequate treatment in captivity resulted in a dangerous infection, and many in his own company assumed he would die. He was eventually transferred to the post hospital in Cairo, where he met Mary Bickerdyke. He lauded the lifesaving measures provided by the male surgeons on duty in Cairo, but he emphasized a strong preference for "*Mother Bickerdyke* as she became known throughout the armies of that area from the Battle of Belmont to the end of the Civil War," for she was "*better than all.*"³⁰ Bickerdyke cared for Adams and his ailing comrades at the hospital for months. Adams noted, "I have seen Mother Bickerdyke sit all night by the cot of a sick and dying soldier. She never seemed to tire, and could do more work than *any two nurses I ever saw*. She made sure that everyone had proper attention and that no special favors were shown. Every sick or wounded soldier was *the same to her*, from General Grant to the newest recruit."³¹

For soldier patients like Adams, Bickerdyke's maternal presence was deeply comforting, providing a rare sense of stability and care amid the brutality of war. Where medical professionals had been unable or unwilling to provide familiar and sufficient care, Bickerdyke filled the void with a combination of skill, discipline, and compassion. Her presence transformed the hospital from a place of fear and uncertainty into a space where soldiers felt truly cared for. In a world where war had stripped men of the consolations of home and family, the presence of a maternal caregiver with both medical knowledge and deep emotional resilience offered a critical form of reassurance. For many, Bickerdyke was not just a battlefield nurse. She was a surrogate mother, an unrelenting advocate, and a source of hope in the most desperate circumstances.

## The Lady and the Lamp: Accounts, Memories, and the Truth at the Battle of Fort Donelson

The Battle of Fort Donelson in February 1862 propelled Bickerdyke into a more active phase of wartime duties, and she accompanied General Grant's troops as they were deployed on their campaign. Along with other medical personnel and troops, Bickerdyke stepped off a hospital steamer in the Cumberland River onto the Tennessee shore as the Union army advanced on the Confederate position at Donelson, which could open the door to overtaking the South's defenses. Just days earlier, the Union victory at Fort Henry catapulted Grant's army and naval officer Andrew Foote's armada to the next fortress of the rebel position. A victory at the border of Kentucky and Tennessee held tactical importance for Grant's forces and solidified the general's reputation for an offensive style of unconditional surrender against the enemy. This was the tactical drive that would make Ulysses S. Grant famous: a string of Union victories that stretched from Donelson to Shiloh to Corinth to Vicksburg.[32]

Bickerdyke arrived on the scene toward the climax of the battle at Fort Donelson, on February 13, as General C. F. Smith's brigade approached the Confederate stronghold.[33] As the overzealous Union generals took the offensive in defiance of Grant's orders to avoid unnecessary engagement, Fort Donelson became the site of disproportionate death for the victorious Union army.[34] Ultimately, the Union's superior forces overtook the fort, despite its advantageous defensive position, but not before a great deal of carnage occurred. Amid the bloody assault, Bickerdyke remembered, "I left the boat and went directly to the hospital, and supposing we would be safe from the enemies [sic] guns, but Gen C. F. Smith made his charge right in front of this hospital . . . and men fell right before our eyes."[35]

At the end of the day's siege, there was "rain and snow, thawing and freezing alternately," as the slushy winter landscape accumulated around the bodies of fallen men as well as those whose lives lay in the balance.[36] Among the first carried back to the hospital tents was Henry Rogers, a "bright young man of 18 summers from Knox College, Galesburg Ill."[37] Though Bickerdyke was not a direct witness to his death, she was deeply affected as she watched his childhood friends carry his lifeless body into the makeshift hospital, laying his young frame gently on the straw.[38] Confident in her devotion, they relied on her to report back to their families should they meet the same fate. Many expressed this trust explicitly, telling her, "If we face the same fate let our mothers know."[39] In the heat of battle, without the luxury of time to consider other arrangements, these young soldiers entrusted Bickerdyke with their final wishes, relying on her to preserve their legacies and ensure their loved ones were informed.

Bickerdyke's ability to minister to the families of the dead and dying extended beyond the orthodox medical practices of the time. As a caregiver without institutional affiliations or accompanying moral imperatives, she could provide reasonable alternatives to the ideal "good death" by standing in as a mother, listening to last words, and conveying news to families back home. Since the beginning of the war, Bickerdyke had worked alongside doctors, observing their procedures and treatments. Yet no amount of medical experience could have prepared her for the weight of Henry Rogers's death. In this instance, the loss was personal: she knew both the deceased and his helpmates from life before the war. This death was not anonymous, and community ties complicated its meaning, stretching the boundaries of what it meant to mourn and bear witness. It was not only about respecting the dead and ensuring their good death but also about providing intentional communication and guidance to aid the home-front community through the pain of individual and collective loss. How families should come to know of their sons' deaths mattered.[40] A personalized notification from a community member who witnessed the deceased's final moments could confirm details, fortify religious hopes, and indicate the continued social bonds that brought community members into traditionally familial grief practices.

Nineteenth-century Americans were not prepared for such a profound disruption of their death and mourning rituals. Historian Drew Gilpin Faust details the *ars moriendi* of Victorian America that pervaded prewar culture and explores how the Civil War shattered those mores, quickly constructing new configurations of mourning. Prior to the Civil War, death customs revolved around private and domestic scenes and spaces. It was expected that death would occur at home, surrounded by family, where the last words and countenance of the departing could be witnessed.[41] In order to be assured of the soul's ascension in those final moments, witnesses needed to observe that the deceased was conscious of their fate, had demonstrated a willingness to accept it, had shown signs of a belief in God and in their own salvation, and had left messages and instructive exhortations for those at their side. In this way, there was an assurance of a good death that gave the surviving kin faith in reunification in heaven.

The Civil War challenged these customs associated with death, leaving Americans to try to restore and revise folkways related to these practices. New rituals did not satisfy those whose lives and deaths were made meaningful by dying under certain faith-building conditions, and many alternative commemorative attempts "almost always failed."[42] With few alternatives, letters became a way to come to terms with and make sense of deaths that occurred far from home, taking the place of family members who would normally be deathbed witnesses. The premature loss of life was tragic, and condolence letters could sometimes provide solace. These letters served as a bridge across the chasm of war, connecting the horror of the battlefield with the familiar rituals of home. In an era when war had profoundly disrupted domestic understandings of death, such letters reaffirmed the comforting mid-nineteenth-century beliefs about life's meaning and purpose, offering a symbolic return to order amid the chaos of conflict.[43] Letters sought to make absent family members virtual observers of a loved one's dying moments. Though not a reliable letter writer herself, Bickerdyke always found a willing amanuensis to share the somber news with the deceased's family; she also gave comfort by telling families that she was there with their loved one, like a mother, during their final moments.

On the night of the first battle at Fort Donelson, Bickerdyke, exhausted from the day's labor, retired to a nearby house where Union surgeons and nurses were staying. That day, she had witnessed the horrors of battle firsthand, watching as young men like Henry Rogers were cut down before her eyes. Despite her fatigue, she embarked on a midnight mission to search for wounded soldiers, braving the darkened battlefield to find those still alive and freezing. Her actions that night became the stuff of legend, immortalizing her as a pioneering Civil War nurse and cementing her reputation in postwar narratives. However, these later memorializations often reflected American tropes about nursing, emphasizing heroism while overlooking the radical nature of her unsanctioned intervention. Bickerdyke later corroborated the event, adding details from her own recollections. Notably, she did so after several memoirs had already shaped the public memory of her actions. Her own written accounts, crafted for personal reflection, offer a counterpoint to the mythology that emerged around her, revealing the tension between her lived experience and the ways that her story was later told.

After the battle, as she settled in to rest for a few short hours, she heard a faint but repeated moan in the distance, drifting through the darkness.[44] The haunting intonations disturbed any notion of sleep and pulled Bickerdyke from her bed to investigate. She descended from her quarters to ask the other boarders about the noise outside, but they assured her that all the wounded had already been brought to hospitals. Unconvinced, she could not shake the certainty that men were still out there, suffering, alone, and left behind. Refusing to ignore the cries, she "started out with a lantern, and canteen, filled with hot milk punch, and an escort, and went in the direction of the moan."[45] Armed with the homeopathic remedies of her mother's kit, the most comforting tools in her arsenal, Bickerdyke went out on a midnight mission to relieve the suffering. She was prepared to help and provide palliative and medical supplies for any potential survivors. Her instincts proved to be right.

In the frozen night, she discovered two Union soldiers, wounded and barely clinging to life, their bodies stiff with cold.

To keep the men alive, Bickerdyke's small detail carried the men to the floating hospital on stretchers.[46] Once the men were safely removed from the dangerous conditions and put aboard the hospital steamer, the *Fannie Bullet*, they were transferred to Mound City, Illinois, near Cairo, for further treatment. In her account, Bickerdyke acknowledged that other medical workers and institutions were needed to save the "two frozen heroes," including the detail and the hospital staff that would receive and transfer the men.[47] Yet this episode also demonstrates how she operated outside standard medical protocol. Acting on intuition rather than orders, she organized and requested support for a rescue mission that others had dismissed as unnecessary. When she returned with survivors, she vindicated her own judgment and enhanced her authority, earning greater trust and respect from those around her.

Bickerdyke's unpublished memoir, preserved in her personal papers, offers a more intimate and understated account of this event that differs significantly from the dramatized retellings in postwar memorial literature. While later narratives cast her midnight excursion in the mold of Florence Nightingale's "Lady with the Lamp," emphasizing patriotic heroism and the improvisational nature of women's nursing, Bickerdyke's own recollection underscores a deeper and more personal commitment. For her, the mission at Fort Donelson was not about spectacle or symbolism; it was about devotion to the dead and dying. She approached suffering with a regimen of care that extended beyond mere rescue. She knew when to revive and when to comfort, instinctively choosing the tool most appropriate for the moment. Above all, she carried a sincere and unwavering desire to alleviate suffering and to ensure that no soldier died alone in the cold, denied the dignity of the "good death."

The nighttime rescue mission at the Battle of Fort Donelson quickly became Civil War lore and was "told and re-told by many writers."[48] The anecdote immortalized Bickerdyke's encounters with Civil War patient care and, over the course of its retelling, began to shape a historical understanding of nursing. In the first wave of narration were the USSC histories, which were less intimate and specific in their details. They framed the story for their purpose: Bickerdyke became an explanatory tool for the institution's actions on the field and its ability to adequately bridge the gap between the home front and the battlefield with committed and knowledgeable caretakers. USSC principles fed the prevailing narrative about the effect of the Civil War, even when recounting Bickerdyke's battlefield actions that occurred before her official affiliation with the USSC. This is an example of the sort of narrative that has downplayed Bickerdyke's actual significance as a Civil War nurse.

The initial accounts of Bickerdyke's battlefield actions were published immediately after the war by upper-middle-class reformers and leaders of the Chicago Sanitary Commission.[49] These were institutional histories that sorted through massive amounts of documentation and attempted to craft them into reliable accounts, albeit with a heroic flair. Sarah Henshaw, an associate manager of the Chicago branch, was tasked with writing a history of the Chicago Sanitary Commission, which eventually folded into the USSC. When she accepted the daunting task, she made it clear that she had grander intentions for her work, saying "that story should not be made a mere statement of facts—it should be invested with what answers to color in a picture, and expression in a countenance."[50] Mary Bickerdyke's extraordinary battlefield actions provided Henshaw with a means for coloring in the picture with her interpretation of the USSC's purpose and success at Fort Donelson.

Henshaw included the account of Bickerdyke at Fort Donelson as an example of the ways that "exultation and sorrow met" at the battlefield and sanitary depots in the initial chaotic days of the war.[51] In Chicago, news of the Union victory at Fort Donelson caused a joyful fervor to rise as "men sung and danced and indulged in all sorts of patriotic gymnastics."[52] The enthusiasm was matched by an impromptu meeting of citizens in Chicago who made plans to gain subscriptions, provide surgeons, and raise funds to provide direct relief at the battlefield. The Union victory, however, did not lessen the staggering human toll of the battle. While supporters in Chicago celebrated, many were acutely aware that their sons, brothers, and fathers remained in immediate danger and in desperate need of aid. Bickerdyke's acts of valor and meticulous care, as described by Henshaw, embodied these hometown longings for both patriotic service and compassionate intervention. As Henshaw reflected, "Zeal without knowledge characterized all these efforts, but it was a zeal which no discouragement could repress, and no failure abate. It was the earliest reliable channel of communication between the soldier and his home, between the loyal woman and her government."[53] This underscores how well-intentioned but untrained volunteers, driven by patriotic urgency rather than medical expertise, filled critical gaps in wartime patient care.

Henshaw's account of Bickerdyke's midnight rescue mission powerfully illustrated the almost reckless zeal associated with those early days of the war. Against all odds on that freezing night after the Union attack on the Confederate stronghold, Bickerdyke desperately worked among the dead and dying, "flitting, singularly about the hillside; like a will-o'-the-wisp," using her light for a "narrower examination of the dead faces, as she stooped down, and turned them toward her."[54] In Henshaw's retelling, Bickerdyke exhibited the same devotion that would have been exercised by mothers back home: she sprang to action, and could not idly stand by as their sons froze, wounded and unattended. Henshaw's history of the USSC Chicago branch conveyed gratitude for the efforts of women who displayed individual patriotism and sacrifice at home. Her inclusion of Bickerdyke's battlefield actions illustrated the extension of local aid societies and their connection to the war's success. While mothers at home provided whatever relief they could muster, Bickerdyke took their cue and applied the same extraordinary level of sacrifice, maternal intuition, and zeal on the field.

Fort Donelson tested how citizens would respond to local battles involving their community-attached regiments. In the initial scramble to provide aid, disparate efforts, such as those from Chicago, struggled to channel individual zeal without knowledge into an organized system capable of efficiently distributing supplies. The result was inadequate and unequal care, as some soldiers were found "just as they had been left by the fortune of war four days before; their wounds, as yet undressed, smeared with filth and blood, and all their wants unsupplied."[55] The genuine efforts of individual communities, state executives, boards of trade, and other benevolent organizations posed a problem that required the machinery of the USSC.[56] The national commission positioned itself as the solution to what it identified as a "sprawl of misdirection" and "waste of means" caused by "independent and spasmodic operators."[57] However, in shaping this narrative, the commission downplayed the significance of figures like Bickerdyke, whose approach to care extended beyond emergency intervention. By focusing on the failures of early relief efforts and the necessity of centralized oversight, these historical accounts often overlooked the long-term, community-driven palliative care that defined Bickerdyke's practice and deepened her connection to the soldiers she served.

The Battle of Fort Donelson propelled the Chicago branch of the USSC into full operation, establishing the Chicago office and storeroom as a mediator between "promiscuous beneficence" of private donors and the national organization's push for scientific management.[58] A storeroom that had been set up in Cairo months before the conflict at Fort Donelson provided a distribution point for the sudden influx of donations. The Chicago branch outfitted an additional hospital steamer with supplies, invited citizens the opportunity to assist with distribution, and sent seventeen volunteer surgeons to reinforce the medical staff in the field.[59] Jane Hoge boarded the steamer, determined to ensure that the supply from Chicago was adequately managed, a commitment that foreshadowed her eventual role as co-administrator of the branch alongside Mary Livermore.

As she continued her work, Hoge facilitated nurse recruitment, raised funds, and solicited donations of hospital goods and food from the many soldiers' aid societies in northwestern townships. Hoge knew Bickerdyke personally and respected her abilities, but the two women existed in different socioeconomic worlds. After the war, when Hoge helped establish Chicago's Home for the Friendless, an early model of a women's shelter and orphanage, she employed Mary Bickerdyke to work on the ground level of the operation.[60] They had a functional professional relationship, but it remained stretched across class lines: Hoge, the wealthy reformer, and Bickerdyke, the industrious worker.

When Hoge published her personal history of the war in 1867, *The Boys in Blue*, her assessment of Bickerdyke's contribution took on a much more practical tone than Henshaw's account. As a witness, Hoge was privy to various aspects of Bickerdyke's performance in the field. To underscore her role as one of the key organizers of "faithful and efficient nurses" to the USSC Western Department, Hoge pointed to Bickerdyke's work at Fort Donelson as a quintessential example of the heroic nursing cadre that she helped to equip in Chicago.[61] Hoge did not exploit the literary potential of Bickerdyke's midnight mission but instead focused on Bickerdyke's duties aboard the commission's hospital steamers and her contribution to healing efforts beyond the singular mission. The steamers acted as dual-purpose supply ships serving the scene of battle and transporting wounded soldiers to various post hospitals for more stable care.

After the Battle of Fort Donelson, Bickerdyke made five trips with wounded men on the steamers.[62] The boat trip from the battlefield to the hospitals in southern Illinois was harrowing, and nurses were required to quickly adapt to the challenges posed by these retrofitted floating hospitals. Men were packed together tightly onto the ship, "obliged to lie as closely as possible."[63] Hoge, who made one such trip herself, commented that "no duty was more exhausting in its character, nor more important in its results."[64] These transition trips could have proved disastrous for the Union army and the USSC if they were not properly attended. The institutions relied on this innovative system of transportation to save the literal boatloads of soldiers who would likely have died in a field hospital. Bickerdyke's ability to both "smooth the passage to the grave, and rob the grim messenger of his stern features" was indispensable to the USSC's success as a medical partner to the Union army's system of care.[65]

Hoge was most impressed with Bickerdyke's fortitude and her "superhuman strength and endurance" to manage those trips and continue on in the work.[66] Hoge's account used Bickerdyke's example of important and well-ordered work to emphasize the efficiency and innovation of the USSC.[67] Her description of Bickerdyke suggested her participation in and compliance with the organization's main values, which sometimes directly conflicted with Bickerdyke's maternal style that prioritized individualized patient care. By all accounts, Hoge sublimated Bickerdyke's episodes of insubordination in favor of reframing Bickerdyke's actions to demonstrate the ideal of White patriotic motherhood and womanhood.

The second wave of memorial literature featuring Bickerdyke and her midnight mission was published in the 1870s and 1880s. It coincided with a rise in professional women nurses as well as the development of training programs for women who were privileged enough to participate. In 1873, three nursing education programs were established: the New York Training School at Bellevue Hospital, the Connecticut Training School at the State Hospital, and the Boston Training School at Massachusetts General Hospital. These programs are widely recognized as the foundation of professional nurse training in the United States based on the tenets of nursing introduced by Florence Nightingale.[68] As a result of this development, memorialists began to draw different meanings from Bickerdyke's actions during the midnight mission. These nursing programs facilitated the institutional growth of the hospital and emphasized the belief that women's caregiving was based on moral expectations rather than monetary compensation.[69] The authors of Civil War histories in the 1870s and 1880s reflected on women like Bickerdyke to find examples of those who embodied a dutiful commitment to the tenets of the nursing profession and who, because of their motherhood and womanhood, did not demand compensation for their extra efforts.[70]

The enduring prototype of Florence Nightingale as the "Lady with the Lamp" served as both a measuring stick for nursing's capacity and a rhetorical tool for those who sought to reinforce traditional gender roles within the profession. Earlier forms of nursing were influenced by family ties that were shaped by resentments, inescapable responsibilities, affection, and choice. Early sick nursing was defined more by a woman's social role—whether as a mother, nun, hired servant, or enslaved person—than by her knowledge of therapeutics.[71] By the 1880s, as medical institutions expanded, nursing evolved into a more distinct profession, sparking public debates about women's professional status. These discussions played out as new models of professionalism emerged, challenging traditional views of caregiving as merely a domestic duty. Historical narratives became a battleground for defining nursing's place in the professional sphere.

Florence Nightingale captured the American imagination as her actions and organizational efforts in the Crimean War were covered by newspapers across the globe. Nightingale is often referred to as the founder of modern nursing, and she contributed helpful treatises and practical instructions on care for the sick and wounded. She challenged the assumption that all women are natural nurses, pointing to London's high infant mortality rate as evidence that, if nursing were instinctual, mothers would have been able to prevent such widespread deaths. Instead, she championed tenets of hospital management, attentive patient care, and special knowledge of disease manifestations.[72] Nightingale framed nursing as a profession best suited for women of reputable moral character, prioritizing virtue and discipline over any preference for maternal instinct.

Before the American Civil War, Florence Nightingale's dignified nobility and careful adherence to statistics, hygiene, and order provided a template for professional nursing.[73] Nightingale produced "persuasive evidence" that documented how military hospitals and procedures caused more harm than good.[74] When she raised her own funds to lead a small group of nurses to Turkey in 1854, there was no precedent for women's work within the British Army. So, she was charged with developing that protocol as well as performing other duties such as cooking, laundry, and supply distribution.[75] She observed the squalid conditions of military hospitals, and the experience shaped her views on sanitation. She successfully instituted reforms in military hospitals, curtailing the enormous death toll from disease among the British forces. After the war's conclusion, she met with Queen Victoria and Prince Albert and gave evidence before a commission tasked with understanding the human toll of the conflict, which resulted in 900,000 deaths among the 1,650,000 soldiers who fought the war. Nightingale's work served as a model for the USSC when it became embroiled in a conflict just five years after the devastation of the Crimean War. In 1859, Nightingale published the instructive treatise *Notes on Nursing*, which further entrenched nursing as a distinctly noble and predominantly female pursuit.

Nightingale became a beloved symbol in America, and her work quickly became part of the nursing and sanitary science canon. Henry Wadsworth Longfellow published "Santa Filomena" in 1857 in *The Atlantic Monthly*.[76] The poem's content was a response to the stirring visuals and accompanying descriptions in the *Illustrated London News*, depicting Florence Nightingale's devoted attention to sick soldiers in her orderly hospital during the Crimean

War. Longfellow immortalized Nightingale's work, causing her to be forever remembered as the "Lady with a Lamp":

> A lady with a lamp shall stand
> In the great history of the land,
>   A noble type of good,
>   Heroic womanhood.[77]

Nightingale's work and the British development of sanitary principles for nursing served as a blueprint for American nursing even before a formal training system was established. Civil War doctors were predominantly men, and strict qualifications were developed and implemented by the United States Army and Medical Bureau.[78] President Abraham Lincoln and his administration braced for the beginning of the Confederate assault and hastily accepted Dorothea Dix's proposal to provide "aid in organizing military hospitals," especially in furnishing nurses and disbursing hospital supplies.[79] Dix was a wealthy New England reformer who had spent the better part of the previous five years in England surveying medical facilities.[80] Dix became the commander of an army of nurses and fully subscribed to Nightingale's vision of benevolent womanhood. Dix was not alone in her quest to build a force of exemplary moral character and action; by 1861, the Lady with the Lamp had become a ubiquitous image of nursing. But Dix's efforts were only one part of the Union army's nursing initiatives, competing with the USSC's more nebulously defined sanitary agents.

For its part, the USSC was intent on showing how it had improved upon the British model. After a year in the field implementing the intricate bureaucratic system, the USSC produced statistical pamphlets that compared the incidence of disease in the United States to that of the Crimean War.[81] The commission's experiments with statistics were yet another nod to Nightingale's contributions to the nursing field, as moral care was intermingled with measurable results. The pamphlets were designed to show the effectiveness of preventative hygiene in camps and hospitals and to encourage the Union army to avoid the certain death they would face without such guidance. The USSC was deeply interested in producing better results for the Union army through a program of scientific management, and its early numbers seemed to indicate success. While the graphs, forms, and guidelines held the organization accountable to its own philosophies, a sentimental public still relished the stories that brought the science to life.

Bickerdyke's Civil War work mirrored Nightingale's in specific ways that inspired American writers in the 1880s. Both women challenged military bureaucracy, took the initiative in reforming hospital conditions, and extended their influence beyond bedside care to supply distribution and logistical planning. Like Nightingale, Bickerdyke challenged existing gender norms, proving that women could play a critical role in wartime medical administration and patient care. Mary Bickerdyke's midnight mission at Fort Donelson was referenced by memorialists and authors to highlight the American manifestation of some of Florence Nightingale's ideas about the nursing profession. Mary Davis Burton's *The Woman Who Battled for the Boys in Blue* (1886) sought to enhance Bickerdyke's image through comparison, secure Bickerdyke's pension, and leverage Nightingale's popular imagery to bolster Bickerdyke's public perception.[82]

Bickerdyke's pension campaign occurred before the Army Nurses Pension Act of 1892 was passed and coincided with the beginnings of Nightingale-inspired nursing institutions. The direct comparison to Nightingale was meant to rally public sentiment and support and generate personal recommendations and connections to legislators. Burton wasted no time rallying public sentiment by advocating for Bickerdyke's recognition. "The world is not rich enough," she rallied, "to neglect the touching story of Florence Nightingale in the Crimea," strongly implying that America had rudely forgotten some of its own Nightingales, most of all, Mary Bickerdyke.[83] Congress passed the bill after facing constant petitions and lobbying from the National Association of Army Nurses of the Civil War, as well as a swell of public support from books like Burton's. The new legislation allowed for a $12 per month stipend for all Civil War army nurses who had been hired by and served the government.[84]

Burton framed Bickerdyke through a comparison to Nightingale, and the interpretation of her midnight mission at Fort Donelson suggested that she was the truer, American counterpart to Longfellow's Lady with a Lamp. Her account, here in its entirety, suggests that Bickerdyke's efforts were even more courageous and sacrificial than Nightingale's:

> From a weird incident that occurred here it may be gathered how courageous and deeply interested Mrs. Bickerdyke was. Through the darkness that wrapt the whole landscape at midnight, a strange light appeared flitting about over the deserted battle-field, where the dead still lay awaiting burial. This was seen by an officer who chanced to be looking out of his tent, and he sent some one to inquire into the cause of the phantom semblance. He was startled on the return of his messenger to learn that it was Mrs. Bickerdyke examining, by the light of a lantern, those who had been left, because she feared that some among them might still be alive. She said that she could not endure the thought that any conscious being was lying out there in the cold

and gloom with the slain. Through that awful field she searched, not with a grief-stricken heart seeking her kindred, which might have inspired her with such fearlessness, but only for humanity's sake. Rarely, indeed, does a woman possess such nerve or self-forgetfulness as this.[85]

Bickerdyke, unlike Nightingale, had gone unrewarded and largely unnoticed for her patriotic and swift actions. Without a national platform or personal wealth, Bickerdyke was unable and humbly unwilling to take the credit for her actions. Though Burton portrayed Bickerdyke as the better, truer Nightingale, she carefully infused Nightingale's theories of nursing so that the reader could identify Bickerdyke's distinct professionalism and competency. As Bickerdyke surveyed the ghastly scene at Fort Donelson, she was able to calmly harness specialized medical knowledge needed to attend to the Union soldiers. She exhibited characteristics that Nightingale demanded in competent nurses: "There is unquestionably a physiognomy of disease as well as of health ... and people never, or scarcely ever, observe enough to know how to distinguish between."[86] Burton's storytelling demonstrates Bickerdyke's special knowledge of physiognomy and her careful attention to the dead. In addition to these basic characteristics, though, Bickerdyke employed extraordinary measures and demonstrated how American nursing during the Civil War was a step above the British brand, partly because of the maternal moral character of the nurses employed. Bickerdyke did not limit her duties to the safety of the hospital but cared for each soldier as though he were her own son.

If Bickerdyke were the truer and better reflection of Nightingale in this era of Civil War histories, then there was value in her professional example for a new generation of women nurses in the United States. Mary Livermore's autobiographical history of the war, *My Story of the War*, visually compared Bickerdyke to Nightingale. Mary Livermore was Jane Hoge's counterpart in the Chicago branch of the USSC and continued to use her upper-class philanthropy for reform work after the war. Livermore's most noted contribution to the effort was the organization of the wildly successful Northwestern Sanitary Fairs that raised at least $80,000.[87] Livermore's description of Bickerdyke at Donelson was unremarkable and largely borrowed from previous authors' accounts. However, the compelling comparison to Nightingale emerged not in her text but in the imagery she used to frame Bickerdyke's contribution.

For her sweeping memoir, Livermore enlisted the talented American illustrator F. O. C. Darley to add visual depth to some of her most stirring anecdotes. One such illustration, "Midnight on the Battlefield," borrowed structural elements from Nightingale's famous depiction in the *Illustrated London News* (see figures 2.3 and 2.4). In the British rendering, Nightingale is centrally positioned, demonstrating command as she shines a light into the dark recesses of the hospital. She stands watch, her lamp a symbol of healing, illuminating spaces that, left in darkness, would surely bring death. In contrast, Darley's depiction of Bickerdyke demonstrated a more intimate scene and emphasized its chiaroscuro. Even with the waning moon in the background, the American scene is much darker without Bickerdyke's lamp. Around her, shrouded in shadow and stripped of individuality, lie the faceless bodies of the Union dead. Only through Bickerdyke's touch, provision, and care do the fallen regain distinction, their features brought to life through her attentiveness. Livermore's description mirrors Darley's artistic choices: "Stooping down and turning their cold faces towards her, [Bickerdyke] scrutinized them searchingly, uneasy lest some might be left to die uncared for."[88] In this instance, as in others before, authors signaled Bickerdyke's special knowledge in physiognomy to demonstrate her adherence to professional nursing practices.

Livermore's interpretation of Bickerdyke's actions infused her philosophy of history and her own memory of and experience in the war. At the beginning of *My Story of the War*, Livermore admitted that her tendency was to periodically destroy her own records, which was not an uncommon practice at the time.[89] However, such practices hindered an accurate historical account of the war and caused her to rely heavily on memories from decades past and to corroborate with other histories. Livermore did not personally witness Bickerdyke's actions at Fort Donelson, but she recognized the value in cultivating an image of an American Nightingale at a time when contemporary culture was defining the meaning of professional nursing.

Mary Bickerdyke's evolving portrayal across two eras of Civil War literary history reveals how her image served both the authors who wrote about her and the audiences who consumed these narratives. Over time, the changing depictions of her work solidified into a persistent myth about her action. The comparison to Nightingale, for instance, resurfaced in Martin Litvin's biography *The Young Mary, 1817–1861: Early Years of Mother Bickerdyke, America's Florence Nightingale, and Patron Saint of Kansas*. Even during her lifetime, revisions to her public image emphasized her maternal authority, boosting her reputation as "Mother." Bickerdyke allowed authors to amplify her legacy, allowing them to recount her accomplishments in ways that reinforced her influence. In turn, these literary and visual portrayals helped her secure financial stability, public recognition, and lasting social prominence.

Bickerdyke's depiction as the American Nightingale contributed to wider cultural debates about women's professional positions in the nursing profes-

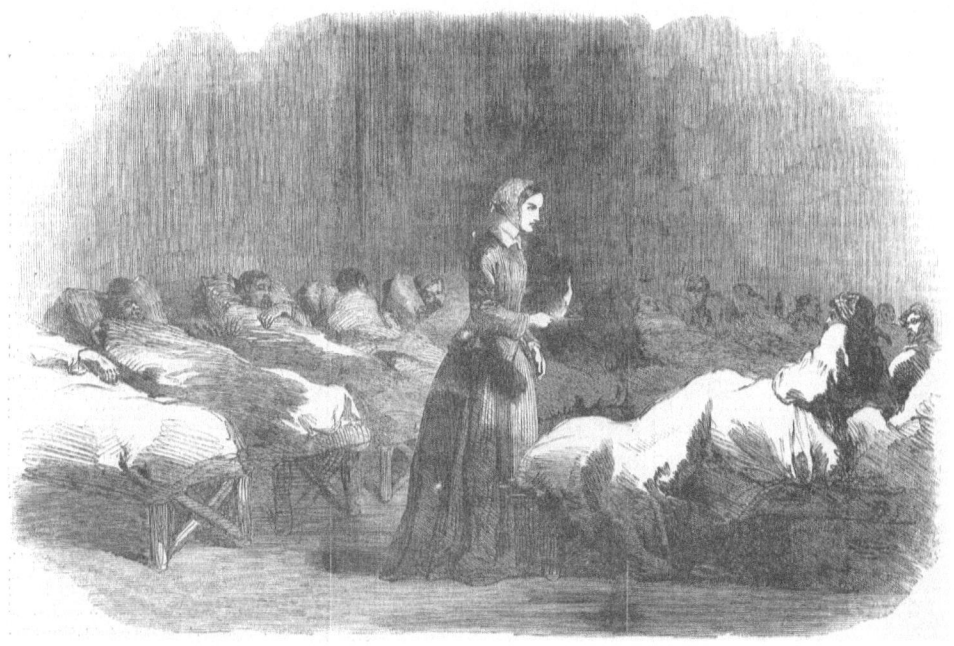

FIGURE 2.3 Florence Nightingale, "Lady with a Lamp." Wood engraving appearing in the *Illustrated London News*, February 24, 1855. © 1890 National Portrait Gallery, London. Used with permission.

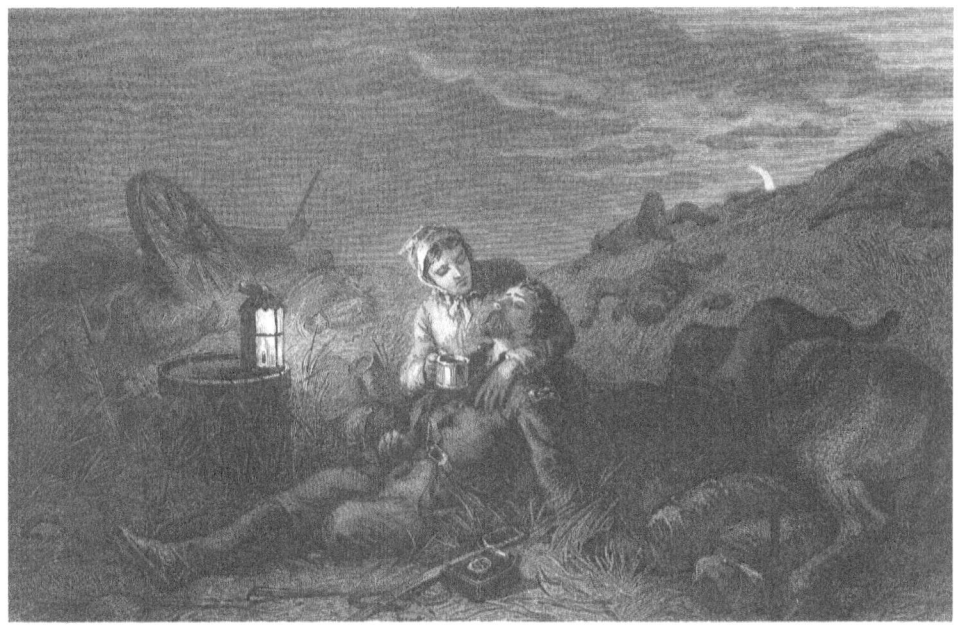

FIGURE 2.4 "Midnight on the Battlefield." The frontispiece in Mary Livermore's *My Story of the War*. Courtesy of the New York Public Library Digital Collections.

sion. From 1866, when Sarah Henshaw began to produce the USSC history, to the time Mary Livermore published her personal memoir in the late 1880s, the United States underwent major shifts when it came to women in medical professions. Professional nursing programs for women disrupted the social order of traditional medical practice and used women's medical heroism and accomplishments from the Civil War as proof of their long-standing competency as medical professionals. Through it all, Bickerdyke did not mind being used as an example, even if the authors of these memoirs used her story for their own purposes. Whatever their purpose, her name was secured in print as a demonstration of women's contributions to the Union victory. However, Bickerdyke's legacy was more than commemorative; it was forged through her relentless work as Grant's army pressed south.

Following the Fort Donelson campaign, Bickerdyke accompanied Grant's forces down the Tennessee River, where she was placed in charge of training incoming nurses and maintaining sanitation and supplies at the Savannah hospital before the Battle of Shiloh.[90] In the weeks after Donelson, she solidified her reputation by marshaling resources and organizing large-scale efforts to support the army.[91] She led a laundry operation to salvage uniforms and bandages from wounded or deceased soldiers, prepared hot meals from USSC stores, and treated common ailments among Grant's troops. Her efficiency and resilience earned her the trust of generals, camp surgeons, and soldiers alike. Unlike many women volunteers who found themselves sent home after failing to meet the army's demands, Bickerdyke proved indispensable, enduring the hardships of life on the march.

In April 1862, Grant's forces clashed with the Confederates at Pittsburg Landing, also known as Shiloh—a battle in which more Americans died in two days than in all the nation's previous wars combined.[92] Among the thousands of wounded at Shiloh, Bickerdyke cared for a mortally wounded soldier from an Iowa regiment. A minié ball had entered near his heart, and the surgeons deemed it too deep and dangerous to remove. Such wounds often resulted in prolonged, agonizing deaths as the bullet slowly made its way toward the heart. Anna Webb-Peck, a nurse at Shiloh, recorded the man's final moments, offering a glimpse into Bickerdyke's ability to comfort the dying. She wrote, "One evening as she was in the room he called to her saying that he felt strangely. She placed her hand on his heart, felt only a fluttering, and she said to him 'Your time has come, if you have anything to say, say it quickly.' He looked up into her face with a smile and said 'Tell my wife to meet me in heaven.' He was gone."[93] In a battle often marked by great men and myths, anecdotes like this, and others untold, demonstrate the revised "good death" experienced by countless unnamed soldiers whose stories rarely make it into the historical records. These small, intimate, and final moments defined the true meaning of Bickerdyke's work. While medical protocols for attending to dying patients had circulated internationally, largely due to Nightingale's *Notes on Nursing*, her instructions largely omitted the spiritual and emotional care that was paramount to Bickerdyke's approach. It was her substituted motherhood and her promise to connect the dying with their living kin that earned her the trust and affection of both soldiers and communities of survivors across the North.

Grant's campaign continued south to the siege at Corinth in late April to June 1862, during which Bickerdyke was assigned to a large hospital in nearby Farmington.[94] She was present at the Battle of Iuka in September and then in October at the Second Battle of Corinth. After nearly a year and a half of unrelenting volunteer service, she took a brief furlough in the winter of 1862 to return to Illinois and care for her own children. During this period of respite, on December 18, 1862, she was officially appointed to the USSC, solidifying her role within the wartime medical effort.[95]

## Specialized Maternal Medical Care: Botanic Interventions and Palliative Care

Before the war, much of Bickerdyke's work fell within the realm of untrained therapeutics in women's domestic health care rather than the emerging specialized knowledge of professional medicine. However, as the war unfolded, her expertise—rooted in botanic remedies and palliative care—became indispensable on both the home front and in the battlefield hospitals. Male doctors, some of whom had trained overseas or attended accredited institutions, were often ill-prepared for the personal and emotional aspects of caregiving, particularly in the face of mass casualties. They increasingly relied on women like Bickerdyke to bridge this gap, entrusting them with the deeply ingrained rituals of death and mourning. Bickerdyke's success during the Civil War demonstrates the critical intersection of traditional caregiving practices and evolving medical advancements. Her work was an operational example of care-switching, where women seamlessly adapted domestic medical knowledge to the structured demands of wartime sanitary science. This transition was not merely practical but also symbolic, revealing how women's healing labor—often dismissed as informal or unscientific—was, in fact, foundational to the professionalization of nursing and battlefield medicine. The Civil War's medical crisis forced a reevaluation of expertise, and figures like Bickerdyke proved that maternal-based care was not only compatible with modern medical practices but, in many cases, essential to their success.

One of Bickerdyke's key responsibilities with the USSC was bridging the divide between the battlefield and the home front, ensuring that care extended beyond the war zone to families and communities. Her advocacy for soldiers did not end with their deaths; it extended to their families, helping to address and fulfill their final wishes. In February 1863, while stationed in Memphis, Bickerdyke employed George Weeks, a former postmaster clerk from Galesburg, to help her with her mounting correspondence.[96] Weeks exchanged letters with Mrs. Abbott, who was caring for Bickerdyke's sons. Abbott's own son, Sherman, died on May 4, 1862, from unknown causes at the front. He had served in the Twenty-Sixth Illinois Infantry, a regiment composed largely of men from Bickerdyke's home county, Knox County.

After Private Abbott's death, his mother used her frontline connections to Bickerdyke to locate his remains so that he could be reburied at home. Death away from home was a symptom of war, but surviving families felt the disruption of customs that tied death and burial to home and domesticity.[97] USSC memoirs often include anecdotes of civilian mothers, fathers, and other relatives traveling to the site of their son's death in an attempt to locate the body of the slain.[98] It was an expensive ordeal to locate, disinter, and transport soldiers' bodies back to their home states. This meant that only families with at least moderate means could afford the luxury of bringing a soldier back home. Poor families were forced to leave their dead on the battlefield as their place of burial, despite earnest desires to bring their bodies home to family burial plots.

The USSC used its vast organization across the North to aid families' attempts to bring their loved ones home, but the organization of this effort was not systematized until the last year and a half of the war.[99] Mrs. Abbott was asking for help from a friend, Mary Bickerdyke, whom she believed might be able to leverage her position and knowledge to locate and send Sherman Abbott's body back to his Illinois home. George Weeks included directions for Mrs. Abbott: "Mrs. Bickerdyke says that you must send the map of your son's grave and she has a friend, a Lieut in the Scouts who will make almost any sacrifice to get the remains but you musn't place two [sic] much confidence in our getting them. But we will do all in our power please don't forget to send the map."[100] Bickerdyke's dictation showed her willingness to help despite the difficulty of the task at hand. It was a glimmer of hope for the grieving mother, mixed with a commitment to honor her request.

Mrs. Abbott's drawing marked the final resting place of her son near the post hospital at Hamburg, Tennessee (see figures 2.5 and 2.6).[101] The burial

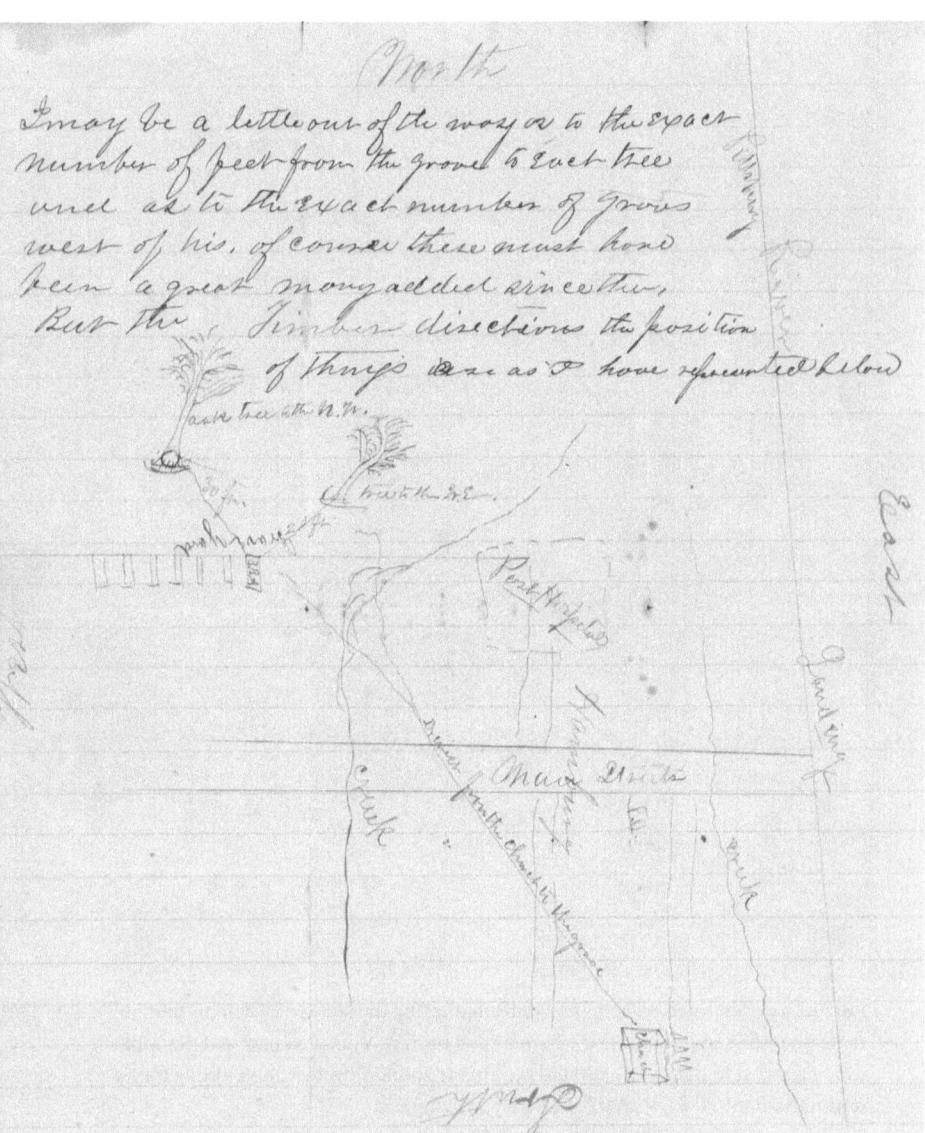

FIGURE 2.5  Letter written to Mary Bickerdyke by Mrs. Abbott. The map is carefully detailed to ensure Bickerdyke's efforts would have the best outcome. A portion of the image is magnified in figure 2.6. Courtesy of the Library of Congress.

spot indicated that Private Abbott died while under care at the post hospital, likely from one of the many diseases that ravaged Union encampments. By the end of the war, Abbott's regiment lost a total of 286 men; 194 of those deaths were from disease.[102] The letters to Mrs. Abbott do not indicate

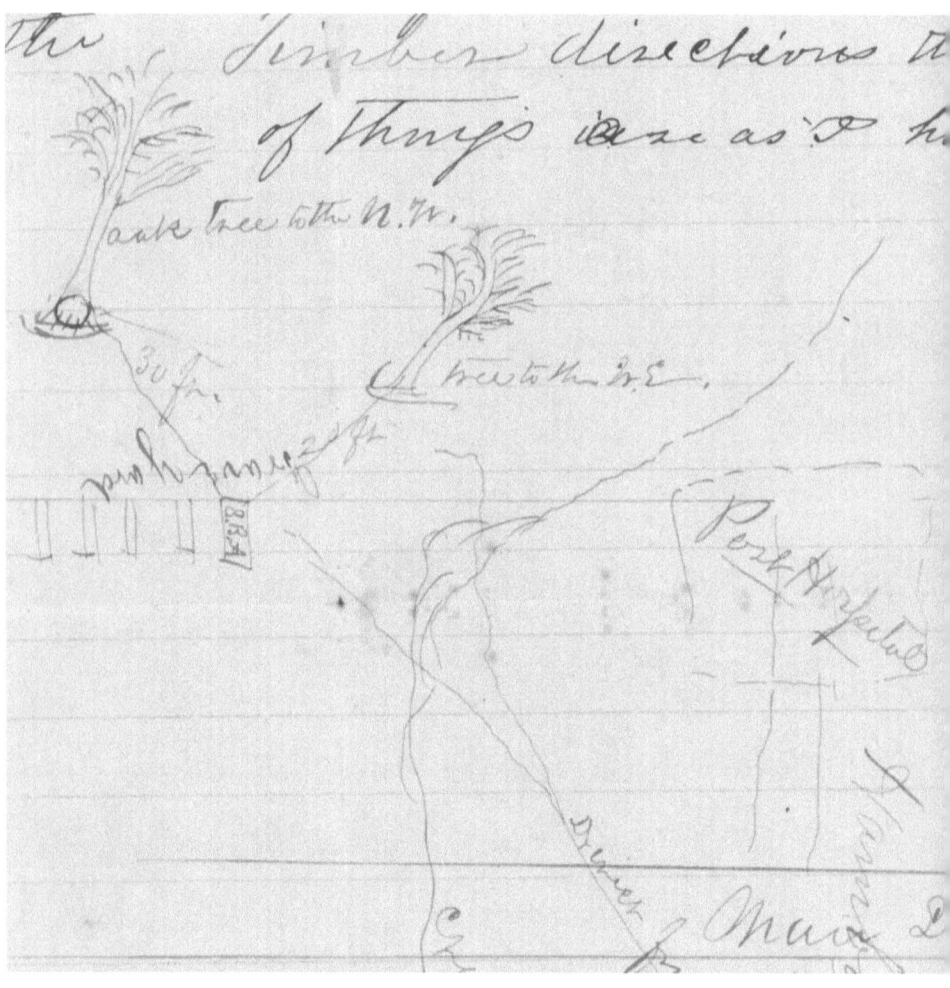

FIGURE 2.6 Sherman Abbott's gravesite, marked by the large trees that his mother remembered as landmarks near where he was buried. A detailed map and description were provided to help Mary Bickerdyke's friend locate Private Abbott's body for its return to Illinois. Courtesy of the Library of Congress.

whether Mary Bickerdyke was present when her son died, but it is unlikely. Still, Bickerdyke's work with the wounded and dying intimated that she had tended to many others like him—men whose deaths, though not in battle, were no less a sacrifice for the Union cause.[103]

Faithfully, Mrs. Abbott returned the request with a detailed map, suggesting she had made a pilgrimage to the gravesite. Close examination of the image reveals the approximate distances from the distinctive trees that surrounded Abbott's gravesite. A towering oak tree was thirty feet to the northwest, and another tree was marked twenty feet to the northeast. The meticulous presentation of the locations and markers around the grave indicates the attentiveness of a grieving mother, taking in as many sensory and scenic details as possible before returning to Illinois without her son's body. Lacking the financial resources to have him disinterred and returned home, Mrs. Abbott placed her trust in Bickerdyke, hoping that the woman who had cared for so many Union soldiers in life could also ensure their dignity in death. Mrs. Abbott, who had been caring for Bickerdyke's sons in her absence, now asked Bickerdyke to do the same for her.

AS THE CIVIL WAR progressed, Bickerdyke's role as a caregiver deepened, expanding beyond the battlefield and into the very structure of wartime medicine. Her experiences at the Battles of Fort Donelson and Shiloh, as well as her work in various hospitals and on hospital steamers, transformed maternal instincts into a form of professionalized care, adapting her knowledge to meet the demands of the war. Bickerdyke's ability to care-switch, seamlessly blending traditional maternal practices with emerging medical techniques, allowed her to navigate the complex and often chaotic landscape of Civil War medicine.

Likewise, Bickerdyke's role as a surrogate mother and her commitment to providing comfort and dignity to dying soldiers extended beyond the immediate battlefield. Bickerdyke served as a crucial link between soldiers and their families, offering solace and support to those grieving the loss of loved ones. Her efforts to locate and mark graves, as well as to facilitate the return of bodies to their home communities, underscored the importance of the revised "good death" in the context of the Civil War.

As Bickerdyke's reputation grew, so did her responsibilities and the scope of her influence. Her official appointment to the USSC in December 1862 marked a new phase in her wartime service, one that would see her take on increasingly prominent roles in the management of hospitals and the distribution of supplies. Armed with the knowledge and experience gained from her early years of service, Bickerdyke positioned herself to be memorialized for the combination of her abilities, maternal authority, and courage to follow her instincts in times of crisis, expanding both private and public notions of a mother's place.

CHAPTER THREE

# She Ranks Me
## Asserting Motherhood in the Civil War (1863–1865)

Mary Bickerdyke's Civil War journey was marked by experiences that transformed and expanded her concept of motherhood. After the exhaustive efforts in 1862, she briefly returned to her biological sons as they transitioned from care in Galesburg to boarding schools. Her visit to her sons produced an internal tension and conflict that persisted throughout her life, causing her to care-switch as she oscillated between roles. Her decision to serve as a Civil War nurse and sanitary agent took her away from her young sons and redefined the narrative of traditional motherly care into a role of remote and removed caretaking. Simultaneously, she became a surrogate mother on the front lines to the young men of the Union army, nursing them back to health and attending to them until their deaths, deepening the bonds of affection that tied the devoted caregiver to her thankful sons. She was a mother at war: at war with herself, at war with the cultural expectations placed on her by an observant community, and, coincidentally, on the front lines. The moment had arrived for her to boldly amplify the significance of her motherhood, showcasing why it was an invaluable asset to the Union army.

Mary Bickerdyke's devotion to the cause of patient care is unquestionable; yet, she did not fit the strict institutional roles that were reluctantly assigned to women by the powerful elite men who ran the United States Sanitary Commission (USSC) and the surgeons of the Union army. Constantly under scrutiny, Bickerdyke was continuously required to confirm her competency as a medical worker and as a favored caretaker of soldiers. The hospitals were regularly inspected and visited by army staff, and it was evident that many men within the military structure were uncomfortable with a female authority figure in the wards. These tensions often erupted into direct confrontations, as in one instance when she recalled being challenged by an inspecting officer:

> The morning work had been done up in most of the wards, I met the Inspector in the amputating ward, He says "Madam what are you doing here we don't allow women in military hospitals. You can be employed as a laundress but you can't be in the wards. I strictly forbid it." I replied, "That's my rank sir" and passed him and left the room.... They watched me about an hour, giving the cooks directions for dinner. In the after-

noon Major Stearns and the Inspector were walking when I passed them, the Inspector said, "Well, I see you haven't left" I replied "No Sir the *Lord* of creation woman obey" from that on I had no more trouble with him.[1]

Her response reveals how she effectively used her maternal identity to validate her medical skills. Her justification for remaining in the wards, despite military protocols that prohibited female medical personnel, was based on a God-given mandate to care for the sick and wounded. God had ordained and called her to work as a mother and caregiver. She decided to leverage her commission through an appeal to the sovereignty of God's dictates that superseded the regulations of the Union army.

Before her USSC appointment in December 1862, Bickerdyke had no official standing or authority to claim other than the command of the Almighty and the favor of the soldiers. These men had decided that her presence as a surrogate mother—cleaning their sheets and attending to their comforts during battle—was both desired and appreciated. Bickerdyke welcomed patients into her personal quarters to examine them whenever she had the time or when she went there to rest, following her motherly instincts.[2] Compassionate care for the dying was an essential health protocol and individualized treatment that Bickerdyke offered in the intimacy of the home setting. In a culture that highly valued the concept of dying well, Bickerdyke occasionally sidestepped efficient triage management and attended specifically to the dying as both a mother and a medical professional.

The year 1863 marked an important shift, not only in the Union's prospects of winning the war but also in Mary Bickerdyke's ability to leverage her distinctive motherhood as a weapon for the boys in blue. As the war progressed, she gained endorsements from traditional avenues of authority. Her efforts in the first part of the war had earned her recognition and notoriety among important men and women in the Union war machine, introducing her to the reformer class of women who also occupied the upper echelons of society. At the same time, Mary Bickerdyke's experiences as an agent on the ground highlight her complex navigation of the racial and class hierarchies that shaped the Union war effort. As a working-class woman, Bickerdyke recognized the value of labor performed by Black refugees and sought to integrate them into her sanitary work, challenging the prevailing attitudes of some Union officials. Her actions, while primarily driven by pragmatism and a desire to care for soldiers efficiently, also had significant implications for the inclusion of marginalized groups within the Union cause.

## "She Ranks Me": Articulating Maternal Authority in the US Military

Mary Bickerdyke reported to the Memphis hospitals after her furlough to Chicago at the beginning of 1863. Her principal achievement from the previous year had been the development of a laundry system to recycle garments from the battlefield and hospital. Prior to her innovation, such garments that were "saturated with blood, and the discharges of healing wounds, and sometimes swarming with vermin . . . had been collected, and burned or buried."[3] Such practices resulted in the excessive waste of materials that the Union army constantly needed, like shirts, undergarments, socks, and pants. At each location where she was stationed after Fort Donelson, Bickerdyke requested a team of Black refugees who had fled to Union lines to help with the work. She then oversaw the laundering operations, ensuring that General Ulysses S. Grant's army always had fresh and sanitary materials. Over the course of a few months, Bickerdyke's "extemporized laundry" saved the Union army and the USSC a huge number of resources.[4]

Laundering tended to be the domain of working-class White women, Black women, and the formerly enslaved.[5] The work was grueling, requiring laborers to scrub garments soaked in blood, sweat, and disease, confronting the physical remnants of war with each load.[6] It was not the type of work suited for the reformer class of the USSC, but they were nonetheless impressed with Bickerdyke's resourcefulness and utility. Mary Livermore marveled at the effectiveness of her portable laundry, which included Bickerdyke's "washing-machines, her portable kettles, her posse of contrabands, an ambulance or two, and one or two handy detailed soldiers."[7] The emphasis on the inclusion of Black refugees, referred to as "contraband" under wartime legal definitions, was particularly significant to USSC reformers such as Livermore and Jane Hoge. Their admiration for Bickerdyke's resourcefulness was not just about the practical benefits of clean clothing and bandages but also about the broader implications of her workforce. Amy Murrell Taylor has examined the role of Black refugees in Union war labor, highlighting how their participation in laundry work for the military became part of what she describes as their "martial route to freedom."[8] By engaging in essential wartime labor, formerly enslaved individuals reinforced their claims to autonomy and citizenship, demonstrating their value within the Union war effort. Bickerdyke's operation, then, was more than just a logistical success; it functioned within a larger framework of wartime emancipation, where labor became both a survival strategy and a path to securing a place in postwar society.

Bickerdyke never wrote about her personal views on equality and citizenship, nor did she hold the institutional power to offer her laundry workers formal employment—she struggled to receive such recognition herself. Her decision to utilize Black labor was, at least in part, pragmatic, driven by the immediate need to complete an overwhelming task efficiently. However, it is also possible that her actions carried a broader significance, demonstrating that these men and women, regardless of race, were vital to the Union cause, just as she was.

This form of labor differed from prewar laundry work in important ways. Under Bickerdyke's leadership, organizing large-scale sanitation efforts aligned with the USSC's dual mission: functionality and reform. For the Chicago reformers, including Livermore and Hoge, Bickerdyke's collaboration with Black refugees reinforced the image of the USSC as a benevolent and forward-thinking organization aligned with the presidential proclamation. Livermore, in particular, highlighted Bickerdyke's efforts to integrate Black workers into sanitation work, framing their participation as both practical and symbolic. By securing recognition from progressive reformers within the USSC, Bickerdyke helped transform a traditionally menial task into purposeful and patriotic labor. In this way, the contributions of working-class White and Black women were not only essential to the war effort but also became tied to the broader ideological support of the Union cause that was shifting by 1863.

In Memphis, the USSC relied on Bickerdyke to continue the sanitation work initiated during the previous campaign. Following a decisive naval battle, the Union army occupied Memphis, and by late June 1862, the city had become Grant's headquarters. Soon after, it emerged as a major medical center in the mid-South, where thousands of wounded and sick soldiers were treated.[9] During her time in Memphis, Bickerdyke served as a hospital matron and worked with various institutions to transform medical settings, striving to replicate the care that soldiers might receive at home. This work was difficult and sometimes disrupted the establishment of order and bureaucracy. Though she clashed with some members of the USSC and individual surgeons, she never lost the trust and admiration of the soldiers she served. Her insistence on holistic healing methods in the face of rapidly changing medical conditions contributed to long-term patient-practitioner trust that would serve her for decades after the war was over.

Bickerdyke settled into Gayoso Hospital, one of eleven Memphis hospitals redeveloped to accommodate at least 6,000 men from the Siege of Vicksburg.[10] Before that, Memphis hospitals were primarily used for wounded soldiers and as sites for long-term convalescence. In addition to her duties as matron at Gayoso, she was tasked with visiting the other hospitals to "fit them up" for proper use. According to Bickerdyke, they were in bad condition. At Adams Block Hospital, she found the cellar "full of clothes that needed washing."[11] Only a month after her arrival, she commenced in large-scale laundry work and "called upon the steward for kettles and help." Within four days, her Memphis team had washed, dried, and ironed "1500 Government Shirts and Drawers; 800 Sanitary Shirts; 520 pairs Sanitary Drawers; 353 pairs woolen Socks; 630 Woolen Shirts; 216 pairs Woolen Pants; 1832 Government Sheets; 542 Government Pillow Cases."[12] By March 1863, Bickerdyke, employing a team of Black refugees, was running a laundry operation that washed garments for all the hospitals in Memphis, in addition to carrying out her hospital duties.[13]

Bickerdyke's labors were directly observed by Jane Hoge and Mary Livermore, who led a team of USSC workers on a tour of Memphis to examine and report on its conditions. They lauded Bickerdyke's work, noting that she was "a woman of amazing energy, full of maternal tenderness to the sick and wounded soldiers, and nursing them through the depths of neglect, squalor, destitution and disease," and her hospital was "the most homelike, cheerful and comfortable in Memphis, and it turns out weekly twice as many convalescents as any other."[14]

Bickerdyke had enlisted USSC support to employ and provide rations for between fifty and seventy recently freed men and women who had been living in Memphis's contraband camps.[15] Her efforts were small but meaningful; the refugee crisis in Memphis was bleak. One hospital ward master, his original spelling and punctuation maintained here, relayed the dire conditions to his wife in late January 1863:

> My heart is bursting with sympathy for poor suffering humanity wich I see every day and I cant releave them. . . . I have often spoaken to you about the refugees that come inside of our lines more or less every day = chiefly women and children = . . . I came to a large coton shed that was used formely for a coton whear house but lately had been used for a goverment stable = well inside of this shed wear about 800 refugees women and children hear they wear poor things with thear gaunt and sickely looking faces with out food or means to buy with no friends to provide for them many of them wear sick with no medical help.[16]

The higher-ranking USSC women were impressed with Bickerdyke's production, but they noted that some Memphis authorities disagreed with Bickerdyke's insistence on Black employment. During their visit to Memphis in

March 1863, they recounted a series of interactions between Bickerdyke and Dr. Bernard J. D. Irwin, who was the newly appointed medical director in Memphis. Irwin did not approve of Bickerdyke's "contraband help, nor of her possessing so much power" and actively worked to undermine her work.[17] The episode's retelling by the USSC women represents Bickerdyke's shift toward an assertive motherhood that demanded the army bend to her solutions.

Bickerdyke's relentless commitment to sanitation and patient care often brought her into direct conflict with military bureaucracy. In early spring, which coincided with the USSC women's visit, she was sent to the smallpox hospital within the Memphis medical complex, where she led an effort to cleanse the facility and reduce its mortality rate. For several days, Bickerdyke worked to purify the facility, whitewashing the walls and reforming the kitchens so that sick men in the hospital were provided with an appropriate diet.[18] While she was away from her laundry operation, Irwin issued a written order stating that "all the contrabands detailed to her service should be sent to the contraband camp by nine o'clock the next morning," effectively dismissing them from her employment without her input.[19]

Upon receiving the notice late in the evening, Bickerdyke wasted no time in mounting a response to preserve the system that she had implemented. Without hesitation, she decided to take the matter directly to the highest-ranking official in Memphis—General Stephen A. Hurlbut. Dragging a reluctant Mary Livermore along, Bickerdyke set off on a harrowing, rain-soaked carriage ride through the war-torn, heavily guarded streets of the former Confederate stronghold to Hurlbut's headquarters. The groggy commanding officer was met with a firm demand from Bickerdyke for written authorization to "keep her detailed contrabands."[20] Without argument, General Hurlbut granted the request. The following morning, when Irwin arrived at the hospital, he was met by a triumphant Bickerdyke, who smugly handed him the general's written order. Initially enraged, the doctor resisted, but over time, he grew to respect her persistence and unorthodox methods. As Livermore later noted, Irwin's hostility stemmed from an "inborn belief that all women were to play 'second fiddle' to him"—a sentiment common among army doctors but one that Bickerdyke rejected.[21]

The instance with Dr. Irwin reflected a broader pattern of gendered authority in military hospitals where women, regardless of their expertise, were expected to remain subordinate to male leadership. However, as Jane Schultz has noted, these conflicts over power and professionalism were not just about gender but also about race. The same hospital structures that sought to limit Bickerdyke's authority reinforced the racial hierarchies that permeated Union medical spaces. Schultz's research highlights how White women in Civil War hospitals often leveraged racial distinctions to assert control over Black workers, even as they themselves were marginalized by male military officials.[22] Northern officers and hospital administrators frequently assigned Black women to menial labor while restricting them from roles as nurses despite their experience and capability. This hierarchy ensured that even as women like Bickerdyke fought for professional legitimacy, they often worked within systems that continued to oppress Black workers. Bickerdyke's insistence on retaining her Black laundry workers challenged this racial order, at least in part. By demanding the authority to keep them under her supervision, she pushed back against the bureaucratic control that sought to remove them from their positions. However, her ability to advocate for their labor did not necessarily translate into an equitable working environment. As Schultz notes, White women's perceptions of Black workers often deteriorated when they shared proximity in the workplace. Many reformers viewed Black women not as colleagues but as subordinates, reinforcing racial distinctions even within supposedly progressive institutions like the USSC.

During her tenure in Memphis, Bickerdyke became bolder in pursuing her preferred courses of relief, and she was more assertive with those who hindered her mission. Her self-efficacy was reinforced by high-ranking military officials who affirmed her productivity and were unbothered by her methods for achieving positive results for the men under her care. For middle-ranking officers, especially those who interfered with Bickerdyke's systems of care, conflict was more likely to occur. Historians who have written about women's entrance into medical professionalism generally agree that an early nineteenth-century emphasis on female moral purity gave credence to the formulation of the idea of separate spheres. Such distinctions encouraged men to use Victorian sexual stereotyping to exclude women from medicine, as well as from other public or professional activities for which they might be distinctly suited.[23] Practicing Civil War surgeons struggled with Bickerdyke's maternal authority, but her apparent confidence in that authority drove her to continue, despite objections from Union surgeons.

The most repeated punchline of any Mary Bickerdyke war story, from contemporary accounts to memorialists to Ken Burns's *The Civil War*, infers maternal authority. "She ranks me," a quip attributed to both Generals Grant and Sherman, encapsulated the way both soldiers and officers deferred to Mary Bickerdyke's actions in the wards. The genesis of this incident seems to be Dr. Linus Pierpont Brockett and Mrs. Mary C. Vaughan's 1867 book,

*Woman's Work in the Civil War: A Record of Heroism, Patriotism and Patience.* Brockett and Vaughan's work was a collection of chapters that presented short biographical vignettes and war stories celebrating the accomplishments of women across the nation who contributed to the Union war effort. The authors began collecting "voluminous correspondence" and conducting "personal observation" of women's contributions in the fall of 1863 and continued to gather information on their chosen subjects.[24] For Mary Bickerdyke's chapter, they likely obtained accounts from Mary Livermore, who was mentioned in the authors' preface and who repeated the Brockett and Vaughan anecdote in her own memoir that was published years later.[25]

The episode began one morning as Livermore accompanied Bickerdyke on her typical rounds to the Memphis hospital. The two women arrived in the late morning to discover that the attending surgeon had not reported for duty, leaving the sick and recovering men without their special diet breakfasts. Mother Bickerdyke sprang to action immediately, preparing "enormous tin pails and trays with coffee, soup, gruel, toast, and other like food" to tend to the neglected men.[26] Livermore and a detail assembled by Bickerdyke set out to complete the surgeon's assigned duty. When the surgeon of the ward lumbered in, "looking as if he had just risen from sleeping off a night's debauch," Bickerdyke responded with an excoriating tirade.[27] She called him out for his inexcusable drunkenness and demanded that he remove the straps from his shoulders that signified his advanced rank. She plainly stated to the surgeon that she would have him dishonorably discharged from the service for his wanton dereliction of duty to the suffering men. Within a week, the man was dismissed from the service. To regain his position and refute his discharge, which came from a woman he outranked, he reportedly appealed to then Major General William T. Sherman. When Sherman asked the dismissed surgeon who was responsible for the charges against him, the man referred to Mother Bickerdyke as "that spiteful old woman."[28] Brockett and Vaughan recounted that Sherman, immediately recognizing Bickerdyke, stated plainly, "Well, if it was her, I can do nothing for you. She ranks me."[29]

In every variation of this story, a high-ranking official in the Union army—in this telling, Major General Sherman—confirmed that Mary Bickerdyke's maternal authority superseded his own military authority. The message is important, regardless of whether the interaction occurred as described by its various acolytes. Some details in each iteration were undoubtedly overstated. For example, if the incident took place in March 1863 when Livermore was in Memphis, then Sherman had already joined General Grant in the Siege of Vicksburg and General Hurlbut assumed command at Memphis.[30]

In Livermore's account, Bickerdyke calls the man a "scalawag," a term that surfaced after the war as a derisive reference to Southerners who supported Reconstruction policies. Additionally, in the 1890s, at least two veterans wrote to Mother Bickerdyke with variations on the "she ranks me" anecdote, claiming the celebrated incident took place at different times in the war and that each of them was present at the general's signature remark.[31] Through the mists of retelling and the elaboration of commemoration, one truth stands resolute: the written acknowledgment of Mary Bickerdyke's maternal authority over military command not only underscores the legendary status of her contributions but reaffirms the enduring power of motherhood within the Union army.

In late 1863, Bickerdyke demonstrated her maternal medical competency in a sanctioned health campaign. While superintending the Gayoso Hospital under USSC employment, Bickerdyke had difficulty obtaining milk for her soldier-patients, which she found to be instrumental in their recovery—a part of their special diet. Bickerdyke complained that "a gallon of water, barely colored with milk, cost 40 cents," causing her to spend an inflated $400 per month on "sham milk."[32] She resolved to solve the supply problem by soliciting donations of live cows and hens from anyone willing to aid her request. This method was anything but the standardized medical protocol of the USSC or United States Army, but it was uniquely designed by Bickerdyke's combination of maternal authority and medical competency. To accomplish her ends in the mission, Bickerdyke welcomed the help of competing benevolent agencies, including the Western Sanitary Commission (WSC) and the Illinois Sanitary Commission.

Bickerdyke exhausted local options to provide adequate diets for those recovering from various illnesses and injuries in Memphis. In the spirit of a mother's self-sacrifice, she had "foraged from the secessionists, had traded with them her own clothing and whatever else she could spare, for the necessaries for her 'boys,' until there was nothing more left to trade."[33] Left without local options, Bickerdyke proposed a plan to canvas Illinois, Wisconsin, and Ohio to obtain donations that would provide a direct and cost-effective supply of fresh farm goods for recovering soldiers in Memphis: at least 100 milk cows and up to 2,000 hens.[34] Memorialists dubbed the event the "Cow and Hen Tour," while the contemporary press saw the campaign as "an opportunity to do good."[35]

Mary Bickerdyke's execution of her "Cow and Hen Tour" demonstrated her willingness to navigate—and even exploit—the rival structures of the USSC and the WSC to meet patient needs. Though Bickerdyke knew the tension between the wartime sanitary institutions, she approached relief with a practical, ends-focused mindset. She was willing to break official alliances and cross institutional lines for the sake of expedient care.[36] If one organization could provide a quicker solution to one of her proposals, she tended to accept the first bidder. Later biographers called Bickerdyke's penchant a desire to "cut red tape," but such an analysis suggests her tacit disapproval of the institutional bureaucracy.[37] The evidence points instead to a more strictly patient-oriented approach to relief and care and an ability to utilize her maternal authority to question faulty protocols. In fact, it could be argued that Bickerdyke was engaging in the most efficient implementation of sanitary science and recognized the futility of such bureaucratic boundaries. In June 1863, James Yeatman of the WSC visited Memphis to survey hospital operations. During his time there, he met Bickerdyke, and she appealed to him to help her begin her campaign to solicit livestock donations, despite her alignment with the USSC. Yeatman wrote Bickerdyke letters of introduction and provided transportation passes to connect her with potential resources.[38] The tour was eventually endorsed by the Chicago Sanitary Commission, but not until mid-August 1863, almost a month after Bickerdyke left her post in Memphis to procure the livestock supplies.[39]

The Cow and Hen Tour created a great deal of excitement in newspapers across Illinois and Wisconsin that lauded Bickerdyke's efforts as "a noble enterprise."[40] The advertisements introduced her more broadly to the public and backed her with the endorsements of the USSC, the WSC, and now, the Illinois Sanitary Commission as well. Under Bickerdyke's proposal, the coalition of organizations called for patriotic and loyal farmers to donate whatever they could for the sake of the suffering soldiers. Telegraphs poured into Mrs. Bickerdyke as large and small donations were shipped down to Memphis: $300 from the Milwaukee Aid Society, "35 to forty cows in this neighborhood," "25 cows furnished here," "thirty three cows and Twenty three calves were shipped today," "18 cows shipped from here that came from Jacksonville and fifteen raised near here—with 23 calves—about 90 fowls also shipt recently."[41] The generosity exceeded expectations and her campaign resulted in over 200 milk cows and 2,000 hens shipped to Memphis to begin the therapeutics.[42]

Observers referred to Bickerdyke's Cow and Hen Tour as "characteristic," citing her unifying efficiency, resolute energy animated for soldiers' benefit, and assertive determination to provide for sick soldiers.[43] The sentiment of Bickerdyke's resourcefulness was coupled with the humorous, preposterous visual of "loyal cows and hens" led by Bickerdyke in a "bizarre procession" as they triumphantly marched to the soldiers' aid in Memphis, suggesting how her ethic and actions defied convention and decorum of middling domesticity.[44] This depiction also revealed some of the tension between the practical and the preposterous in how female leadership was perceived during the war. Even as Bickerdyke's logistical genius and boldness won admiration, her ability to wield authority remained wrapped in the language of maternal instinct and eccentricity, rather than the professionalism and pragmatism it demonstrated. Her Cow and Hen Tour embodied the contradictions of women's wartime labor—both indispensable and irreverent, deeply necessary yet framed as an amusing spectacle.

### Her Boys: Motherhood at Home and at War

To survive as an independent wage earner, Bickerdyke had little choice but to continue working. The Civil War presented both an economic opportunity and a profound risk—its benefits were uncertain, but the alternative was the potential for financial instability. Some psychoanalytic interpretations of her prolonged maternal absence during and after the war overlook the material realities that shaped the lives of poor, female-headed families.[45] Scholars have noted that widowed families were often broken up by economic hardship. Despite community support, public and private relief efforts, and waged labor, many mothers still faced the painful decision of sending their children to orphanages or indentured placements in order to secure a means of survival.[46] For Bickerdyke, leaving her two young sons was not an act of cruelty or a subconscious response to trauma; it was a pragmatic choice dictated by necessity and opportunity.

On the other hand, Bickerdyke's sudden and distant employment choice raises explanatory questions because her actions did not exactly fit the understood model of independent female wage earners. Why, for example, did she leave for Cairo, Illinois, and continue there without any contracted employment or wage? If the decision to leave her young sons was purely financial, it stands to reason that she would have secured a contract before committing to an extended leave. Alternatively, Bickerdyke viewed her ability to help mitigate a medical disaster in Cairo as an interview process; if she could prove her worth, work ethic, and skills, then she could be successfully folded into an organizational structure and compensated. Bickerdyke joined other women whose positions and possibilities were substantively different from her own. Notably, Mary Safford and Eliza Porter, who were present at the Fort Defiance camps and early sanitary efforts in Cairo, assumed voluntary roles as middle- and upper-class women who could freely offer their time and services for the causes of the Union.[47]

At the end of 1863, after a productive year and now firmly situated in the USSC's employment, Bickerdyke took her second and final furlough of the war to visit her sons and help them settle into new living and school arrangements. After a short-lived experiment to keep her sons in Galesburg with their older half-sister, presumably until Bickerdyke had enough money to make a more suitable provision, the boys spent most of the war in various boarding school institutions and placements in the Midwest. This decision highlighted the reality that Bickerdyke's employment provided her sons with access to educational opportunities they might not have otherwise had. Her exposure to the middle-class values embedded in the USSC may have encouraged her to pursue formal education for her sons. Many of her colleagues and the men in positions of power around her had benefited from the privileges of wealth and education—advantages that she, as a widowed mother, was determined to secure for her sons.[48]

According to the USSC's official history, the salaries paid to the women were meant to remunerate "wear and tear and inevitable expense ... covering, in some degree, the pecuniary loss that must accrue to any family where the eye of the mistress is not over her household."[49] This rationale reflected the deeply ingrained assumption that women's primary duty was domestic management and that paid work was an exception rather than an entitlement. The USSC framed its pay structure as progressive, suggesting that compensating women at rates comparable to men was a fair and "just arrangement of a practical generation." The pay for male agents ranged from $40 to $100 a month, while that for female agents, from $30 to $100 a month.[50] Bickerdyke accepted a starting salary of $25 per month, which was less than the published remuneration.[51] By 1865, Bickerdyke had her pay increased to $50 a month, the lower end of a male agent's monthly pay.[52] The USSC approach to wages mirrored broader class and gender hierarchies of the period. Middle-class reformers, who often did not rely on their wages for survival, could afford to view women's pay as supplementary rather than essential. Working-class women like Bickerdyke, however, had no such luxury. Her compensation was not merely a symbolic acknowledgment of her labor; it was a necessity for maintaining her household and securing her children's future.

Her level of pay by the end of the conflict proved, to some extent, that Bickerdyke was proficient at her job and valued by the organization. Apart from her compensation, the constant demands and volume of work from the

USSC gave her an opportunity to repeatedly demonstrate her ability to meet complex logistical tasks. As an USSC agent and later as a nurse, she received invaluable medical and administrative education that she would have been denied in the gender-restrictive halls of formal medical institutions. Further, she was publicly recognized for her achievements in newspapers, through published histories, and in the word-of-mouth laudatory remarks from her thousands of soldier-patients. Her time in the army provided professional and intellectual freedom, for the first time since her marriage, to pursue employment that suited her growing skills and offered her the opportunity to exercise leadership as a woman in a profoundly male-dominated realm of professionalism. She was able to embody some iteration of Sarah Josepha Hale's revolutionary encouragement for wage-earning mothers to cultivate their intellect and pursue the satisfaction of a chosen professional life.[53] In other words, the Civil War instilled in Bickerdyke the belief that her motherhood was an important part of her identity that could be leveraged for her economic and professional advantage while also allowing her to operate successfully outside those cultural demands.

When Bickerdyke was hired to work for the USSC, it was clear that she did not belong to the same social class as her female coworkers in the institution. She was characterized by her lower class and was consistently noticed for her lack of refinement. This became an idiosyncratic style to embrace and embody through her actions: she *was* the "cyclone in Calico" imagined by Nina Baker in the 1950s; she *was* the "prairie-plough in the thunderstorm" that endeared her to USSC reformers like Jane Hoge. Her class became her calling card. Moreover, it made her accessible and empathetic to thousands of soldiers under her care. Her class distinction meant that her motherhood legitimized her claim to medical competence. Those under her care valued her pragmatic and familiar approach to caregiving. But pure pragmatism only got her so far because to operate within a regimented institution like the USSC, she needed to embrace some middle-class conventions to accomplish her professional goals. Literacy and correspondence were key components of middle-class behavior, sensibility, and social interaction in Civil War–era America. Men and women became well known and gained esteem for their ability to communicate information, share ideas, and comment on contemporary society.[54] During the war, Bickerdyke's lack of confidence in her letter-writing abilities caused her to employ creative solutions and solicit the help of another writer to dictate her correspondence to USSC headquarters, various donors and aid societies, and the military personnel with whom she worked.[55]

In contrast, Mary Livermore's involvement in Civil War organization and activism was quintessentially upper middle class. Born in Boston as a direct descendant of Puritan immigrants to the Massachusetts Bay Colony, she was educated at a Massachusetts female seminary, married a minister, and relocated to Chicago a few years before the war. She was fiercely intelligent, and her desire for education was met with opportunities for cultivation from a young age. She was reform-minded and became a member of the Republican Party, an abolitionist, a women's rights activist, and a temperance advocate. At the start of the Civil War, she was given a leadership position with the USSC because of her social standing and education. For those under her supervision, such as Mary Bickerdyke, she demanded industrious work and effective communication. For her part, Bickerdyke confidently provided skilled labor, and she constantly tested the boundaries of acceptable communication. The two women did not always see eye to eye—Livermore's calls for frequent reports and formal interactions clashed with Bickerdyke's reliance on informal, results-driven action. Their relationship revealed the tensions between working-class pragmatism and middle-class professionalism, highlighting how class distinctions shaped women's experiences within the USSC.

In March 1864, Livermore was growing impatient as Bickerdyke neglected to write letters to various aid societies that had given donations, noting that "the ladies will rather think you ungrateful, or that I have been remiss in forwarding the money to you."[56] For Livermore, as for other middle-class women, such correspondence was a sign of dignity, respect, and a general philanthropic spirit.[57] She regularly registered her disappointment with Bickerdyke but was also resigned to Bickerdyke's bad habits: "Remember me in love to Mrs. Porter, tell the boys what we are doing, take good care of yourself, and if I thought it would avail anything, I would add, write! Write!! Write!!! Or get somebody else to."[58]

The persistent problem of Bickerdyke's epistolary negligence went beyond some personal quirk. It revealed a real gap in education between Bickerdyke, a lower-class domestic worker, and the middle-class women who were more typically assigned to professional positions during the Civil War. For their part, women like Mary Livermore, Jane Hoge, and Eliza Chappell Porter were schooled in the Victorian norms and trained to constantly engage in correspondence to keep up with those expectations. Bickerdyke was evidently self-conscious about her penmanship and writing ability, and it often meant that she simply decided against writing.

Bickerdyke was constantly compared to her fellow sanitary agents and colleagues, but 1860 census data draws a clear contrast between Mary Bickerdyke's

TABLE 3.1  1860 US Census data comparison of Chicago Sanitary Commission workers

| USSC Employee | Head of House Occupation | Place of Birth | Number of Servants | Real Estate ($) | Assets |
| --- | --- | --- | --- | --- | --- |
| Livermore | Unitarian clergy | Massachusetts | 1 | — | — |
| Hoge | Merchant | Pennsylvania | 3 | 8,000 | 1,000 |
| Henshaw | Captain US Army | Connecticut | — | 7,000 | 2,000 |
| Porter | Presbyterian clergy | New York | 1 | 3,000 | — |
| McCagg | Lawyer | New York | 6 | 140,000 | 50,000 |
| Bickerdyke | Botanic physician | Ohio | 0 | — | 100 |

socioeconomic status and that of other prominent men and women of the Chicago Sanitary Commission (see table 3.1). At the war's outset, Bickerdyke owned no real estate and possessed $100 in assets. In contrast, her constant field companion from the Chicago office, Eliza Chappell Porter, the wife of an army chaplain and mother to two Illinois soldiers, listed $3,000 in real estate in 1860 and employed one household servant.[59] The two women were friends and amicable coworkers in the field, but their differences, not only financial, were noted by battlefield observers: "The mildness of [Porter] was an offset to the positiveness of [Bickerdyke]; the noiseless efficiency of the one, to the turbulent energy of the other. The culture and social position of Mrs. Porter gave her ready access to officers."[60] The two women, united in cause, took varied approaches to their sanitary service, and it resulted in a markedly different reception by the soldiers on the field.

While Porter's social position gave her clout with the officers, Bickerdyke was uninterested in building rapport with the higher-ranking men and women unless it directly benefited the common soldier in some way. Jane Hoge, a Chicago reformer, described Bickerdyke as a woman who was fiercely loyal to the rank and file and had little regard for hierarchy when it came to care: "A pythoness, if her precious boys, as she called them, were assaulted . . . woe be to the man, no matter what his rank, who trampled on the rights of the 'Boys in Blue.'"[61] USSC President Henry Bellows agreed that Bickerdyke had attained "undying renown throughout the northern armies as preeminently the friend of the private soldier."[62] Bickerdyke's reputation was staked on her commitment to the common rank-and-file soldier, to those men whose lives mirrored her own.

Bickerdyke's own limited literacy and aspirations for her sons' success motivated her decision to pursue a more rigorous education on their behalf.[63]

Bickerdyke removed her children from the care of the Galesburg community and placed them in a Chicago boarding school. When James was old enough to enroll in secondary school, the boys were moved to Beloit, Wisconsin, where James attended Beloit College and Hiram enrolled in the Beloit public schools.[64] During this time, the boys were placed with a woman named Laura Hayward, who housed, fed, and cared for them in exchange for payment. The practice of placing children with farmers became so widespread that between 1850 and 1900, one-fifth to one-third of farm homes included children who were not the biological offspring of the adults in the household.[65] Her remote work, which broke the norms of nineteenth-century motherhood, allowed Bickerdyke to provide important aspects of care.

While Bickerdyke sought to provide financial and educational stability for her sons, she frequently struggled to make timely payments to their caretakers. What she envisioned as a means of securing greater opportunities for her children often introduced unforeseen challenges and emotional strain. As a teenager, James found himself repeatedly reminding his mother to cover overdue expenses for essential goods and services, including winter coats and boots, to meet their growing needs.[66] At age 16, James kept his mother's books, so to speak, and implored her to pay for their care on schedule. When he failed to hear from his mother, at one point for almost five months, he pleaded with her: "Don't fail to send the money. I wish you would send Mrs. H's money which you promised her over 8 weeks ago. You now owe her some $150 and [we] hope you will come up and see about it."[67] The strain revealed the emotional burden placed on her sons, who were forced to navigate both economic precarity and the absence of their mother in ways that blurred the lines between childhood and adulthood.

The conundrum of Bickerdyke's care-switching between professional and personal motherhood found ways to both benefit and harm her sons. While James and Hiram were placed in prestigious learning environments, they also faced the stress of financial instability and the emotional toll of prolonged parental absence. With their only living parent stationed on the front lines of a dangerous war, they were left to navigate uncertainty largely on their own. Bickerdyke tried to reassure them that she had their situation under control, but her inability to dependably deliver on her promises did not promote confidence in either of her children. In a letter addressed to both James and their caretaker, she sought to earn their trust: "I do not forget my dear boys tho I do not always send [payment] to them as promptly as I should like to. I know what the arrangements are about Hiram and am not afraid of him being turned out of school because his tuition isn't paid. They know I'll do as well as I can—My son, don't worry! You can trust your mother's planning and tho I cannot see the end from the beginning, I cannot but think my plans will ultimately succeed. So, don't worry!"[68]

Her reassurances were rooted more in hope than certainty and highlighted the tensions between her professional ambitions and the sacrifices they demanded of her family. Bickerdyke's decision to enlist her time and services to the Union army signaled both the making and breaking of her home circle. It simultaneously promoted and deteriorated her motherhood. She sacrificed proximity and traditional maternal presence to pursue professional fulfillment, believing her service would ultimately secure a better future for her sons. While they benefited from educational opportunities, the emotional consequences of her absence played out in their fractured relationships that would take years to repair. In many ways, Hiram and James were forced to share their mother with the soldiers she had claimed as her boys.

After she returned to the front from her March 1864 furlough, Bickerdyke's repeated encounters with familial devastation in the midst of war began to take their toll. One visit to a hospital for Black refugees deeply unsettled her, as she witnessed immense suffering in overcrowded and unsanitary conditions. The experience compelled her to write to her young sons, sharing grim details of what she had seen:

> We went into one room where several families were crowded together and on a box in one corner was laid out a poor little boy eleven years old who had died in the morning. His mother was lying sick on a bed near him and there were several sick in the same room. About two hours afterward, we were in the cemetery, and there we saw the father who had come alone to bury his boy, the sixth child he had lost. Five were buried side by side and as there was not room for more this little boy was laid in the grave of his sister eight years old.[69]

Writing such a letter to her adolescent sons served multiple purposes. She offered them a stark reminder of the daily realities of her work, while also pointing to suffering that was far more acute than their distance from her could ever cause. On a personal level, it may have been a form of emotional release for her and an attempt to process the horrors she encountered by sharing them with those closest to her. More significantly, it functioned as a tool of instruction, exposing James and Hiram to the brutal inequities of war and reinforcing the sacrifices she made by remaining on the front. By detailing the immense loss experienced by others, particularly Black refugee families, she may have hoped to instill in her sons a sense of gratitude for their own relative security, however precarious it might be. At the same time, the letter implicitly justified her absence, illustrating the urgency of her mission and the profound need for her work. Though Bickerdyke could not be physically present for her children, she used letters like these to remind them—and perhaps herself—that her labor was not only necessary but meaningful. Her letters to James and Hiram sought to impress on them the weight of war's tragedies. Her work placed her in direct contact with the systemic neglect that shaped the experiences of African Americans seeking freedom.

Black refugees fleeing into Union lines were regularly met with inadequate and negligent medical care. Historians have suggested that the federal government was unprepared to manage African Americans' health needs during and after emancipation.[70] But as was the case in other instances, Bickerdyke's focus remained on the immediate, personal impact of death rather than the broader governmental failures, although such failures in medical and sanitary care were obvious, as this encounter demonstrated. The sorrow and grief associated with such heart-wrenching stories only served to remind her of a shared human experience. It was "touching to see" a grieving mother dress and prepare her deceased infant girl in preparation for burial. She attended the quaint funeral, watching as the mother wept and "planted a bunch of flowers upon the little grave." Seeing the death of so many children, she wrote to her boys, "I could not but contrast their conditions with that of my own dear boys."[71] Bickerdyke was not a wealthy woman, but she understood her relative privilege as a woman employed by a national organization.

Though she was never a champion for any sort of racial justice, she was not blind to the suffering of those around her. That Bickerdyke would include these stories in her letters to her sons indicates her intent to do what many Civil War soldier-fathers did for their sons: instruct them on the realities of death.[72] Those on the field who saw such horrors and suffering were taught by death, and they did not waste opportunities to educate the next generation on how to manage its inevitabilities.

## Letting Mother Go: Maternal Expediency versus the USSC

In the last year and half of the war, Bickerdyke was constantly on the move, following the Union army of Tennessee's Fifteenth Corps under Generals William T. Sherman and John A. Logan through the Atlanta campaign.[73] As the army pressed deeper into Confederate territory, she adapted her work to the shifting needs of the battlefield. She managed diet kitchens, distributed sanitary stores from multiple relief agencies, and ensured that hospitals remained stocked with essential supplies. Her authority came not from rigid institutional structures but from the trust she had earned among the soldiers she served. Bickerdyke's commitment to *maternal care* remained the cornerstone of her service, but she wielded it pragmatically. She exercised influence first through the cultural legitimacy of motherhood and, when necessary, through the official backing of the USSC. Yet, she was not beholden to any single institution. Her loyalty was not to the USSC or the army bureaucracy, but to her protocol of soldier care.

This flexibility defined her wartime leadership. She collaborated with any organization that could help her accomplish her goals, prioritizing expediency over bureaucratic allegiance. If the USSC provided the resources she needed and facilitated her initiatives, she cooperated; if they imposed obstacles, she found ways to circumvent institutional constraints. Bickerdyke's ability to navigate multiple layers of military and relief administration was a testament to her ingenuity and her unwillingness to compromise on the needs of the men she cared for. To the USSC, she was often a liability: she was unruly, ungovernable, and unpredictable. To the soldiers, she was indispensable.

Bickerdyke was a fierce advocate for soldier welfare and did not hesitate to intervene when it best served the men under her care. Her reputation as a protector of the rank and file gave her the confidence to challenge injustice when she saw it. While military discipline was an essential part of army life, she viewed excessive punishments as an abuse of power, especially punishments that jeopardized a soldier's health. Soon after she began traveling with the Fifteenth Corps, Bickerdyke witnessed one such case of extreme disciplinary action and took it upon herself to report it "to the Proper Authorities." Early one morning, she witnessed a soldier tied up for so long that "his hands had become *black* from want of circulation."[74] Disturbed, she inquired about his case and learned that his offense was missing in his company's roll call. His punishment, seemingly far harsher than his crime warranted, also included being forced to march "double quick with a heavy piece of timber on his shoulder" and being denied a meal.[75] While the officer in charge likely saw the sentence as an example for other soldiers, Bickerdyke made her disapproval clear: "Being here to look after the interests of soldiers who are in health as well as those who are sick, and believing that in this case of this man there was uncalled for *harshness* exercised, I have felt constrained to make this complaint to you, in the hope that you will not pass it unnoticed."[76]

Bickerdyke clearly internalized her authority as an expert in matters of wellness, so when military decisions intersected with her realm, she was prepared to defend her position as a health professional. She generally deferred to military rules and understood protocol and hierarchy, but she did not waver in her demonstrated competency and authority that stemmed from her role as a capable maternal medical practitioner. It was her duty, not only as a professional but also as a mother, to advocate for soldiers and report on the perceived abuses within the military system. In this way, the roles of mother and medical authority necessarily converged to alleviate patient suffering.

Bickerdyke and her USSC colleagues on the front, including Eliza Chappell Porter, were chiefly responsible for distributing food, maintaining cleanliness through laundry services for the camp, and managing hospital supplies as they were delivered to various post hospitals and soldiers' homes. Additionally, ministering to and nursing sick soldiers was a central part of their duties. USSC agents were excluded from the same authority granted to army surgeons, but the practicality of battlefield care and convalescent therapeutics often put these female agents in the position of primary physician. Historians have made compelling arguments about the advantages of this system and the accountability that this protocol promoted amid battlefield chaos.[77] However, the standardization of care did not typically include preventative sanitation or end-of-life assistance, focusing more on the direct treatment of diseases or injuries.

As had been the case in Memphis, not all medical professionals accepted Bickerdyke's authority, a predictable reaction in the male-dominated medical field. Despite her proven effectiveness, some doctors remained resistant to the presence of women in hospital settings, dismissing their contributions as overly emotional or lacking scientific rigor. While Bickerdyke had contentious run-ins with such figures, many physicians deeply respected her work and remained friends with her after the war, publicly acknowledging her contributions to battlefield medicine.[78] At the same time, hostility toward women's participation in medical matters persisted. Some Union doctors clung to a strict, gendered hierarchy that relegated women to subordinate roles, particularly in hospital administration. Bickerdyke faced her share of complaints from those who viewed her assertiveness as an encroachment on male authority. This resistance was formalized in "Special Order No. 21" issued by two assistant surgeons in Chattanooga, which directly targeted Bickerdyke and Porter. The order stated that the women's "province in this hospital is the *special* and *extra* diet kitchen, and you are ordered to confine your operations, herein, to the discharging of your duties in this kitchen"; the order further noted that they should discontinue their visits to "other Departments of this Hospital."[79] The special order issued by the Chattanooga doctors did little to deter Bickerdyke in her future dealings. Instead of retreating, she intensified her efforts, forging new partnerships with aid agencies outside the USSC to secure medical supplies and hospital stores. The order, intended to limit her influence, only reinforced her determination to work around bureaucratic barriers rather than within them.

As she encountered moments of institutional failure, she continued to push against any bureaucracy that stifled direct aid. This, in tandem with her growing reputation as "Mother" and her popularity among soldiers, suggested a style of advocacy that was atypical within the hierarchical structures of authority. Her bold, independent actions, however, did not sit well with her principal employer, the USSC. E. B. McCagg, president of the Chicago branch of the USSC, maintained strict expectations for his employees and made clear his vision for how sanitary agents should conduct themselves. In a report reprinted in the *Bulletin of the Sanitary Commission*, McCagg emphasized that "the distributing agents are more often than otherwise men of education, accustomed to the comforts of home, and refinements of social life."[80] To McCagg and the other architects of the USSC, its agents were representatives of a national institution. They were expected to embody middle-class efficiency, maintain dignified decorum, and assert authority as educated men positioned at the forefront of emerging medical science.[81] In other words, they were everything that Mary Bickerdyke was not.

Bickerdyke's instinct for soldier care often clashed with the rigid structures of institutional authority. Her ability to identify and address urgent medical concerns was unquestioned among the men she served, but the hierarchical systems governing wartime relief did not always recognize her expertise. A particularly frustrating episode during the winter of 1864 underscored the extent to which gendered bureaucracy could obstruct even the most basic efforts to preserve soldier health. After a long and difficult winter on the march South, disease ran rampant, and scurvy threatened the success of Sherman's plans to overtake Confederate forces and end the war. The crisis prompted requests to the USSC for a massive number of vegetables to provide sources of vitamin C to combat the disease, with onions, potatoes, and sauerkraut being the most common supplements.[82] General Grant commented that "the supply of vegetables and sanitary stores sent last winter saved his army, and that he looked to the same instrumentalities to save it in 1864, in a region stripped of everything by the contending forces."[83] Bickerdyke was assured that the vegetables were being procured and transported to the South by the Chicago branch of the USSC. According to Mary Livermore, thousands of dollars in vegetable donations were earmarked, with more on the way.[84] More than two weeks after that promise, Bickerdyke had yet to receive a shipment that was sufficient to meet the growing need. Sanitary agents exchanged anxious correspondence in the field as they witnessed the effects of a lack of nutrition among the troops.[85]

As it turned out, the supply was not the problem. It was, instead, a bureaucratic transportation logjam triggered by gendered notions of authority. The Union army and the USSC brokered a deal with the railroads that afforded the USSC one car per transport to deliver supplies. In extraordinary or emergency situations, like the growing nutrition crisis in Tennessee and Alabama, railroad operators required a "proper medical certificate" to increase the number of cars for the necessary supplies.[86] The coded language meant that in some instances, health solutions hinged on the willingness of a male surgeon to sign off on the plan. Even though Bickerdyke was charged with vegetable distribution and her male superiors agreed with her proposal, she lacked the power to deliver the vegetables effectively and efficiently to the army because she did not have the bona fides to sign the paperwork. The entire affair infuriated Bickerdyke, and while she was unable to change this rule, she began to lodge her complaints more regularly with the system and turned to other institutions and donors that allowed her to exercise her medical competencies for soldier health.[87]

Male surgeons eventually assented to the need for increased vegetable rations. On April 11, 1864, surgeons in Tennessee issued a certified statement indicating that the condition of the troops rendered "the issue of vegetable rations absolutely necessary to arrest a growing tendency to scorbutic disease, and the consequent preservation of the general health and physical efficiency of this command."[88] The pressure mounted for the USSC to follow through with a large delivery, and it put Bickerdyke in charge of distribution. Bickerdyke immediately made her way to USSC depots to await the promised vegetables, but by April 18, it was evident that there was a delay in delivery and the vegetables were at risk of decaying in the sanitary rooms across the North. Even with the urgency required, the USSC "evidently [did] not cooperate with her."[89] Bickerdyke and Porter waited several days, for hours at a time, on a train platform in Tennessee for promised vegetables that never arrived.[90]

Bickerdyke was not quiet about her frustrations over the vegetable debacle. Much-needed medical care in the form of basic nutrition was denied to scores of soldiers because of a technicality and hesitance to rely on a woman's word. The refusal to prioritize the shipment was a glaring example of how institutional rigidity and gendered authority could obstruct even the most fundamental aspects of soldier care. Intent on resolving the issue, Bickerdyke and Porter "determined to go again to Nashville to learn the cause of the delay as [they] knew that all the transportation needed had been promised by Genls Grant and Sherman."[91] When they arrived, the response they received from the USSC did not satisfy Bickerdyke. The USSC claimed it could not spare transportation until the hospitals were supplied and that it was unwilling to interfere with such work. Rather than accept the USSC's decision, Bickerdyke insisted that its leadership accompany her to the transportation office, where the quartermaster could confirm her work and attest to the legitimacy of her request.[92] She and Porter continued to push against the commission's protocol while simultaneously complying with its bureaucratic requirements, maneuvering within the system until the long-promised transportation was finally arranged—three weeks late.

Bickerdyke's grievances reached the home office in Chicago. McCagg, in a state of obvious annoyance at Bickerdyke's lack of cooperation with the USSC, scribbled out a hasty note to Bickerdyke. "Dear Madam," he wrote, "Mr. Richards of this City has just returned from Huntsville and has made us great trouble by reporting that our Sanitary matters are very badly managed there and at Nashville and telling many stories which he says . . . you gave to him."[93] McCagg was unhappy with Bickerdyke's behavior and lectured her, saying, "It seems impossible that an agent of the commission would injure it before and without making known to the commission itself the trouble."[94] McCagg was concerned that "strangers," such as the man mentioned in the letter, armed with knowledge of disunity within the USSC, might act to undermine its mission. He feared perceived incompetence, and Bickerdyke's willingness to speak critically of the commission put her at odds with the bureaucracy.

Bickerdyke continued to disrupt McCagg's rigid sense of order, ultimately leading to her dismissal from the USSC less than a year after the vegetable incident. Frustrated by institutional inefficiencies and motivated by the pressing needs of war, she began using USSC funds to travel and solicit donations for an independent project, an "institution for the benefit of soldiers orphans."[95] To McCagg, this misappropriation of USSC resources was a final affront. He justified her termination in no uncertain terms: "Refusing to give up her project no resource was left but to dismiss her. She is too largely controlled by her impulses, and has too little judgment or care . . . that she should under no circumstances remain in our employ."[96] The official resolution stated that Bickerdyke had made clear that she would be "obtaining subscriptions for soldiers' orphans," which was "incompatible" with the mission of the Chicago branch of the USSC.[97] If the mission of the USSC was singular in its focus, Bickerdyke's actions demonstrate her philosophy of care that extended beyond the war's conclusion. Though the USSC might dissolve after the war's end, Illinois families would be left to suffer its grievous consequences. As a widow herself, she intimately understood the long-term hardships that awaited soldiers' families—realities that the E. B. McCaggs of the world could not, or would not, fully grasp.

Bickerdyke's dismissal highlights the precarious nature of White middle-class motherhood within institutional structures. While soldiers revered her as the beau ideal of a wartime mother, her real-life assertion of authority clashed with the rigid expectations of maternal virtue—at least in the realm of professional employment. Her leadership and defiance were tolerated as long as they served the needs of male-dominated institutions, but once she stepped beyond the prescribed boundaries of acceptable maternal care, her position became untenable. Notably, Bickerdyke's dismissal from the USSC is missing from the secondary literature on her life. Any characterization of her as "untruthful" or "ignorant," as McCagg had labeled her, would have undermined the dominant narrative of pure-hearted sacrifice, devotion, and service. Her discharge did not align with the idealized version of motherhood that later biographers sought to preserve, and so it was quietly omitted from her legacy.

Despite threats to her employment, Bickerdyke leveraged alternative support networks to secure the supplies she needed, demonstrating her resourcefulness and resilience. Frustrated by the USSC's inability to meet demands, she turned to the Christian Commission, private donors, and her connections within the United States Army to procure essential goods. Even before McCagg dismissed her from the USSC, Bickerdyke made it clear that she intended to "co-operate cordially with the Christian Commission" in her work, requesting favors, transportation passes, and even clothes for herself.[98] On April 1, 1865, Dorothea Dix, the superintendent of women nurses for the Union army, retroactively certified Bickerdyke's position as an official nurse in the employment of the Medical Department of the United States.[99] While she could no longer draw a wage from the USSC, other organizations recognized the value of her work, willingly bypassing the USSC's decisions to ensure she received compensation and position her for a pension for her service.

Two themes emerged from Bickerdyke's Civil War service that shaped the rest of her personal and professional trajectory. The first was an affirmation of her authority derived from her effectiveness as a mother-caregiver. She gained a reputation as a fierce advocate for individual soldiers, aiding them in whatever way seemed most practical. She was, indeed, the "prairie-plough and the thunderstorm," as she tirelessly and persistently broke through institutional barriers to provide holistic care.[100] The war emboldened women who cared for soldiers and who felt they possessed a "special dispensation" to relieve suffering with their helping hands, willing service, and informal household training.[101] Women proved their place in the professional realm. Women nurses and female institutional agents of all persuasions asked themselves some version of the question: "How shall we get on when the war is over and there are no more 'boys' to be looked after?" It was women like W. A. Laurence and Mary Bickerdyke whose answers to that question were clear. Mrs. Laurence wrote to Bickerdyke saying, "I don't regard the war as over yet. The fight is over but the war includes more than mere fighting and our war is not over till no more boys are likely to be left to suffer."[102] The war was only the beginning of a longer mission to translate the competence of household training into professionalized care where it was needed.

The second major theme of Bickerdyke's wartime experience was her remarkable ability to navigate the challenges surrounding death and dying. While Civil War nurses routinely encountered death, Bickerdyke's correspondence with professionals and community members reveals a deep commitment to alleviating suffering. Though she had witnessed death outside war, the relentless exposure during her service strengthened her sense of purpose, compelling her to continue this work throughout her life. Her experience across multiple hospitals and battlefields, along with her role in corresponding with grieving families, equipped her with the skills to serve as a lifelong caretaker. She blended conventional medical knowledge with holistic therapeutics, adding her own unpretentious approach to guiding the dying through their final moments. While she fought tirelessly for patient recovery, she did not shy away from death's inevitability, instead offering comfort by being present at soldiers' bedsides. Her war experiences reinforced a lifelong lesson: death was inescapable, but health and healing were attainable for those who understood and could share that knowledge. In both life and death, Bickerdyke possessed a rare ability to provide solace and care.

Mary Bickerdyke's Civil War service not only defined her career but also reshaped cultural understandings of motherhood, caregiving, and women's roles in public life. Her service record stretched from Cairo, Illinois, in June 1861, to the Grand Review of the Armies parade in Washington, DC, after the Union's victory, and to Camp Butler in Springfield, Illinois, where she was mustered out with the last Illinois troops in March 1866.[103] She ran a

Memphis hospital for over a year and followed both Generals Ulysses S. Grant and William T. Sherman during their long southward campaigns. She witnessed nineteen battles on land and by river steamer, campaigned for funds and goods in the North, and attended to the victims at the notorious Andersonville Prison after the war concluded. Few individuals accomplished as much as Bickerdyke, and remarkably, she did it all for a modest wage that went directly to the care and education of her sons.

On the battlefield, Bickerdyke became both a tangible source of comfort and a symbolic maternal figure to thousands of soldiers. War commentators evaluated her, widely publicized her national maternal impact, and determined that the soldier-sons "were dear to somebody, and she would be a mother to them."[104] The adoration that she gained from the men under her care led to her adoption as Mother Bickerdyke. Her job and the reputation that developed from it signaled more than just a professional calling—it represented a new civic motherhood. As Bickerdyke associated with middle-class reformers and embraced the moral imperatives of middle-class mothers as an employee of the USSC, she was thrust into a social, cultural, and economic maelstrom that allowed her to refine her maternal identity and consistently challenge the typical gendered structures of the public sphere. Throughout the war, Bickerdyke persistently asserted her maternal authority in the face of procedures, red tape, and conventional modes of military authority—conscious of her difference but confident in her ambitious redesign of motherhood. As her relationships with her biological sons suffered from distance and perhaps even occasional regret over her professional choices, her adopted sons provided almost constant reassurance and comfort throughout her life.

In Mary Bickerdyke's maternal sacrifice, she found reward by leveraging her abilities as a mother to serve other people's sons. As the war reshaped the nation's understanding of professional opportunities for women, Bickerdyke was suddenly able to rewrite her own narrative of what working motherhood meant. She could make decisions that both abandoned culturally accepted maternal ideals in the home and fulfilled them in new ways through a civic and professional motherhood. While her journey yielded personal consequences, a newfound professional efficacy as a national mother produced an individual freedom to act, learn, and grow in ways that domesticity did not offer. Breaking the home circle was Mary Bickerdyke's only viable option to become the "Mother" of Civil War fame.

CHAPTER FOUR

# Mother-Guardian
## Negotiating Institutional Care after the Civil War

The suffering of the Civil War did not end with the Confederate surrender at Appomattox in April 1865. Surviving soldiers faced long journeys home, navigating the slow process of mustering out, collecting their pay, and attempting to reintegrate into civilian life. This transition proved daunting, as hundreds of thousands of families—and virtually every community, North and South— grappled with the profound social and economic upheaval left in the war's wake. Throughout Reconstruction and into the Progressive Era, the national government, local institutions, and private reformers struggled to build infrastructure to support veterans and their families, addressing lingering disease, undiagnosed trauma, and the widespread grief of an entire generation. Like many who had served in wartime caregiving roles, Mary Bickerdyke found it both impossible and irresponsible to return to a civic life that ignored the ongoing needs of those who had endured the hardships of war.

In Chicago, upper-class reformers like Mary Livermore recognized the growing need for social services for women and children, collectively investing thousands of dollars in charitable institutions such as the Home for the Friendless. The organization initially housed approximately 100 temporary boarders at any given time and counted 385 children in 1865, many of whom were driven to the charity by the circumstances of the war.[1] Destitute and desperate single mothers turned to the Home for the Friendless for shelter, food, and support. In a similar fashion, orphans were temporarily accommodated at the home until they could be placed with and adopted by a worthy and competent family.[2]

As matron of the Home for the Friendless in the immediate postwar years, Bickerdyke witnessed firsthand the overwhelming needs of threadbare mothers and orphaned children. The daily influx of families seeking shelter, food, and stability underscored the lingering effects of war and reinforced her earlier commitments to caring for soldiers and their loved ones. For Bickerdyke, this work was an extension of her wartime service, a new means of employment in her field, and a continuation of her evolving maternal role that expanded beyond the battlefield into broader social reform. Her sense of responsibility toward vulnerable children soon took on a more personal, hands-on form. In 1867, Mary Bickerdyke formalized this commitment through a contract of indenture for Emma Liegenspeck, a young orphaned German immigrant.[3] The agreement stipulated that Emma would "live in the family of the said party of the second part [Mary Bickerdyke], until she arrives at the age of 21 years," and that Bickerdyke would provide for her English education, clothing, training, treatment, and other needs related to child-rearing.[4] For all intents and purposes, Bickerdyke temporarily adopted this young woman and took legal responsibility for her over the course of five to six years until she reached adulthood.

The singular indenture document in Bickerdyke's archive is the only known reference to Emma, and there is no indication that she lived with or accompanied Bickerdyke after the contract was signed. Given Bickerdyke's own transience during this period—moving between advocacy work for the Illinois Soldiers' Orphans' Home, a brief tenure at the Home for the Friendless, and her eventual relocation to Salina, Kansas, in 1868—it is likely that the indenture served as a legal mechanism to release Emma from institutional care and facilitate her placement in another household where she could work as a domestic servant.[5] This case illustrates Bickerdyke's willingness to circumvent bureaucratic obstacles to provide guardianship and advocate for practical solutions for those who needed them most.[6]

Not all the orphans who passed through the Home for the Friendless were able to receive this treatment. The institution's managers likened their efforts to distributing "five barley loaves and two small fishes," acknowledging that demand for services far outpaced the available resources. The money to provide the charity to a growing number of indigent women and children was largely reliant on generous benefactors or internal institutional reforms, hardly a stable funding model.[7] With what it could collect, the Home for the Friendless sought to provide a "morally healthful place of resort" and an "inviting place of refuge for dependent and *worthy* females."[8] By referring to the business as a "home," the managers exerted a domestic sphere of influence over its inhabitants, making it a place of discipline and training predicated on moral teaching and maternal training. This setting encouraged the matrons, who served as official matriarchs within the institution, to instill contemporary values in the patient population while also providing the warmth and familiarity of a strong maternal presence. The initial actions of the board of managers and the staff at the Home for the Friendless reflected the pre–Civil War cultural ideals of feminine behavior, and they attempted to apply their Christian moral standards to the women who entered their home. In this sense, motherhood and institutional guardianship were intertwined, while public services substituted for proper instruction that had previously been rooted in private domestic settings. The fusion of moral instruction with institutional charity resonated with a public anxious about rising poverty and delinquency, reinforcing a selective approach to aid distribution that would extend from orphanages to Civil War pensions in the decades to come. From childhood to old age, Americans continued to wrestle with how to translate the moral authority of the home into a public ethic, balancing benevolence with control in the nation's expanding social infrastructure.

By the early 1900s, liberal government provision for Civil War combatants opened the door for increased aid for women affected by the loss of household income and recognized women's ability to run their households independently of male leadership. Until that time, Mother Bickerdyke attempted to fit the prescription of maternal care that she fostered during the war into institutional models and frameworks that existed in the war's wake. The Civil War caused a crisis in American welfare that prompted an essential question at all levels of government and in public life: Who should be responsible for the long-term care of soldiers and their families? The answer was an often-contested public matter that eventually formalized a maternalist welfare state by the turn of the century. Bickerdyke's case, however, demonstrates that some advocates wasted no time in enacting the process of relief, stepping into quasi-public roles before formal structures existed.[9]

Before the state made larger reforms around ideologies that "exalted women's capacities to mother and extended to society as a whole the values of care, nurturance and morality," women empowered by their Civil War professionalism worked out these ideas in their local contexts.[10] Bickerdyke quickly put her tested nursing skills to use and exercised her newly developed social connections to extend her maternal competence into social services and welfare before those debates were resolved in the public square.[11] Bickerdyke's institutional interventions and situational red tape cutting preceded the larger maternalist reform, signaling women's grassroots efforts to create their own versions of maternal welfare at local levels, leveraging and manipulating developing institutions as governments slowly addressed questions of state-supported care.

Mary Bickerdyke immersed herself in a range of experimental institutions designed to support soldiers and their families, unwilling to wait for local or national authorities to address the mounting social welfare crises left in the wake of the Civil War. Her postwar efforts reflected the evolving and often improvised nature of America's early welfare systems, which lacked cohesive governmental oversight. As with Emma Liegenspeck, Bickerdyke continued to advocate for guardianship, although its meaning fluctuated throughout her postwar career. For her, guardianship—whether legal or informal—was an extension of her professional maternal duties, shaped by her wartime experience and reinforced by her widely accepted title of Mother Bickerdyke. Crucially, Bickerdyke's status as a Civil War nurse and USSC agent legitimized her authority in caregiving roles that might otherwise have been restricted for working-class women. Her war service conferred trust in both her maternal morality and professional competence, allowing her to navigate institutional structures with remarkable fluidity. In a period when guardianship was gaining legal recognition as a form of state-sanctioned parental authority, Bickerdyke's ability to step into both official and unofficial caregiving roles demonstrated her capacity to care-switch—a skill that allowed her to move between bureaucratic systems, institutional settings, and personal advocacy while maintaining her core mission of care. Unlike many of her contemporaries, who remained confined to singular roles within charitable institutions, Bickerdyke leveraged her wartime credentials to expand the possibilities of maternal care, ensuring that her influence extended well beyond the battlefield.

## The Extension of Palliative Care: Protecting Soldiers' Orphans through Institutional Guardianship

After the Civil War, social reformers and state governments struggled to agree on the best solution, whether institutional or otherwise, to manage the influx of children in need of welfare provisions.[12] One of Bickerdyke's first projects after the war was to garner statewide support for the establishment of a home for Illinois soldiers' orphans. Her involvement signaled an extension of the palliative care practices formulated during the war. Caring for deceased soldiers meant acknowledging their last wishes and providing meaningful support to help their families continue their livelihoods. Individuals such as Mary Bickerdyke identified gaps in support and encouraged the state to intervene by establishing relief institutions for affected families. The creation of the Illinois Soldiers' Orphans' Home in 1867 fulfilled Bickerdyke's immediate goal of providing for soldiers' children and reinforced a precedent for state-sponsored child welfare, signaling a shift from private charity to public responsibility.

States had a patriotic commitment to families who had sacrificed for the benefit of the nation's preservation.[13] In the wake of the Civil War, this sense of duty reflected the moral and political belief that the state bore responsibility for those who had ensured the Union's survival, extending the notion of military service into an obligation for postwar social welfare. Civil War orphans had unique needs and, more importantly, were deserving of special care and protection.[14] Their vulnerability was not only material, marked by the loss of parental support, but also symbolic: their fathers' sacrifices demanded recognition through tangible forms of state care, transforming welfare into a moral obligation rather than mere charity. One Illinois newspaper admonished its citizens that the consequences of collective abandonment could be devastating to society: "If now neglected, these children must grow up in ignorance and wickedness, and be taught, by a terrible experience [the loss of a father], the ingratitude of a country for which their fathers sacrificed their comfort, their property and their lives."[15] The press framed orphan care as a test of civic virtue, urging both the state and its citizens to respond decisively to avoid moral and social decline. In many states across the North, different iterations of orphan care were initiated in response to the call to guard and protect this class of children.[16]

The effort to establish homes for soldiers' orphans emerged as a critical social welfare initiative during the Civil War, reflecting broader concerns about the long-term care of veterans' families. The need for a soldiers' orphans' home was first brought before the United States Congress in 1863. Each state had its own legislative process and timeline for introducing a localized version of such an institution; Pennsylvania and New York were early adopters of state-based systems providing this specific service. Accomplished and capable women were typically behind the creation and implementation of these parental-substitution institutions, but male legislators and benefactors from each state provided the legal and financial accreditation to get the organizations off the ground.[17] This collaboration between reform-minded women and policymakers highlights the gendered dynamics of social welfare work—women shaped the mission and daily operations of these institutions while men controlled the mechanisms of funding and legitimacy. When Illinois finally found ways to meet its funding goals and settled matters among its stakeholders, the Illinois Soldiers' Orphans' Home was built in Normal, Illinois, in 1867 (see figure 4.1).[18]

Bickerdyke played a direct role in the initial fundraising efforts for the Illinois Soldiers' Orphans' Home, petitioning for supplies on behalf of the state government. Her involvement in establishing the institution reflected her broader commitment to extended soldier care, which included their children. However, she did not adhere strictly to any singular institutional model. Despite her advocacy for the home, she frequently circumvented official proto-

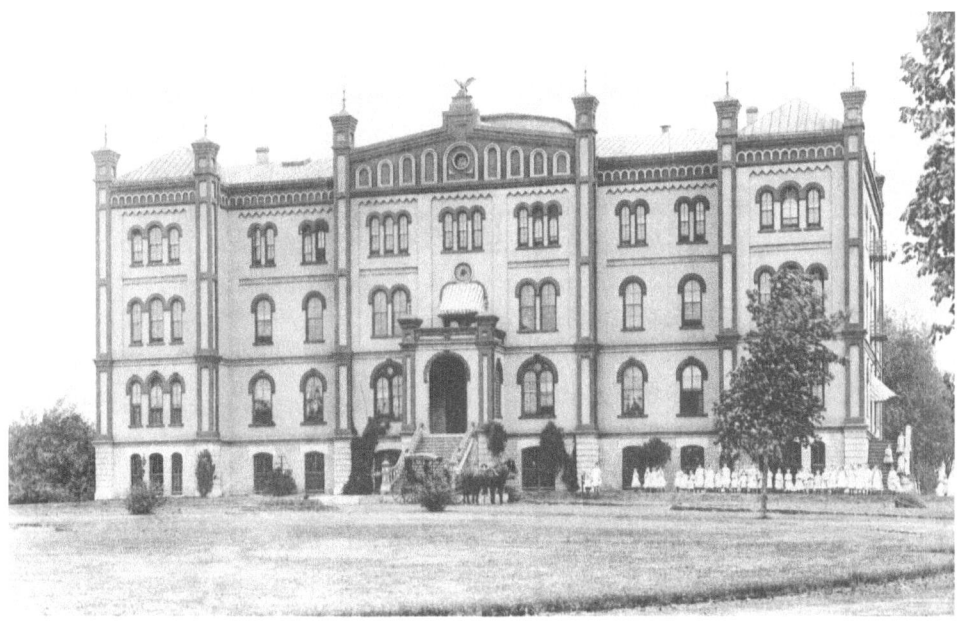

FIGURE 4.1  The Illinois Soldiers' Orphans' Building in Normal, Illinois, whose administrative offices opened in August 1867. "ISSCS-Buildings_00045A," photo collection box 1, folder 1. Courtesy of the McLean County Museum of History, Bloomington, Illinois.

cols, personally placing orphans with families through the "putting out" system when she believed it was in their best interest. She also inserted herself into traditionally male-dominated aspects of organizational development, influencing fundraising efforts, teacher and matron assignments, and even decisions about the home's location.

Publicly, the creation of the Illinois Soldiers' Orphans' Home was the province of powerful Illinois men eager to publicly demonstrate their dedication to fallen soldiers and their families. Even before the guns fell silent, state leaders began to anticipate the social and financial responsibilities that would accompany peace. As the Civil War was still being waged across the South, the Illinois General Assembly recommended a "tax for destitute families of soldiers, schools for soldier's [sic] orphans, and a state sanitary bureau" to prepare for the postwar reality in early 1865.[19] Governor Richard Yates entreated the state's citizens to support the measure and invoked their patriotism and collective obligation to the general welfare of their neighbors: "No State is worthy of its sovereignty, and no government the respect of its people, who will not protect and nurture the children of its soldiers.... Illinois! The first upon the roll of honor among all the States, shall she not be among the first to emblazen [sic] her proud historic record by setting apart a liberal and unfailing endowment for the support and education of the indigent orphans of the soldiers of the State?"[20] The home was proposed as a tangible expression of gratitude from the state to its citizens for their sacrificial service, but in an embarrassing outcome for the governor and the home's advocates, the initial tax measure did not pass. A private subscription plan was not sufficient to cover the high costs associated with construction of the building and the daily needs of inhabitants and employees.[21] As a result, the Illinois Soldiers' Orphans' Home was indefinitely stalled and exposed the tension between public ideals and practical commitment.

Mary Bickerdyke enthusiastically responded to the governor's call for fundraising help while she was still on the front. During General William Sherman's "March to the Sea," Bickerdyke found herself in the company of sympathetic Illinois soldiers and officers who enthusiastically contributed to the benefit of their fallen comrades' families. However, efforts to raise money as a current employee of the USSC represented a conflict of interest for the leaders of that organization. The USSC considered her actions a violation of competitive benevolence and discouraged localized fundraising or aid efforts that might interfere with their mission or otherwise cause confusion.[22] In the view of the USSC, a centralized, bureaucratic effort was the best and most efficient solution to soldier relief and aid, and its proponents rebuffed any state efforts to undermine the national project. The work of competing institutions exposed complicated expressions of allegiance, patriotism, and state versus national authority in the North during the Civil War.

When Bickerdyke's supervisors at the USSC caught wind of her fundraising efforts for the Illinois Soldiers' Orphans' Home, it was the final straw for her employment. E. B. McCagg, president of the Chicago branch of the USSC, had been suspicious of Bickerdyke's occasional rule-breaking escapades and voiced his complaints to her as well as his colleagues. News of her Illinois trip where she combined a personal furlough with a visit to the legislature and openly championed a bill to establish "an institution for the benefit of soldiers orphans," confirmed his suspicions that she had gone too far.[23] The frustration reached its peak when, upon her return to the field, she applied to the USSC for transportation with the intention to do USSC work, "but at the same time to solicit funds for the object indicated in her Bill."[24] The request crossed the line for McCagg. Her extra-institutional project embodied the "competitive benevolence" the USSC most feared, threatening its vision of centralized, controlled wartime charity. With a mixture of exasperation and moral indignation, he moved to end her service. McCagg rationalized his decision to fire her in cutting terms, spelling out the situation to the USSC Western Department secretary: "She is doubtless a capable and very efficient nurse in the extreme fronts but she is ignorant ... and untruthful and I could not consent so far as my consent was necessary that she should under any circumstances solicit contributions in money while acting as our servant."[25]

McCagg corroborated that the initial bill to the Illinois General Assembly to fund the state's home for soldiers' orphans was largely the result of Bickerdyke's advocacy and testimony. Her dismissal from the USSC did not deter her continued efforts; instead, it reaffirmed her belief that institutional bureaucracy should never stand in the way of urgent humanitarian work. Mary Bickerdyke spearheaded a guardianship movement in the state of Illinois just as other Civil War women in similar positions had done.[26] Providing a home for these children was a further extension of Bickerdyke's commitment to palliative care and support for Civil War soldiers and their families to mitigate the stinging consequences of wartime loss. In Bickerdyke's estimation, the project was too important and morally essential to her duty as a mother to abandon for the sake of an institution's rules. Without hesitation, Bickerdyke quietly accepted her discharge from the USSC and shifted her focus to other institutions that aligned more with her mission to ensure homes for soldiers' orphans in Illinois. Her dismissal vanished from the official histories of the Sanitary Commission, as if the institution preferred to forget the woman who defied its rules but carried its mission further than its bureaucracy allowed.

After her release from the USSC, Bickerdyke found that the United States Christian Commission was willing to sponsor her continued battlefield efforts and her simultaneous state fundraising activities. Her work with that organization lasted through the end of the war, after which she returned to Illinois and engaged in debates about the implementation of the orphans' home. In September 1865, a Springfield newspaper noted that "Mrs. M.J. Bickerdike [sic], who was present, stated that the Christian Commission had authorized her to offer the 'Home,' sanitary stores, cooking ranges, and other articles to the value of $1,500, and that the goods were already on the way to this city."[27] The public announcement of her donation underscored her ability to needle multiple institutional affiliations to achieve local humanitarian goals, demonstrating how her personal credibility and moral authority often outpaced formal organizational structures. Bickerdyke's persistent work and cross-institutional solutions helped to bring the Illinois Soldiers' Orphans' Home to fruition.

Mary Bickerdyke occupied a unique role in the organization's funding efforts, and her position superseded the more typical county agent tasked with canvasing citizens for donations. Illinois Governor Richard Oglesby and the former governor, Richard Yates, wrote letters of introduction for Bickerdyke as she worked to convert United States Army and Christian Commission wartime properties to potential sites for the home. The state officials addressed the sitting president of the United States and the secretary of war while Bickerdyke traveled to Washington, DC, to convince ranking men of the government to issue orders to convert "all the public property of the Government now in use or which have been in use in this state for hospital purposes, temporary Barracks, etc during the War."[28]

While in Washington, Bickerdyke petitioned the quartermaster and surgeon general for surplus war supplies that could be allocated to the Illinois Soldiers' Orphans' Home.[29] After appraising the men of her general mission, she asked for authorization to procure "teams to farm one thousand acres of land as follows: (12) twelve Horses, and (12) twelve mules, and (6) six wagons" and "Bedding sufficient to furnish beds of three thousand persons ... Towels, Ranges, Cooking Stoves and Kitchen furniture for three thousand inmates."[30] Bickerdyke found assets that were readily available for repurposing, which resulted in money saved for the state. Bickerdyke's request was enormous, but her goal was to provide long-term resources for an institution that would function properly as a home where the inhabitants were not confined as inmates. Instead, it would furnish children in need of sustenance, training, and the comforts of a home environment. The board and Bickerdyke eyed Normal, Illinois, as the site for the institution's campus and accompanying food sources, which could occupy a large plot of land on the west side of town.[31] Because of successful organization and campaigning for donations, the Illinois Soldiers' Orphans' Home was built in Normal in 1867. As soon as the first buildings opened, applications poured in from across the state, prompting the organization to establish a branch home in Springfield for the overflow of residents while the main campus was still under construction.[32]

Hundreds of Illinois families anxiously awaited and relied on the organization's inauguration. Between the institution's incorporation in February 1865 and its first official placement in August 1867, Mary Bickerdyke was acutely aware that the delayed opening created a gap in care. She received letters from friends across the state who expressed the urgent need for indigent children to be placed in an environment with a compassionate guardian while they waited for admission to the home. During that interim, Bickerdyke researched the placing-out system, also known as the family system.[33] This practice of placing children in the homes of caring families, where they would be raised to adulthood, was at least perceived as "respectable in its intent and motivation" and appeared to the general public to be an amenable solution to the growing problem of urban poor and soldiers' orphans, especially those who could not wait for the state to iron out its system.[34]

Yet the family system carried profound risks. Indentures through the placing-out system lacked accountability and vetting, which sometimes led to abusive situations and produced outcomes that were the opposite of what its proponents desired.[35] Bickerdyke deemed the family system a worthy alternative to the unpredictable wait caused by the red tape that blocked families from benefiting from the Illinois Soldiers' Orphans' Home project. Working in concert with friends she met both during the war and during her employment with the Home for the Friendless in Chicago, Bickerdyke helped coordinate the placement of several orphans and spent considerable effort ensuring that their assignments were hospitable, humane, and industrious.[36]

Her brief tenure as an advocate and fundraising agent for the Illinois Soldiers' Orphans' Home proved to be similar to many of her other institutional entanglements during her professional years. Bickerdyke used and supported the organization to the extent that it allowed her to pursue her solutions for the long-term care of Civil War patients and, in this case, for deceased soldiers and their families. The home's operations proceeded without her direct involvement, but its success was predicated on its foundational mission to honor the Union army's fallen soldiers from Illinois and provide support and welfare to their surviving kin. Powerful men in state and national governments trusted Bickerdyke's judgment to provide competent care solutions based on her maternal authority. When she moved from Illinois to Kansas, her institutional allegiances shifted once again, and Bickerdyke dedicated new efforts to the successful commissioning of a veteran's colony in Salina, Kansas.

## Go West, Young Man . . . and Follow Mother

Any modern traveler might recognize Salina, Kansas, as a small but necessary pit stop before the long, flat, and sparsely populated drive on Interstate 70 toward Colorado. In the late 1860s, the small but growing town served as a junction for rail lines coming west from Topeka and south toward Wichita, fulfilling a similar pit stop function. A booster advertisement promised that

"Salina and Saline County have a present prosperity greater, and a future prospect brighter than any other part of the State—than any other part of the great west, even.... Those who come here, and make the proper effort, *all thrive*."[37] The promise, of course, was impossible to keep, but it drove many Civil War veterans and some families to settle there in the late 1860s. The allure of the West did not always result in newfound riches or the establishment of the mythical independence associated with the frontier. Westward settlement was an attractive option to many Civil War veterans and their families who believed that a new start might allow for peaceful labor and the opportunity to acquire property after the tumultuous years of enlistment.

Bickerdyke moved to Salina to test new modes of economic independence, setting her sights on a temperance hotel, an establishment that aligned with her vision of providing both moral and physical sustenance to travelers and locals. This endeavor reflected what historian Lindsey Peterson has termed "paragons of permanency and order," as Union veterans sought to stabilize frontier communities by promoting institutions that reinforced free labor ideals and respectable domesticity.[38] Bickerdyke strategically positioned herself within this effort, leveraging her wartime reputation to secure business partnerships. She corresponded with the president of the Chicago, Burlington, and Quincy (CB&Q) Railroad to establish her business location and procure free transportation for soldiers and their families relocating to Salina. Another investor loaned $10,000 to Mrs. Bickerdyke "for the use of the veterans who would come West under her chaperonage."[39] Her "chaperonage," more functionally a maternal guardianship, provided moral safeguards against the unknown of the West. Bickerdyke advertised financial assistance to Civil War veterans interested in resettlement in Salina.[40] Beyond running a business, Bickerdyke's efforts aligned with a broader national narrative in which Union veterans positioned themselves as the rightful architects of western settlement, framing their migration as a continuation of the Civil War's mission. By advertising financial assistance for veterans interested in resettlement, she played an active role in this process, facilitating westward migration while reinforcing the notion that veterans and their families deserved priority in claiming new opportunities. Applicants from as far away as Massachusetts asked Bickerdyke for transportation funds for their families and for furnished goods.[41]

As she ventured toward Kansas, her sons were under the care of Mrs. Laura A. Hayward in Beloit, Wisconsin. Mrs. Hayward conveyed James's and her own disappointment at Bickerdyke's prolonged six-month absence.[42] In a moment of candor, Hayward acerbically wrote, "Now I know very well you have your *hands, head* and *heart* ful [sic] with your children in Chicago but you realize you have two children here who are *ragged* and *destitute* of many things, who have been looking for something from you these many days, as it was with such a *promise* you left us."[43] Hayward's letter was followed by a scrawled note from James on the back: "I hope you will attend to our wants and Mrs. H. before you attend to any body else."[44] James, who had been without his mother for years, knew that she still had a material duty to provide him with the bare minimum essentials of daily life. Even more, he articulated a clear sense that his own needs and desires were—or at least should have been—subservient to those of the other sons and children whom his mother attended.

It is apparent from multiple letters that Bickerdyke did not provide reliable payments to Hayward, which prompted James to feel "very anxious about the money affair."[45] Besides the stress caused by a lack of money, James resented learning more about his mother's activities from public discourse than from her directly. "I hear in the Papers that 'Mother Bickerdyke' has left Chicago for Kansas. I hope I shall have the chance to follow if that is the case," he wrote incredulously.[46] James's letters, written by a teenager full of earnest expressions of love and homesickness, call into question the nobility of Bickerdyke's care-switching ventures. They reveal the complexity of her fluctuating motherhoods as the human toll of her decisions became increasingly apparent. Despite the protests from her sons and their caregiver, Mother Bickerdyke's Kansas project pressed forward.

By 1870, a large contingent of single working-age men and young families had moved to Salina. Through her influence and advice, as many as "three hundred families" settled in central Kansas between 1867 and 1869.[47] This estimate, though inflated compared to reality, brought attention and credit to Bickerdyke's advisory role in the town's migration boom. One former patient wrote to Bickerdyke in 1868 and requested guidance from the trusted Mother Bickerdyke. He explained, "My object in writing to you is to ascertain something about the Country in which you reside. I have some Idea of going to Kansas and would prefer going where I know some person. I saw your name in print in the Union Pacific R.R. Guide. I am glad to hear that Temperance Hotels are taking the place of Rum Mills in the West. Please send me one of your town papers if you have any."[48] Already motivated to move west for new opportunities, veterans were reassured to know they might be met by likeminded individuals whose reputations for strong morality preceded them. In the potentially chaotic environments of the "Wild West," potential inhabitants sought a sense of familiarity and decorum in their desired locale. If "Mother" thought the place fitting for a soldier's homestead, then it must be.

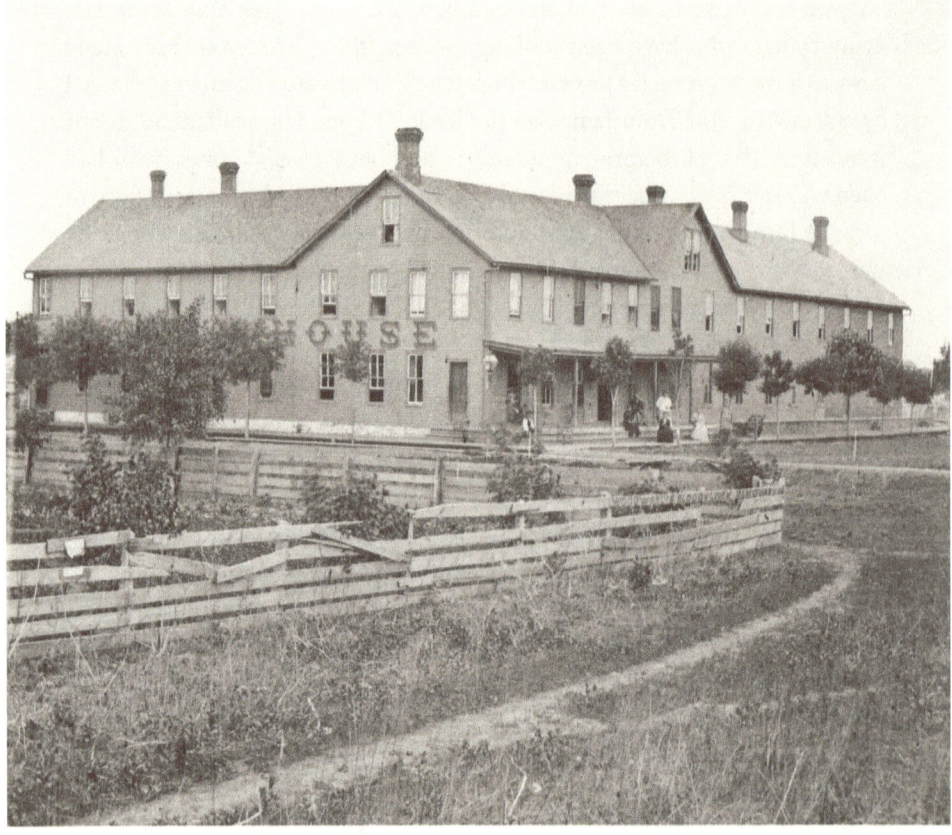

FIGURE 4.2 Bickerdyke Hotel in Salina, Kansas, stereograph. The hotel had changed ownership by the time the photo was taken in 1879. Courtesy of the Kansas State Historical Society.

Once Bickerdyke established her temperance hotel at the railroad junction, she set up the business to accommodate weary travelers, simultaneously engaging in "missionary work" (see figure 4.2).[49] In establishing a temperance hotel, Bickerdyke aligned herself with the growing temperance movement's reformist aims to create non alcohol-free environments and a moral refuge designed to counteract the perceived dangers of saloons, transient male labor, and frontier disorder. While her hotel was in operation, she housed famous guests such as Susan B. Anthony, who commented that Bickerdyke's hotel was a welcome respite with a "clean, sweet room and uninhabited bed."[50] In addition to the hotel, Bickerdyke positioned herself within the community to provide moral guardianship to the hundreds of impressionable young men who sought work and a home in Salina. The American Tract

Society of Chicago sent her monthly religious pamphlets, "papers, little books, tracts, etc" to distribute to guests and veteran migrants in her Salina hotel.[51] She created a suitable home atmosphere in the developing town and used the relational equity she had established to provide moral and spiritual influence, instruction, and help in the process of building a reputable and upstanding community. The potentially rowdy town of independent-minded men looked to Mother Bickerdyke for spiritual guidance, maternal care, and the warm meals that she provided.

Bickerdyke helped to organize community aid in Salina after the "Indian raids of 1868" disrupted the White emigrants who presumed ownership of Indigenous lands in Kansas through their settlement. With the development of Salina as a Western settlement, the local Cheyenne and Arapahoe were forcefully displaced from their hunting grounds and became frustrated with the dishonest and objectively unfair trade deals proposed by the new inhabitants of their ancestral lands. In August 1868, as a result of that irritation, a small band of Cheyenne attacked a group of settlers, causing some White settlers in Salina and surrounding communities to respond with both fear and retaliation. One member of local settler law enforcement spurred a generalized panic among the citizenry when he "returned to Salina believing that the entire Cheyenne Tribe was then at his heels."[52] The situation instigated periodic raids and retaliatory attacks on Salina citizens and their new community in the fall of 1868. In the final account, only fifteen to twenty Cheyenne men were involved in the initial raid that resulted in the displacement and unnecessary destitution of up to 1,400 White settlers by January 1869.[53]

The local government was forced to issue rations to the leaders of Saline County to feed its many citizens in sudden need. Due to mismanagement and waste, authorities squandered the supplies, leaving Salinians in dire conditions, with some nearing starvation. Observing the inappropriate prosecution of aid distribution, Mother Bickerdyke intervened in the impending local disaster and earnestly requested more rations and blankets from the US War Department in November 1868.[54] Soon after, General George Armstrong Custer, General William Tecumseh Sherman, and other Fort Leavenworth officers traveled to Bickerdyke's hotel to have dinner and discuss plans to protect the settlers from further disturbances.[55] She hosted the men at her temperance hotel, and the setting facilitated collaboration between a civilian reformer and top military leaders, signaling the urgency of the crisis and the respect Bickerdyke commanded across social spheres. Sherman and Grant ultimately acquiesced and provided the needed personnel for security and funds for more supplies. Newspapers praised Bickerdyke's maternal guardianship and productive concern for her community, publicly congratulating her on her efforts to protect and provide: "She deserves much credit for the prompt, persistent, and never can-be-put-off manner in which she captured and enlisted the sympathies of the 'powers that be.'"[56] Bickerdyke would not allow continued mismanagement to devastate the people she had helped convince to relocate their livelihoods to Kansas. She assumed personal responsibility for the continued well-being of her soldiers and the place that they now called home.

After her aid work was affected by the growing Kansas veteran community, Bickerdyke's reputation continued to be bolstered by national newspaper coverage of her wartime maternal efficacy. In Chicago, her former colleague Mary Livermore became publisher of a newspaper, *The Agitator*, whose byline often read: "Healthy agitation precedes all true reform."[57] Grounded in the egalitarian framework of the Universalist denomination, Livermore drew on her professionalism to stand firm in her activism for women's rights during the Civil War.[58] In 1869, Livermore published several stories that began to feature Bickerdyke's wartime heroism and peculiar style. The anecdotes eventually found their way into Livermore's memoirs, but the initial newspaper stories had the effect of embedding ideas about Mother Bickerdyke into the popular consciousness.

At least one hundred newspapers across the country reprinted stories touting "The Heroine of Hospitals: Mother Bickerdyke." Several episodes from the war were shared, but as in this one, Livermore continued to shape the public perception of Bickerdyke as a woman undeterred by even the most extreme challenges. Livermore's circulated story described Bickerdyke as a "titan" and "indefatigable," highlighting her efforts in terms that underscored both her superhuman resolve and her deeply personal connection to the men under her care. These soldiers, Livermore wrote, could speak of her only "with tears and benedictions," a sentiment that further solidified her reputation as a singular maternal force in the war's aftermath.[59] Her persistent presence in popular media allowed her to maintain influence in postwar veteran communities, reinforcing the idea that her maternal guardianship had not ended with the war but had simply evolved to meet the needs of aging soldiers and their families. The ongoing public retelling of her exploits strengthened her authority, allowing her to care-switch seamlessly from wartime nurse to postwar advocate, using her well-established identity to rally support for veterans' aid, pensions, and institutional reforms.

Years after the "Indian raids," the Kansas frontier was struck by another disaster that required large-scale aid. In the mid-1870s, the Kansas grasshopper plagues ravaged the plains. At its broadest extent, the plague engulfed nearly one-quarter of the North American continent. It consumed an area extending from the Rocky Mountains to the Mississippi River and from 200 miles north of the Canadian border to northern Texas. The plague was perhaps the single most serious sustained environmental crisis in Great Plains agriculture during the nineteenth century.[60] Like the raids that preceded it, the plague forced Western settlers to evaluate and recalculate the extent to which both state and local governments were obligated to relieve their citizens in times of disaster. For those left in desperate need, figures like Bickerdyke emerged to meet the emergency, shifting seamlessly between institutional advocacy and direct aid, embodying the roles of both maternal guardian and pragmatic problem-solver. Her ability to care-switch allowed her to step into the void left by ineffective government responses, ensuring that those who were most vulnerable were not forgotten.

Kansans described in haunting detail the effects of the grasshopper plague. One woman standing at her front door "found the air filled with whizzing grasshoppers, producing as they struck the side of the house, or fell in the drying corn field nearby the noise we had heard."[61] She went on:

> The blue sky turned black at midday as the full-grown insects, at once began to devour every green thing left growing at that time of year. The cabbages were gnawed clean down to the roots. Red peppers did not phase them, leaves as well as green and ripe peppers seeming a favorite relish. The sweet potato vines vanished. They ate the tomato leaves, but only nibbled at the fruit. After eating all the green things the females began depositing their eggs in the paths, roads and in the firmer portions of the fields, drilling little holes to the depth of an inch or more, and filling them with little sacks of eggs. These holes honeycombed the ground, the grasshoppers working away so closely that it was difficult to walk in the paths without crushing several at every step.[62]

The cycle of devastation repeated itself: attack, egg-laying, hatching, and another wave of attack, leaving crops in ruins. Desperate farmers dug trenches and deep post holes, forcing the wingless nymph-stage grasshoppers to fall into them and die before they could mature and take flight to destroy more food.[63] Despite their relentless efforts, the insects' sheer numbers overwhelmed many, turning vast stretches of farmland into wastelands.

The plague robbed families of their stored and incoming winter's food and demoralized farmers who had spent years attempting to create arable farmland in the harsh prairie environment. Affected Christians were convinced that some sort of apocalyptic judgment had been cast upon their land, punishing them for some undisclosed sin. The secretary of the State Board of Agriculture wrote to the Kansas governor to report that the grasshoppers had left at least twenty-six counties "absolutely unable to provide for their own destitute" and that, out of a total population of 66,104, at least 12,089 were destitute.[64] With entire communities on the brink of starvation and no means of recovery, the crisis forced the government to step in as a benevolent protector and as the last hope for survival.

The catastrophe caught the attention of reformers in Kansas as well as those across the country. Among others, Mary Bickerdyke advocated for an interdependent, community-centered political intervention to provide relief. In Great Bend, Kansas, she had contemplated establishing a farming homestead with her two sons, but the plague disrupted her family's plan to finally settle together as James started his teaching career. This pestilence, "worse than [the] Egyptian plague," afflicted her potential home and caused her to seek direct aid for that community. Nevertheless, the newspaper lauded her efforts as "philanthropist personified" as she arrived with two carloads of food and clothing with "three car loads more" on the way. Perhaps even more important than this benevolence was her direct involvement as she distributed the aid: "A committee is appointed who report to Mother Bickerdyke and her assistants the needs of the applicant whereupon Mother B, if satisfied that the parties applying for aid are really worthy, directs to have their wants supplied."[65] Other newspapers across Kansas applauded the continuation of her efforts: "In the list of names who the love of God has bless'd, Mother Bickerdyke's will not be far from the top."[66] Despite new crises, she remained the steadfast force that communities turned to for stability, guidance, and protection. Her response to the disaster reaffirmed that her guardianship extended beyond the Civil War—she continued to embody a living, breathing institution of care, stepping in where government aid faltered and ensuring that no one under her watch was left behind.

Because Bickerdyke developed associations with railroad magnates during her Civil War service when she assisted with the transportation of war materials, she was able to translate those relationships to relief for Kansas citizens. Bickerdyke arranged for approximately 200 railroad carloads of supplies to be shipped to Kansas, attempting to restore that which the plague of grasshoppers had stolen. In McDonogh County in western Illinois, Bickerdyke worked with the mayor of its county seat, Macomb, to collect supplies for plague relief. She looked to allocate the abundance of Illinois to the scarcity in Kansas, urging Illinois to exercise "the best qualities of human nature—Sympathy and Charity."[67]

With her insistence, the supplies were distributed under Bickerdyke's personal supervision alongside other institutional and governmental measures also meant to provide aid. Bickerdyke, while relying on the railroads and government for supply provision, felt that she alone was best suited to manage the distribution to those most deserving of relief.[68] The charity that Bickerdyke best understood and advocated, in concert with local governments and institutions as necessary, relied on the goodwill and moral aptitude of private citizens who acted out of their Christian duty as fellow citizens.

Bickerdyke's interventions during times of crisis showcased her ability to mobilize resources and advocate for government assistance when communities faced dire circumstances. Her actions underscored the importance of interdependent, community-centered approaches to relief efforts and the vital role of private citizens in providing aid and support. In the first decade after the war, Bickerdyke remained a visible force in the public arena, and her endeavors underscored the social and political need for the professional skills that women had cultivated during the Civil War.

The events described in this chapter highlight Bickerdyke's dedication to the well-being of veterans and their families; they also demonstrate the development of her social capital and influence. Her successful advocacy for the Illinois Soldiers' Orphans' Home, her ability to attract settlers to Salina, and her effective mobilization of resources during times of crisis all served to enhance her reputation as a respected leader and maternal figure forged by her wartime experience. As a result, Bickerdyke's sphere of influence expanded, allowing her to make an even greater impact on the lives of those she sought to support.

Mary Bickerdyke's experiences as a mother-guardian in the post–Civil War era informed her continued work as a nurse and advocate. As the nation entered a new phase of growth and development, Bickerdyke's commitment to providing care and support to those in need would lead her to take on new challenges and adapt her approach to the evolving demands of veterans.

CHAPTER FIVE

# Mother-Nurse
## Care-Switching Between Private and Public Motherhood

Bickerdyke's public career did not end with the Civil War. Buoyed by the widespread admiration she had earned for her tireless devotion to soldiers, she entered the postwar years determined to translate her wartime authority into new professional opportunities. The steady employment and income she secured during the conflict had given her both practical experience and financial independence, enabling her to support her children. Yet the end of the war also forced a reckoning: the hospitals had closed, the army had disbanded, and the work that had defined her public identity was no longer available. Rather than retreat into private life, Bickerdyke adapted to extend her maternal persona, which had been cultivated in the hospitals, into emerging arenas of postwar need, focusing especially on the welfare of veterans and their families. At the same time, she redirected some of her energy toward the domestic responsibilities that had long been eclipsed by her wartime service. In doing so, she carved out a distinctive postwar path, one that blurred the boundaries between public service and private duty, and allowed her to remain a visible and influential figure well into the 1870s. Bickerdyke's postwar career exemplified her ability to care-switch, navigating between institutional caregiving, entrepreneurial ventures, and deeply personal nursing roles. No longer employed within the structure of war, she sought new avenues to provide structure and stability to the men she had once nursed, following them westward as they rebuilt their lives. Recognizing the railroad's expansion into Kansas as an opportunity, she leveraged her reputation and soldier loyalty to recruit veterans and their families to resettle in Salina, where she envisioned a community anchored in moral and economic support.[1] That Kansas venture morphed into other opportunities where Bickerdyke spent time as a private nurse to veterans in the West. And then in the mid-1880s, Bickerdyke was thrust once more into the private sphere of caregiving and provided palliative care for her stepdaughter in her final days. In engaging with this traditional domestic care, she briefly restored the home circle she had left behind during the war, returning to the intimate responsibilities of mothering through end-of-life care.

These varied efforts were not solely about settlement or survival; they were about sustaining the multiple meanings of motherhood she had cultivated during the war while also reaffirming her role in private, familial care. In Salina, the temperance hotel provided weary travelers with shelter, but more importantly, it extended her moral guardianship over a frontier town in need of order and care. In cultivating her private motherhood, she attended to her stepdaughter's final days and demonstrated how caregiving transcended institutional settings and included deeply personal acts of care. Through these experiences, Bickerdyke continued to redefine maternal authority, proving that her wartime mission had not ended with the last battle but had evolved, moving fluidly between public duty and private responsibility, and between the care of soldiers and the care of family.

## Working it Out: Independent Employment after the War

In the years immediately following the American Civil War, Mary Bickerdyke made several attempts to apply her skills to institutional efforts that provided relief to suffering men and women.[2] She aided in the establishment of the Illinois Soldiers' Orphans' Home in Springfield, participated in the moralizing work and mission of the Home for the Friendless in Chicago, and attempted to coordinate and rally state and national relief for Kansans during the Indian raids of 1868. In each of those instances, she operated alongside these various institutions, as she had during the Civil War under the United States Sanitary Commission (USSC). But as was the case during her employment with the USSC, Mary Bickerdyke struggled to adapt to the restrictions imposed on her by the ranking men in each respective organization. These frustrations revealed the widening gap between Bickerdyke's sense of efficacy, which was grounded in direct, maternal authority, and the bureaucratic frameworks that increasingly governed charitable and medical work in the postwar era. To manage this internal conflict, Bickerdyke became adept at care-switching. She recognized the developing norms of professionalized nursing and yet still functioned outside those norms when she felt her maternal training was better suited. She operated as a private nurse on her own terms, dictating her own conditions of employment and implementing her maternal medical competence outside the constricting standards of the evolving medical profession.

As Bickerdyke transitioned into postwar life, she needed to employ new strategies to sustain herself financially while maintaining the authority she had built as Mother Bickerdyke. No longer drawing a salary from institutional caregiving, she sought to leverage her wartime reputation to carve out an independent role in the expanding frontier economy. Her efforts in Salina reflected a bold attempt to merge economic self-sufficiency with her established identity as a maternal figure, positioning herself as both a business owner and a guardian of the community. Newspapers as far east as Vermont recognized the boldness of Bickerdyke's plans at Salina, with some even framing her efforts as revolutionary: "Mrs. Bickerdyke, who followed Sherman through his entire campaign, taking care of sick soldiers, has built a large hotel at Salina, Kansas, which she intends to manage entirely herself. If women are to have a place in this world they must get right out of the old grooves and do new and grand things. We have looked through the eye of a needle long enough. It is time for 'The Revolution.'"[3] The press coverage acknowledged her ambition and tied her work to broader movements that advocated for expanded roles for women in society. By managing her own hotel, Bickerdyke asserted a form of sovereignty, creating a space where she could continue to exercise authority over health and care outside traditional institutions. Her efforts signaled that caregiving could be both a public service and a means of personal agency, challenging conventional ideas about women's economic and professional limitations.

In 1870, she received a letter from the esteemed Henry W. Bellows, formerly the president of the USSC (see figure 5.1). Bellows wrote in response to a business proposal that Mary Bickerdyke had sent to the prominent clergyman and lecturer. While the specific details of Bickerdyke's potential venture remain a mystery, Bellows's response to her plan revealed, in plain language, the difficulties women faced when wishing to undertake their own professional endeavors in fields of work that had been considered the province of men.[4] "My dear Mrs. Bickerdyke," the letter began. "This is a beautiful plan—not only on paper, but in conception. It might be carried out, but it probably will not be."[5]

Bellows went on to enumerate the reasons that he thought Bickerdyke's plan would be unsuccessful, which boiled down to this: (1) You need a man of character to guide the enterprise. (2) You need more money, and probably a "judicious man" to lead in finding that capital. (3) You, Mrs. Bickerdyke, are not a man.[6] Bellows's evaluation and rejection of her proposal was anything but subtle. Like many men of his generation and upper-class station, he thought that "women are too good and kind, (when they are good and kind at all) to be prudent, judicious, foreseeing and to earn the confidence of capitalists."[7] And though Bellows believed in Bickerdyke's "devotion, humanity, and earnestness," he also believed that "we all have our sphere—you, yours and I mine."[8] For Mary Bickerdyke and other enterprising women in her generation, owning and operating a business, no matter how brilliant the business might be or how much good it might accomplish, would mean that she was occupying space outside her designated sphere.

*Mother-Nurse* 115

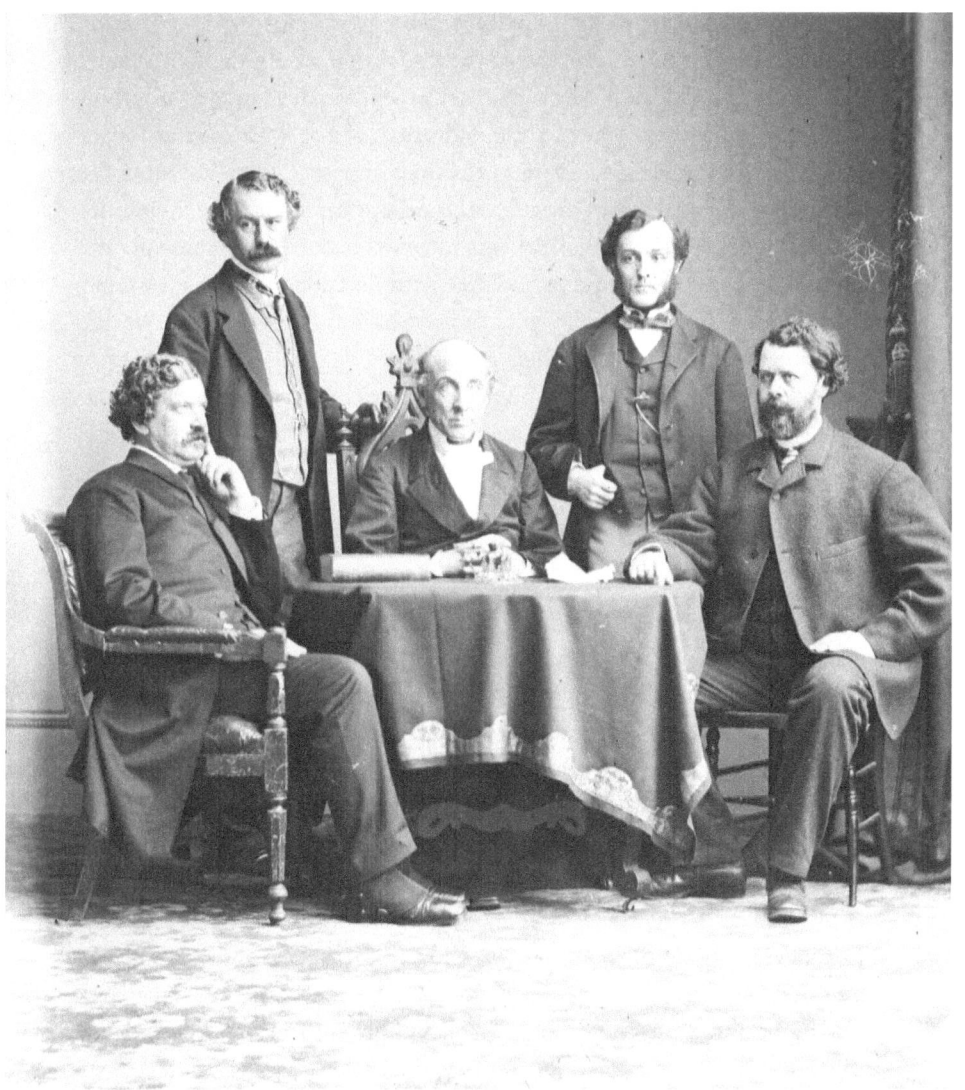

FIGURE 5.1 Leading organizers of the United States Sanitary Commission. The commission's president, Henry Bellows, is seated at the center. Notably, they were all affluent men. Photograph taken by Mathew Brady. Courtesy of the Library of Congress.

Mary Bickerdyke's resistance to nineteenth-century institutional norms stemmed from more than her rejection based on gender but also from her deliberate challenge to bureaucratic constraints, as she embraced a rogue pragmatism to cut through red tape and prioritize direct aid to those in need.[9] The considerations of how to operate as a professional in a highly restrictive and culturally determined workplace prompted women with specialized skills to employ creative solutions so they might engage in their chosen occupation. During the Civil War, nurses eschewed "medical models of professionalism [as] a protest against male authority... that flourished as long as nursing was in its transitional, preprofessional phase."[10] The attempts that they made to operate within the rules of the game and to initiate their entrepreneurial skills were, like Bickerdyke's business plan in 1870, generally met with little to no support, and sometimes with derision. This was especially true for women like Bickerdyke who did not have the privilege of a wealthy benefactor or relative to fund their pursuits.[11] The limitations imposed on Bickerdyke and other skilled but poor women of the late nineteenth century helped shape occupational decisions that sidestepped the gendered restrictions of institutions. For Bickerdyke, this meant venturing into private employment in areas that were obviously in need of skilled medical laborers. Outside the purview of men who held strong opinions about women's abilities as masters of their own labor and skill deployment, women could operate more freely, implementing their skills as they saw fit in privately arranged situations.

Bickerdyke did not attempt to do everything entirely on her own and recognized that her efforts to provide moral guardianship as "Mother" to veterans was a tall task. Early in the Salina experiment, Bickerdyke attempted to recruit an administrative assistant and asked for a recommendation from Reverend George Duffield, a citizen of Galesburg, Illinois—her hometown—and a member of the American Bible Society. Duffield vetted a willing prospect to serve Bickerdyke as a "helper," as well as a "teacher, amanuensis, and adjutant generally," in the management and administration of the Salina project.[12] The candidate was a young woman whose merits were compared to those of the most esteemed ladies in Galesburg and other Knox College graduates who possessed natural abilities and strong character suited to the task. By the late 1860s when Bickerdyke made the request, Knox College was considering combining its separate women's college with the main campus. The prospect of having an educated and organized helper to allow Bickerdyke to continue with her ever-widening enterprises must have promoted a great deal of hope and pride in Bickerdyke, whose Civil War accomplishments and honor had afforded her such an esteemed luxury.

The young woman corresponded briefly with Bickerdyke, and they negotiated finances and opportunity costs. The potential amanuensis anticipated the "noble and useful life" that she might have under Bickerdyke's employ in Kansas.[13] The potential ghostwriter was familiar with Bickerdyke's professional missions, and the letter indicates Bickerdyke's respectability in the community. Unfortunately for Mary Bickerdyke, the arrangement fell through, and she was forced to take on her own secretarial responsibilities after quickly giving up the search.[14] Bickerdyke missed the opportunity to have a helper, and within the first few years of her time in Salina, her business plans failed. She had hosted famous Americans from across the country who stayed at her hotel and gave rave reviews, but she was ultimately forced to transfer ownership to another Salina businessman.[15] Though Bickerdyke had struck out independently on a business venture and convinced families to move across the country to join her, the administrative aspects of her labors suffered. Her lack of literacy and amateur business skills caused her hotel to slowly lose profits.

After leaving Salina, Bickerdyke moved frequently, taking on various benevolent endeavors and odd jobs. While the press occasionally revisited her wartime heroics, she largely operated outside the public eye—though not necessarily by choice. Rather, she was navigating the difficulties of reasserting her authority in a world that no longer revolved around battlefield caregiving. Without the institutional structure of war to legitimize her role, she relied on personal connections and her reputation to maintain influence. In several instances, she solicited her sons to handle her "clerical work" when she engaged in larger and more public-facing tasks.[16] When Kansas citizens called on her for aid, Bickerdyke answered, mobilizing relief efforts with the same urgency she had once brought to military hospitals. During the Kansas grasshopper plague of 1875–76, for example, Hiram accompanied his mother and handled correspondence when she took her aid campaign to Washington, DC. She spent a few months petitioning for donations, meeting with acquaintances from the Civil War and utilizing her name recognition to gain an audience with those she had not met during the war, such as famed nurse and reformer Dorothea Dix. As she wrote to prominent figures like President Ulysses S. Grant, she enlisted trusted representatives to advocate on her behalf, ensuring her voice remained present in the corridors of power even when she lacked direct access. In this postwar landscape, she was not fading into obscurity. Rather, she was actively adapting, finding new ways to assert authority and wield influence in a shifting system of care.

Around the time of his mother's trip to advocate for Kansas aid during the grasshopper plague, James dictated a letter that was signed with his mother's name.[17] Out of the many letters in her archive, this is one of very few that expresses a candid and strong political stance. In the letter, J. R., signing under his mother's name, chastised Kansas legislators for their failure to act on behalf of Kansas citizens suffering from privation. The letter calls out the "rascality" of the senators' behavior, calling them "nothing but Skalewags [sic] and Office Seeking Speculators [sic] who live upon offul [sic] and should be exposed."[18] The severity of this language was entirely uncharacteristic of Bickerdyke. Though pragmatic and frank, she deliberately maintained a tone befitting a respected maternal figure in other correspondence, avoiding inflammatory rhetoric that might jeopardize her credibility. This departure in tone reveals that she did not always exert strict control over ghostwritten correspondence. If those she enlisted to help her fell within her trusted circle, like her son in this instance, they had some flexibility to insert their own interpretations of Mother Bickerdyke's words and sentiments. J. R.'s demand for public excoriation of Kansas senators in the *Chicago Tribune* did not align with his mother's approach to the government's failure to act. Within this letter, it is more plausible that the harsh language reflects J. R.'s feelings and not his mother's.

The day after that scathing letter was drafted, Mary Bickerdyke wrote a note in her own hand in response to a Kansas sufferer. While she maintained her disappointment in the state's representatives, her critique was tempered by empathy and a focus on direct relief. Writing with characteristic compassion, she reassured the recipient of her concern for their family's well-being and expressed hope that aid would soon arrive from alternative sources. She promised assistance and noted that she had recommended the family's case "to Barton County.... [T]hey will probably be up sometime next week. They have a great many [delicacies] such as fruit Pork."[19] At the end of the letter, Mother Bickerdyke mirrored J. R.'s observation that the state government was neglecting its responsibility to aid its own citizens. She wrote, "The corn was entirely destroyed by grasshoppers so far the Legesaturr [sic] of Kansas has done nothing for her people and something must be done as quick as possible."[20] Though both letters addressed the same crisis, their starkly different tones underscore the importance of determining authorship and perspective in Bickerdyke's archive. While J. R.'s version leaned into public condemnation, Bickerdyke's own response focused on immediate, actionable solutions, demonstrating her commitment to a multi-institutional relief effort rather than political reproach. This contrast reveals the complexities of using ghostwriters in her advocacy and highlights how her authority was sometimes mediated, if not outright reshaped, by those who wrote on her behalf.

Mary Bickerdyke's case represents that amanuenses were often employed because of the author's illiteracy and lower education. The ghostwriter, whomever it might be, allowed Bickerdyke to maintain a steady stream of correspondence as she tried to keep up with relief projects. Her aim was to find trusted men and women to represent the respectability that she worked toward in her postwar professional endeavors. Through her adherence to middle-class norms like robust letter writing, Bickerdyke could establish a level of prestige that allowed her to continue her work. Without a ghostwriter, her productivity and the visibility of her contributions suffered. With a ghostwriter, as seen with J. R.'s letter, her work could be easily politicized and discounted as an inappropriate expression for a woman to take. Overall, representing herself and building professional opportunities after the war involved risk, as reliance on ghostwriters simultaneously enabled Bickerdyke to meet middle-class expectations of prolific correspondence and sustain her relief work, while also exposing her growing reputation to distortions of tone and authority that could complicate how her efforts were received.

## Postbellum Private Nursing and the Long Transition of Medical Sovereignty

Throughout her postwar career, Bickerdyke deliberately pursued a professional path that allowed her to apply her expertise in palliative care, offering long-term support to terminally ill patients in private settings. Unlike the emerging hospital-trained nurses of the 1870s and 1880s, whose roles were increasingly defined by hierarchy, discipline, and institutional subordination, Bickerdyke continued the Civil War–era model of relational, maternal-based care.[21] She extended the values of the "maternal and comforting presence" that had at least neutralized the austere hospital environments of the Civil War and continued to apply the "language and actuality of fictive kinship," which provided familiarity and security to patients undergoing medical treatment or nearing death.[22] By working independently, she preserved her authority as a caregiver, free from the constraints of hospital protocols that prioritized obedience over individualized patient needs. This arrangement was especially crucial in regions lacking a robust medical infrastructure, where private nursing filled gaps in care.

The rise of professionalized nursing schools coincided with broader transformations in American health care, particularly in the treatment of terminally ill patients. Modern palliative care is often traced to the hospice movement of the 1970s, popularized by Elisabeth Kübler-Ross. Yet, its principles—relief of suffering, holistic support, and patient autonomy—are deeply rooted in nineteenth-century traditions.[23] Bickerdyke's work exemplifies this continuity, demonstrating how informal, experience-based caregiving persisted alongside the institutionalization of medicine. Her reputation reflected the public's enduring trust in traditional home-based care. As one contemporary observed, she was regarded as a "modern Madonna, the mother of man, the woman whose breast has pillowed more stricken heads and closed more dying eyes than any other in all the world, perhaps."[24] She was a maternal model whose compassionate presence eased the suffering of countless patients.

Despite these persistent traditions, the late nineteenth-century hospital environment increasingly mirrored the rigid structures of Civil War medical institutions, where nurses like Bickerdyke had once fought to humanize care. Death in hospitals became an impersonal process; doctors, lacking critical care protocols, often withdrew from terminal patients, relegating them to secluded wards where their decline would not challenge the institution's claims of medical progress.[25] Hospitals, seeking legitimacy in the eyes of a skeptical public, emphasized scientific efficacy over the relational aspects of caregiving, further marginalizing the role of private, home-based nurses.[26]

Bickerdyke resisted this shift, advocating for the compassionate end-of-life care that had defined her wartime nursing. Her approach was neither unskilled nor incidental—she operated as a palliative care clinician, not merely as a comforting presence. Her rejection of emerging medical hierarchies reflected a broader struggle between traditional community-based care and the professionalization of nursing. While the Civil War had normalized deaths outside the home, many Americans still preferred to spend their final moments under the care of familiar, trusted caregivers rather than in the increasingly clinical and impersonal confines of hospitals.[27] Mary Bickerdyke fulfilled that request and refused to compromise her values even after the war was over.[28]

Bickerdyke's work as a private nurse highlights her ability to navigate both institutionalized, empirical nursing practices and her preferred relational approach, which emphasized maternal medical competency. Her flexibility in adapting to different care settings demonstrates how nineteenth-century nursing remained in flux, shaped by competing models of professionalism and deeply ingrained expectations of women as caregivers. Unlike the 20,000 women who served in Civil War hospitals, the nurses trained in formal programs of the 1870s and 1880s followed a more standardized model.[29] For those who were not fit to operate as professional nurses after the war's conclusion, care-switching was necessary. Private nursing employment was not subject to the scrutiny of institutional protocol. Indeed, private nursing allowed Bickerdyke to implement palliative care practices that aligned with her values and the desires of patients who sought a "good death" under the attentive care of a maternal figure. Private nurses, then, addressed a gap in hospital care, and the dying became the province of untrained nurses and of mothers, who the nursing field had also spurned.

As formal nursing schools became more established in urban centers, uncredentialed yet highly experienced nurses like Bickerdyke found themselves in an ambiguous professional category. Older women, often widows, transitioned into private caregiving roles, drawing on decades of practical knowledge. In the western United States, where hospitals remained sparse, private nurses played a vital role in patient care, bridging the gap between folk traditions and emerging medical science. Though dismissed as "untrained," these women were, in reality, practitioners of a long-standing medical tradition that blended empirical observation, pragmatic eclecticism, and maternal authority.[30]

For Bickerdyke, like many others, the need to generate income combined with a passion for caring for others motivated them to continue as home caregivers who served a patient population that was not yet recognized as worthy by established hospitals. During her time in the West, Mary Bickerdyke's selection and diversity of clientele demonstrated her ability to provide a variety of care as a visiting nurse or live-in caretaker. Despite the concerted efforts of medical professionals to limit the specialized medical knowledge shared with the public, women caregivers like Mary Bickerdyke were confident in their medical abilities and augmented their knowledge through medical guides and advertised therapeutics.

The work of unofficial medical professionals like Bickerdyke and other private nurses contrasted sharply with the growing authority of hospitals after the Civil War. As doctors gained influence in the late nineteenth century, increasing professional specialization reinforced that hospitals were the primary sites for advanced medical care.[31] However, public trust in these institutions developed gradually, as many people associated the clinical setting more with death than with healing. Historian Charles Rosenberg argues that hospitals began to replace homes as the primary locations for treating serious illness and managing death during the Civil War.[32] This shift was propelled by surgical advancements and public acceptance of germ theory and antiseptics, which fostered confidence in hospitals as spaces for healing. Yet, this transformation did not fully take hold in the American consciousness until at least the 1920s. As hospitals solidified their status as scientific institutions, the newly trained nurse emerged, displacing home nurses whose informal expertise was deemed inadequate for professional medical practice. These trained nurses supplemented their basic sanitary knowledge with formal instruction in anatomy, physiology, chemistry, and bacteriology.[33] Meanwhile, Bickerdyke and other private nurses continued working outside institutional settings, demonstrating the persistent demand for traditional home-based care even as the medical profession sought to redefine its boundaries.

Around 1876, after her intense involvement in providing aid during the grasshopper plague in the Midwest, Mary Bickerdyke moved to California. As she settled into the new culture and climate of California, she began offering her services as a private nurse. As she had during the war, she specialized in terminal illnesses and took on long-term and difficult cases. Nursing chronically or terminally ill patients was often done at home as hospitals began employing attendants who were less expensive health care professionals without formal nurse training.[34] Doctors and hospital stakeholders believed that the terminally ill could receive adequate, if less sophisticated, care and did not wish to overcrowd their facilities with dying patients. The dissociation from hospital procedures and oversight allowed these attendants to perform their duties with a level of authority and relative autonomy. Attendants and nurses for hire like Mary Bickerdyke were essential players in the medical profession before the establishment of hospice and palliative care departments precisely because of their lack of formal training or licensure. In western or rural areas, like San Francisco in the 1880s, private nursing was necessary to address the shortage of orthodox medical professionals in those regions.

In 1879, Bickerdyke traveled to Storey County, Nevada, a region energized by the booming gold and silver rush towns of Gold Hill and Virginia City, situated between Reno and Carson City. There, she reconnected with several former soldiers, including at least one who had specifically requested her care. Among them was Theodore B. Janes, a former private in the Wisconsin Cavalry who, in a letter, had been referred to as one of Bickerdyke's "boys" during the war.[35] That label was significant to Mother Bickerdyke, who took seriously her long-term responsibility to the men she met and served during the war. While in Storey County, Bickerdyke stayed with Reverend Rush Eastman, the pastor of St. Paul's Episcopal Church, and his wife Charlotte.[36] While she was in their home, she nursed the Eastman's young daughter Eleanor in addition to Mr. Janes.

Both of Bickerdyke's patients, the one-year-old Eleanor as well as Theodore Janes, died in 1879.[37] Eleanor's surviving sister later recalled the deep meaning of Bickerdyke's care for the surviving family members. She reminded Bickerdyke: "You tottled little baby Eleanor on your knee, and sang again and again to her that old nursery tune on which you said you had brought up so many babies, and which we have never to this day forgotten."[38] The tenderness she showed to the infant and her family reflected the maternal care she had once provided to her own children. She instinctively applied the same nurturing skills, offering comfort even in a time of profound loss.

For Janes, who was dying of tuberculosis, Bickerdyke made a dressing gown that he could comfortably wear during his illness.[39] Without a wife to care for him, he would have needed to rely on outside caretakers to attend to him in the intimate moments of physical helplessness as he approached death. For both the nurse and the patient, this intimate form of care echoed their wartime bond. Bickerdyke had known Janes as one of her "boys," a surrogate son shaped by the shared trials of war. As an extension of her wartime services, providing end-of-life care to her "boys" felt like the culmination of her patriotic duty to care for her wartime patients throughout their lives and deaths. She was, in this sense, truly able to perform her traditional maternal duties by attending to the dying sons of war as they passed from life to death. For the terminally ill, particularly those without immediate family support, private nursing ensured dignity and familiarity in their final days. Bickerdyke's work highlights how private caregivers bridged the gap between traditional domestic care and the emerging medical profession, preserving a model of intimate, patient-centered treatment that institutional medicine struggled to replicate.

After Janes's death, Bickerdyke traveled to Carson City to care for a man named William J. Magee. She stayed with Magee and his family for at least four months, providing specialized care that his wife Lottie had sought for her ailing husband and the father of her four school-age children.[40] His illness had left him unemployed for at least eight months, creating both financial and emotional strain on the family. Unlike her usual patients—Union veterans—Magee had served as a corporal in Lieutenant Colonel Robert S. Gould's Sixth Battalion, Texas Cavalry, fighting for the Confederacy.[41] Bickerdyke, widely known as a mother to "boys in blue," rarely extended her care to former Confederate soldiers, making this case an exception. Perhaps driven by financial need or because she was sought out specifically by the Magee family, Bickerdyke nevertheless applied "great care" to Magee's case. After months of work between Bickerdyke and Lottie Magee, Bickerdyke seemed optimistic that the Confederate veteran would recover from his illness.[42]

The contrast between Mr. Janes and Mr. Magee suggests that while Bickerdyke primarily cared for Union veterans, she did not entirely exclude former Confederates from her postwar nursing practice. Though publicly remembered as a woman with "a mother's self-sacrificing devotion, and the high patriotism and benevolence which exist in her nature," she also navigated the pragmatic realities of nursing as a widowed woman in the 1880s. Her work exemplified both the entrepreneurial nature and the contingent possibilities of nursing during this period, as private nurses adapted to shifting professional landscapes and financial necessities.[43] For the next two years, Bickerdyke continued offering her nursing services to men and women across California. She traveled impressive distances to take on various cases in the region, sometimes up to 400 miles from her home base in San Francisco. She wrote to her older son in Kansas to keep him generally apprised of her work and whereabouts but seemed satisfied with the autonomous and adventurous nature of her newfound niche as a private nurse for hire. In March 1881, she wrote from Sacramento that she was "taking care of a sick Lady" and would accompany her to "San Louis [sic] Obispo" via train and steamer. Later that year, after returning to Reno, Nevada, to complete her nursing assignments, she endured a "hard spell of nursing in Contra Costa Co." with a particularly challenging patient, whom she described as a "rebel."[44] The decentralized nature of health care in the western United States required Bickerdyke to remain mobile, responding to requests as they arose. Despite the physical demands, she reported that she "kept pretty busy at nursing," a testament to both her resilience and the steady demand for experienced private nurses.[45]

The long transition of medical sovereignty from home to hospital over the course of the nineteenth century required Americans to engage in creative solutions to get the care they desired or expected. Many communities remained skeptical of institutionalized medicine, preferring trusted local practitioners or forming their own aid networks, such as the Black women's relief societies in Chicago.[46] Bickerdyke's career demonstrates how individuals navigated these changes, offering transitional solutions that preserved elements of traditional caregiving even as the medical profession sought to redefine its authority. Her ability to shift between institutional and private care settings speaks to the broader complexities of medical professionalization and the contested nature of authority in nineteenth-century nursing.

## Completing the Home Circle: Motherhood through Personal Palliative Care

Mary Bickerdyke found her professional stride in California and Nevada, applying her nursing skills while expanding her network across the region. Though she appreciated the blooming trees, fresh citrus groves, and the presence of veteran communities, she remained deeply tied to her family.[47] By this point, her sons and stepchildren were scattered across the country: James (J. R.) had settled into a teaching and administrative career in Kansas, Hiram had moved with his wife to the ranchlands of Montana, and her stepchildren remained primarily in Cincinnati and Covington, Kentucky. While Hiram remained elusive in his correspondence, J. R. and her stepdaughter Mary "Mollie" Bickerdyke kept up with their mother through letters. It is hard to determine whether her stepdaughter preferred to be called Mary or Mollie in most public contexts. In her correspondence with her stepmother, she primarily defaulted to go by Mollie, which may have been a reversion to a childhood name.[48] Bickerdyke often urged them to visit or even relocate to California, particularly out of concern for their health, as both had struggled with illness. In early 1882, Bickerdyke expressed to J. R. that she wished for Mollie to come to California due to her poor health.[49] Though she found fulfillment in her work as a private and traveling nurse, Bickerdyke viewed her family as her most important patients and longed to care for them in both sickness and health.

Her concerns about her children's health were warranted. Within a few years of initial consultation and inquiry about concerning symptoms, Mollie's health began to rapidly deteriorate. As she approached her forty-second birthday in July 1886, Mollie urged Bickerdyke to visit her in Cincinnati, where she was boarding with another family who provided lodging and some assistance with her health issues.[50] Around this time, it became evident that Mollie was in the early stages of breast cancer. Mollie sent her stepmother several letters detailing her symptoms, treatments, and overall outlook, always expressing her desire for Bickerdyke's presence as she relied on the care of relative strangers in the interim. She continued writing for as long as she was able, keeping her stepmother informed of both progress and setbacks. By the spring of 1887, the setbacks had become more frequent and alarming. In a worried tone, she wrote, "Last week my breast had a very numb feeling. The medicine does not physic me as much as it should. One of my troubles for years has been constipation. The Doctor says I am very hard to work on but said I could send you word I was getting along nicely. I am reduced a little in flesh."[51] Mollie's letter revealed her growing doubts about the effectiveness of her treatment, as her personal experience of her illness did not always align with the doctors' reassurances. This lack of confidence in her medical care likely reinforced Bickerdyke's decision to travel to Cincinnati and tend to her stepdaughter personally.

As the weeks progressed, Mollie's local friends assisted her in writing the letters to Bickerdyke because Mollie was "unable to use her arm on account of the swelling and pain."[52] Mollie's friend described in graphic detail the plaster dressing and redressing of Mollie's breast that had been "cut off to enlarge the opening that the cancerous growth may have more room to come out." The grueling treatment process prompted long spells of vomiting, headaches, and a "fearful pain attending the pulling of the plaster from the inflamed surface."[53] Mollie was withstanding pain from the disease as it grew swiftly out of control and challenged her physically: "Two other places on her breast . . . seem ready to open. One of them has an ill-smelling, watery pus oozing from it, and the odor from it keeps her constantly nauseated."[54] After the report in this letter, Bickerdyke determined to end her tenure in California to nurse her stepdaughter in Covington, Kentucky.

Mollie and Mary Bickerdyke understood that breast cancer was a complicated disease that required the intervention of specialized doctors. Medical professionals with years of training and specialized knowledge about diseases were on the rise in the 1880s, spurred by improvements in how professional knowledge was shared during the Civil War.[55] Unfortunately, Mollie Bickerdyke would not benefit from some of the advances in breast cancer treatment, such as the radical mastectomy, which would not be pioneered in the United States until the 1890s by Dr. William Halsted.[56] Her local doctors prescribed therapeutics to the best of their abilities, but in many cases, a cancer diagnosis was the equivalent to a death sentence. The general helplessness of doctors in these cases led some family members, like her stepbrother J. R., to believe that his mother and other healing methods could be "worth a half a dozen doctors."[57]

The homeopathic care of nurses was popularly seen as superior by family members whose loved ones were in dire circumstances. People frequently turned to extraordinary cures, often advertised in local newspapers, in hopes of finding relief. When faced with terminal illnesses, many believed that every possible remedy should be explored. One such treatment, Swift's Specific, claimed to be an "entirely vegetable" cure, with patient testimonials asserting that it could "cure cancers by forcing out the impurities from the blood" (see figure 5.2).[58] It promised to be an age-old curative, derived from Black doctoring traditions.[59] In the post-emancipation environment, culturally tested medical solutions gained popularity, and White consumers were willing to cross the racial divide to heal themselves and their family members. Across the country, men and women clung to the success stories of ordinary people from their local papers during their own medical crises that seemed otherwise hopeless.

Mother-Nurse 127

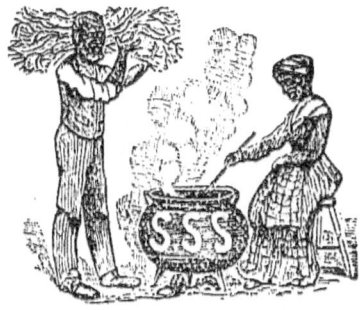

FIGURE 5.2
Advertisement for Swift's Syphilitic Specific published in newspapers across the United States. This image appeared in *The American Israelite* (Cincinnati) on July 30, 1886. Swift Specific Company was incorporated June 13, 1879. The only medicine manufactured by the company was the famous S.S.S. Remedy, also known as Swift's Specific for the blood.

## Swift's Specific

Is nature's own remedy, made from roots gathered from the forests of Georgia. The method by which it is made was obtained by a half-breed from the Creek Indians who inhabited a certain portion of Georgia, which was communicated to one of the early settlers, and thus the formula has been handed down to the present day. The above cut represents the method of manufacture twenty years ago, by Mr. C. T. Swift, one of the present proprietors. The demand has been gradually increasing until a $100,000 laboratory is now necessary o supply the trade. A foreign demand has been created, and enlarged facilities will be necessary to meet it. This great

### VEGETABLE BLOOD PURIFIER

CURES

Cancer, Catarrh, Scrofula, Eczema, Ulcers,

Rheumatism, Blood Taint,

hereditary or otherwise, without the use of Mercury or Potash
Books on "Contagious Blood Poison" and on "Blood and Skin Diseases" mailed free.
For sale by all druggists,
THE SWIFT SPECIFIC CO.,
N. Y. 157 W. 23d St.      Drawer 3, Atlanta, Ga.

Throughout the nineteenth century, doctors steadily increased their authority by legitimizing their expertise through science and reinforcing their control through institutional mechanisms such as licensing, which ensured professional autonomy while limiting competition from alternative healers.[60] This growing medical dominance often clashed with popular trust in traditional and homeopathic remedies. Companies like Swift's Specific continued to thrive in the 1880s, despite lacking endorsement from medical professionals and promoting outdated understandings of disease. Their success reflected the persistent public demand for alternative treatments, particularly among patients who remained skeptical of the emerging medical orthodoxy. Mollie Bickerdyke, for example, consulted doctors but struggled to understand or

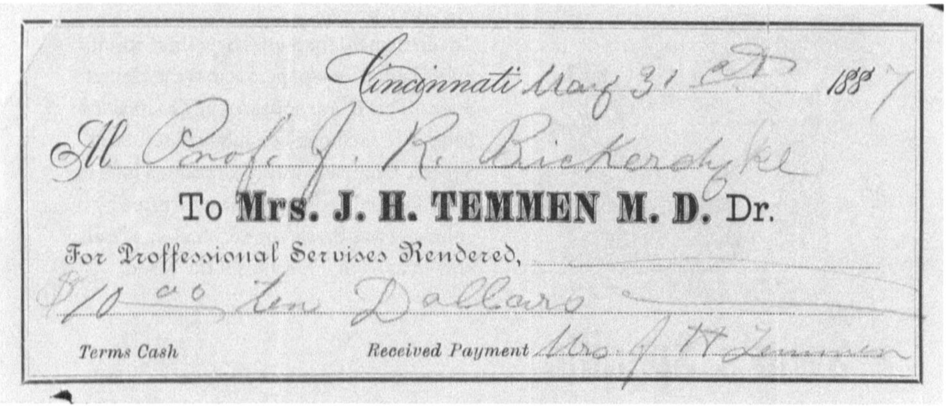

> Cincinnati May 31 1887
>
> M Prof. J. R. Bickerdyke
>
> To **Mrs. J. H. TEMMEN M. D.** Dr.
>
> For Proffessional Services Rendered,
>
> $10.00 Ten Dollars
>
> Terms Cash    Received Payment Mrs J H Temmen

FIGURE 5.3 Receipt for Mrs. J. H. Temmen, MD, a Prussian immigrant and self-proclaimed cancer specialist in Cincinnati. Though women were largely excluded from formal medical certification, Temmen positioned herself as an oncologist, leveraging the support of Cincinnati's German community. Mollie Bickerdyke's decision to seek care from a female physician highlights the limited professional opportunities available to women in medicine and the networks of trust that allowed them to practice, despite institutional barriers. Courtesy of the Library of Congress.

trust their prescribed treatments, particularly bloodletting and circulation therapies, which left her physically drained. Her friend wrote to Mother Bickerdyke, noting that Mollie believed "that her Dr. hoped to bring away the disease through the blood. She misunderstood her for the physician says that she never entertained such an idea but expected to draw it out just as she is doing. I have no idea how long she thinks it will take to effect a cure."[61] This misunderstanding reveals a fundamental disconnect between patient and doctor, likely stemming from differences in medical literacy, communication styles, and the broader tension between patient expectations and professional authority. Mollie's confusion highlights the challenges many patients—especially women—faced in navigating evolving medical practices, where personal experience often clashed with the doctor's clinical approach.

The Bickerdykes's inclusion of Mrs. Catharine E. Temmen, MD, as Mollie's primary cancer doctor indicates both the nature of their social politics and their resourcefulness in recruiting a care team that could address Mollie's specific needs (see figure 5.3). Dr. Temmen was a Prussian immigrant, and not much else is known about her.[62] In the 1870 census, Temmen was listed as a housekeeper, suggesting that she had either not applied her medical training to professional practice or had not yet completed her training.[63] Considering her specialization in oncology and the attitudes of American surgeons toward women professionals before the late 1880s, it seems most plausible that Temmen trained while she was still living in Prussia. Although Germany's certified physician training for women was a couple of decades more advanced, no German university allowed the full matriculation necessary for subsequent certification.[64] Temmen most likely audited some courses at German universities before immigrating to the United States and settling in Ohio. This would have given her the confidence to advertise her services as a cancer specialist.

Although Temmen was listed as a physician in city directories for a decade and claimed specialization as an oncologist, she was no more formally recognized as an oncologist than Bickerdyke was acknowledged as a palliative care nurse by the medical establishment. Yet, both women positioned themselves as competent medical authorities within their respective fields. For female practitioners like Temmen and Bickerdyke, a medical certificate was both an unattainable and, in many ways, unnecessary bureaucratic credential, as their expertise was built on practical experience rather than institutional validation. The Temmens immigrated from Prussia and Hanover before 1857, prior to the birth of their first child. All six of their children were American-born, and despite the rise of nativist movements in the 1840s and 1850s, the family successfully assimilated, operating two businesses from their Cincinnati home and employing a domestic servant.[65] Subsequent waves of German immigration to the United States in the 1880s sparked another nativist movement in cities across the country; however, Cincinnati had cultivated a safe-haven community of German culture that included four German newspapers, various German societies and celebrations, and German churches. It was because of this that a woman physician was able to practice in an otherwise male-dominated field.

When Mary Bickerdyke finally arrived in Covington, Kentucky, to nurse her stepdaughter, the situation was already grim. The palliative care that Mary Bickerdyke could provide did not include any miracle cure and did not address the cancer that had consumed her stepdaughter's body. It was, instead, a regimen similar to those she had administered as a nurse in the Union army and as a private nurse in California. For example, Mother Bickerdyke recruited the help of another attendant to assist with the around-the-clock care that Mollie required.[66] Mother Bickerdyke did not desire to claim a spot as a martyr caregiver; she understood her own physical limitations and her need to rest. The palliative and critical care tasks that Bickerdyke implemented were deceptively simple. She oversaw the patient's hygiene, feeding, medication schedule, housekeeping, and laundry for two months while Mollie's health declined and neared the end of her life.

Because Mollie was both family and, in every meaningful sense, her daughter, the correspondence between family members concerning care arrangements provides insight into the family and community processes surrounding end-of-life care. As the primary caregiver during Mollie's final days, Mother Bickerdyke took charge of the necessary procedures and tasks to ensure her stepdaughter could face death without the burden of practical concerns. Mollie's memorial assured mourners that "her preparations for death were made as calmly as for a journey, and having arranged her temporal affairs, she quietly resigned herself to the guidance of Him who hath conquered death and robbed the grave of its terrors."[67] Such a transition signaled Mother Bickerdyke's familiarity with the process of funerary arrangements and her ability to navigate all the associated details with ease. In mid-May 1887, Mollie's cancer doctor still held hope that Mollie might survive the cancer, but Mother Bickerdyke sensed otherwise, intuiting that her stepdaughter was "failing every hour."[68] Around this time, Mother Bickerdyke encouraged J. R. to make his way to Cincinnati to be present for his stepsister's death, as was the custom. Once he arrived, Bickerdyke coordinated responsibilities among family members: J. R. managed financial matters and correspondence to inform relatives of Mollie's condition, while her stepson Robert and his wife retrieved the medicines and poultices from the doctor for Mollie.

In a final letter, Mollie Bickerdyke dictated a touching message to Mother Bickerdyke to be read after her death. The letter took on the persona of a resurrected soul, addressing her stepmother from beyond the grave. It started, "You did not think that you would so soon come to hear from me. Mother Dear how I love you and how will I ever be able to thank you for the many sacrifices you have made for me when I was in my helpless condition mother dear I am all right now and free from pain."[69] Mollie was quick to reassure her stepmother that she had felt well served and cared for in her time of greatest need and suffering. The words signaled her gratitude and served as an acknowledgment of those who had been with her until the end. Mollie reflected stalwartness in the face of impending death, remaining obedient to its final call on her life. Mollie reassured her surviving family and provided each member with encouragement. To Mary Bickerdyke, Mollie affirmed her stepmother's expert care and the usefulness of her ability to provide palliative care when healing was no longer a viable option. Mollie assured her, "Mother everything was done perfectly as I would wish and I am satisfied everything was done for me that could possibly be done but the time had come for me to leave earth and I had to obey the summons."[70] The letter represented a lasting expression and positive assessment of Mother Bickerdyke's duties, both as a mother and as a palliative care nurse.

When Mollie Bickerdyke died on July 26, 1887, she was with Mother Bickerdyke, and "her brothers were permitted the pleasure of easing her path to the grave with loving attentions, and the suffering of her last days was most tenderly lightened."[71] The quest for a "good death" has spanned centuries, and Mollie Bickerdyke's death occurred in a time of transition regarding what it meant to die well.[72] Much like her beliefs about nursing practices, Mother Bickerdyke held to older conceptions of the "good death" and continued to emphasize those values even as other Americans began to accept newer ways to die well. Family attendance at Mollie's bedside in her final hours was, by her estimation, the best way to die.

An extensive memorial booklet was produced and published for friends and family and is the only existing comprehensive biography of Mollie Bickerdyke. The memorial booklet contains thoughtful details about Mollie's life. It spoke of her active membership at Trinity Church, where the funeral was held, and of her beautiful singing voice, which often led the congregation.[73] Besides those few details, it heavily emphasized the maternal role that Mother Bickerdyke played for Mollie. After her biological mother died, the memorial booklet explained, "she was blessed in childhood with a 'second mother'—one who has for years belonged to the nation, and is to-day known and revered throughout the United States as 'Mother Bickerdyke.' Close ties of affection bound this mother and daughter through life, which years of separation had no power to sunder."[74] It was as if the family felt it necessary to justify Mother Bickerdyke's absence from the family and frame it as patriotic rather than negligent, lest anyone think otherwise. The booklet told of the suffering that Mollie had long endured, but in her time of greatest need, "the cry of her heart was for 'Mother'"—and Mother Bickerdyke came instantly from her distant home in San Francisco prepared to enter the contest with death, and if possible, seize from his dreaded grasp her beloved daughter. All that love, skill, and means lavishly expended could do, were employed to save her live, but in vain!"[75]

The producers of the memorial booklet consulted with the family and emphasized how much they trusted in the effective combination of mother's love and medical skill. In the memorial, the glowing tribute made to Mother Bickerdyke absolved her of any blame for her stepdaughter's death and importantly suggests that her skills were not lacking in any way. Even though Mother Bickerdyke and her family were reliant on her specialization in palliative care, they took obvious efforts to justify those measures to others who might not have the same values. The memorial was sent to friends and acquaintances across the country to both publicize and reiterate their approval and satisfaction of the care process taken by *their* Mother Bickerdyke.

In the aftermath of Mollie's death, the family recorded the costs associated with her care and arrangements. A majority of Mollie Bickerdyke's medical care was funded by her stepbrother, J. R. Bickerdyke. The receipts that still exist in Bickerdyke's archive show that the family did "lavishly expend" for Mollie's care, sparing no expense (see figures 5.4 and 5.5).[76] Mother Bickerdyke had just begun to receive her pension for her time in the army and would not have been able to fund the care on her own. Instead, she began a pattern that would continue into her later years, relying on the relative financial stability of her eldest biological son, J. R. Without a doubt, J. R. loved his stepsister and seemed eager to help in any way that he could, paying for at least three doctors, room and board, ice, and the granite monument purchased upon Mollie's death. As he was on his way to Mollie Bickerdyke's bedside after his school entered the summer term, his mother instructed him to prepare $500, as she had already spent over $100 in her time with Mollie.[77] There was an unspoken acknowledgment between the mother and son that the burden of paying for Mollie's care and death would fall to them as the most secure members of the family. As has only become truer since the turn of the twentieth century, the Bickerdykes understood that the business of dying was no small cost and required cooperative communication among family members and community organizations to ensure an amicable outcome. There is no record that J. R. ever complained about the exorbitant expenses incurred by Mollie's care and death; he had become accustomed to at least partially funding his mother's endeavors. It is possible that his financial contribution, in this case, was meant to supplement and legitimize his mother's efforts at palliation.

In this palliative care case, Mary Bickerdyke faced the added difficulty of dealing with her own personal grief. The separation of duties between the mother and the nurse was not altogether clear, but this was the first instance in decades where she nursed her own family members in their final moments. After Mollie passed, Mother Bickerdyke did not initiate much correspondence with friends or family, but she received many condolences from friends across the country who had received the booklet that J. R. had helped to distribute. After spending decades away from her children, the months that she spent with them during and after Mollie's illness helped her decide to reorient her life to be closer to her surviving children.

BILLS PAYABLE MONTHLY.
TRANSIENT BUSINESS, CASH.

Covington, Ky., July 26th 1887

Mr. L. R. Bickerdyke

To WILLIAM H. HUNT, M. D., Dr.

MADISON ST., BET. SEVENTH AND EIGHTH.

To Medical Services and Medicines to Sister, Mrs Bickerdyke

from July — 1887, to July 26th 1887.

$48.00

RECEIVED PAYMENT, Wm. H. Hunt

W. B. CARPENTER & CO., PRS.

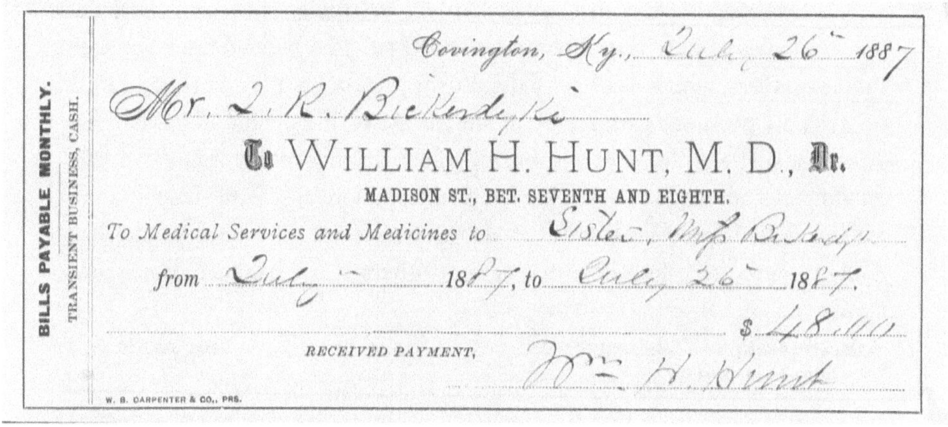

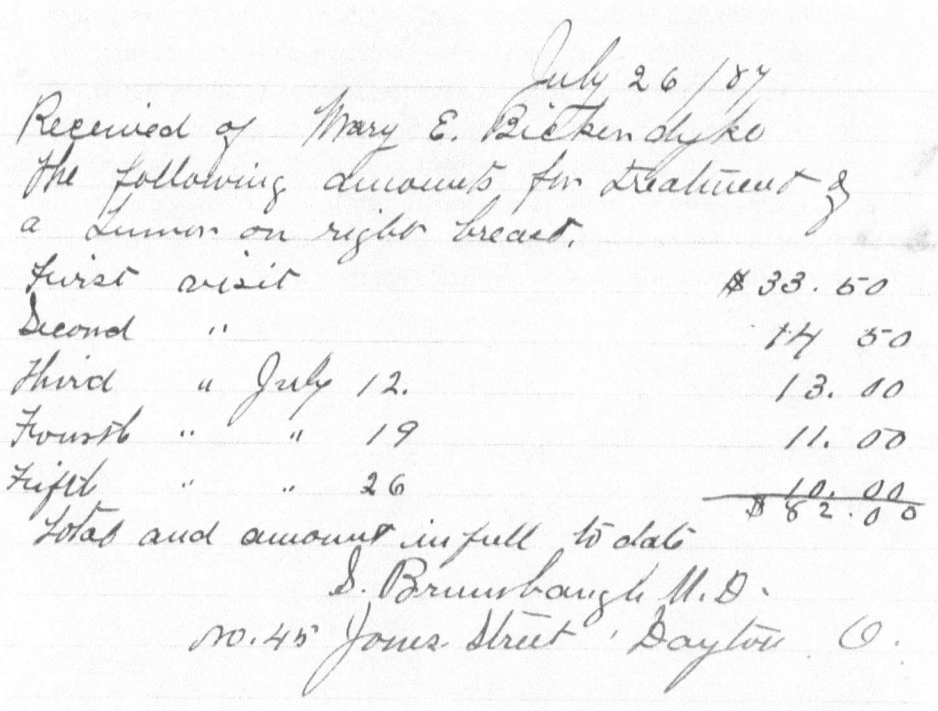

FIGURE 5.4 Receipt for doctor employed in Mollie Bickerdyke's cancer care in the final months of her life. It reflects the care and main therapeutics administered while Mother Bickerdyke was with her stepdaughter, from May to July 1887. Courtesy of the Library of Congress.

July 26/87

Received of Mary E. Bickerdyke
the following amounts for treatment of
a tumor on right breast.

| | | | |
|---|---|---|---|
| First visit | | | $33.50 |
| Second | " | | 14.50 |
| Third | " | July 12. | 13.00 |
| Fourth | " | " 19 | 11.00 |
| Fifth | " | " 26 | 10.00 |
| | | | $82.00 |

Total and amount in full to date
S. Brumbaugh M.D.
No. 45 Jones Street, Dayton O.

FIGURE 5.5 Receipt from Dr. Brumbaugh enumerates the multiple visits made to Mollie Bickerdyke for treatment of "a tumor on the right breast." Courtesy of the Library of Congress.

The loss of Mollie forced Mary Bickerdyke to confront the complexities of her dual roles as both a mother and a "Mother." The blurred lines between these identities, which had been a defining feature of her life's work, now took on a deeply personal significance as she navigated the profound yet familiar grief of losing a child. The outpouring of condolences from friends and acquaintances across the nation served as a testament to the far-reaching impact of Bickerdyke's legacy, but it also underscored the sacrifices she had made in dedicating herself to the care of others at the expense of her own family.

In the wake of this tragedy, Bickerdyke found herself at a crossroads. She was aging, and the time spent with her family during Mollie's illness had awakened a realization that the bonds of family, which she had so often set aside in the pursuit of her calling, were threatened by the passage of time. The decision to reorient her life and prioritize attention toward her surviving children marked a turning point in Bickerdyke's personal and professional journey—one that would require her to reconcile the competing demands of her personal and professional lives.

As she embarked on the final chapter of her life in Kansas living with her oldest son, Bickerdyke carried with her the hard-earned wisdom of a lifetime spent in service to others. The lessons she had learned about the power of compassion, the importance of advocacy, and the resilience of the human spirit continued to guide her as she sought to balance her roles as a mother and a care professional. In the face of loss and change, Bickerdyke's promise to care for those in need remained constant, a testament to the indelible mark she left on the lives of countless individuals and the nation.

CHAPTER SIX

# Special Acts of Justice
## Mary Bickerdyke and Pension Claims

In the postwar period, Bickerdyke's continued advocacy for veterans' rights and pension acquisition demonstrated her commitment to lifelong care and cemented her importance in the evolving landscape of nineteenth-century American social welfare policy. Her personal and professional involvement in the pension debates of the late nineteenth century situated her within national controversies over the expansion of government benefits and the role of the state in providing for former soldiers. The emphasis placed on Bickerdyke's maternal qualities in historical narratives highlights her compassionate nature but obscures the full scope of her professional competence and assertiveness. Thus, Bickerdyke's pension advocacy for herself and then for others offers a case study in the intersection of gender roles, veterans' rights, and the expansion of government support in post–Civil War America, providing valuable insights into the social and political transformations of the era.

Mary Bickerdyke's pension claim as a Union army nurse should be seen as a precursor to the maternalist welfare state that emerged more fully in the early twentieth century. Congress recognized the value of her labor through the passage of a "special act" and emphasized that her maternal reputation contributed to that decision. As a result, the federal government acknowledged the worth of maternal labor and set a precedent to support women who performed compassionate care during wartime. This recognition set a foundation for future legislative reforms aimed at protecting and supporting mothers. Additionally, widespread backing for Bickerdyke's pension—from both ordinary soldiers and influential politicians—highlighted a shifting cultural appreciation for women's vital contributions in professional spaces. The campaign for her pension and the subsequent work for soldiers' pensions required Bickerdyke to draw on the same tenacity, compassion, and resourcefulness that defined her wartime service. Moreover, her official recognition through the congressional special act allowed her to contribute to shaping the nascent welfare state, ensuring that those who had sacrificed so much to the country would not be left behind.

An exploration of Mary Bickerdyke's post–Civil War personal pension campaign and subsequent veteran pension advocacy adds to a body of scholarship that reexamines the intersections of gender, social welfare, and political culture in the late nineteenth century. This chapter builds on the work of Theda Skocpol and Patrick J. Kelly, which explored the development of the American welfare state in the decades following the Civil War. The expansion of veterans' benefits in this period laid the groundwork for the modern American welfare state, and women's activism shaped the contours of emerging social policies and program administration that benefited both male and female war veterans.[1] Situating Bickerdyke's story within a broader context of health activism and emerging maternalist policies demonstrates that these historical processes reach back to the Civil War. Molly Ladd-Taylor's influential *Mother-Work* and Elizabeth Gardner Masarik's *The Sentimental State* recognize the ways in which women's maternal authority and moral suasion helped legitimize and expand the scope of America's social welfare policies.[2] This chapter's analysis adds to those works by examining Bickerdyke's ability to traverse formal institutions and informal care networks after the Civil War. Mary Bickerdyke's employment as a pension attorney and pension guardian allowed her to leverage her legacy as a "Mother to the boys in blue," offering insight into the dynamics of larger social processes at the individual level while underscoring the complex and often contradictory ways in which gender shaped politics.[3]

Among Bickerdyke's treasured possessions was a carefully preserved card adorned with a decorated cross (see figure 6.1). The card contained the words from Bickerdyke's favorite hymn, "Must Jesus Bear the Cross Alone?" It says in part:

> Must Jesus bear the cross alone,
> And all the world go free?
> No, there's a cross for every one,
> And there's a cross for me.[4]

The lyrics of this hymn encapsulated Bickerdyke's personal beliefs and professional ethos, which stressed the importance of both individual responsibility to promote good and a collective mandate to alleviate human suffering. Despite the biblical narrative of Christ's journey to his crucifixion, "Must Jesus Bear the Cross Alone?" echoed a growing populist evangelical hymnody that spoke to the political and social realities of welfare gaps in the American experience.[5] As the Civil War population aged, a new crisis loomed over the nation and its government: Would sacrifices and suffering of veterans lead to destitution, or would local supporters rally and advocate for just rewards for their service to the nation? The answer for Bickerdyke as a pension advocate was firm: the cross of old age and disability was not meant for

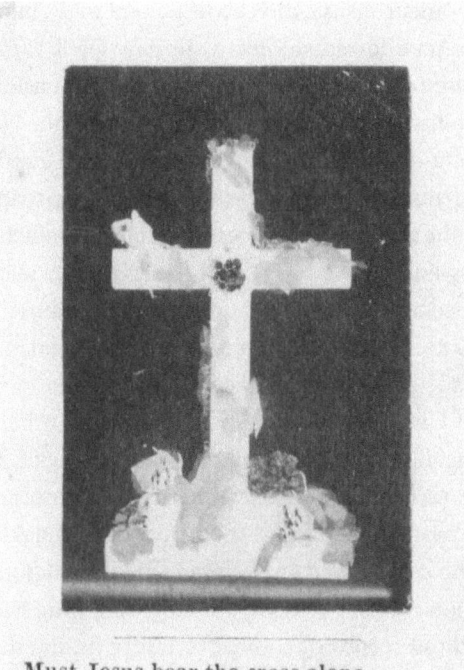

FIGURE 6.1
Mother Bickerdyke's memorial hymn card. Courtesy of the Library of Congress.

Civil War soldiers and nurses to bear alone. Her work, both for herself and for others, highlighted the limitations of formal institutional support in the late nineteenth century and the critical importance of personal, maternal care in filling the gaps left by government aid.

## A Special Act of Justice: Mary Bickerdyke's Personal Pension Battle

A series of legislative acts passed after the Civil War produced national controversy over large-scale social provisions for veterans. Congressional measures slowly increased exceptions to pension awards for soldiers who could prove disabilities that were "incurred as a direct consequent of . . . military duty."[6] In 1879, the Arrears Act allowed soldiers with new Civil War–related disabilities to receive a lump-sum award for all the missed pension payments since the end of their military duty.[7] Between 1880 and 1910, the US government appropriated over one-quarter of its spending to pension distribution. Some argued that vast expansion of benefits would encourage patriotism and a willingness to enlist in the army during present and future conflicts, but others argued that Congress had gone too far in its liberality. In 1887, President Grover Cleveland vetoed a proposed pension expansion, claiming that the projected new expenditures would be "almost appalling" and expressing that "generous laws [had] been passed to relieve against the incidents of war" for the neediest of Civil War veterans.[8] Cleveland and others worried that veterans might exaggerate even minor injuries, retire early from productive work, and live off government income. Despite these protests, Congress continued to push for more benefits, and the Dependent Pension Act of 1890 eventually passed. The law allowed any veteran who served honorably for ninety days in the Union military to apply for a pension if he had since become disabled, even without record of combat or injury during the war.[9]

Amid this complex and evolving landscape of veteran pension legislation, Mary Bickerdyke embarked on her own journey to secure the recognition and compensation she had earned through her tireless service during the Civil War. As a woman who had played a crucial role in the war effort, Bickerdyke faced unique challenges in navigating the pension system, which did not officially compensate women nurses until 1892. Drawing inspiration from the groundbreaking efforts of other female Civil War professionals, Bickerdyke's arduous pension application process exemplifies the struggles endured by veterans, particularly women, as they fought to secure the financial support they deserved.

The inspiration and catalyst for Mary Bickerdyke's formal pension reward was another Civil War nurse whom she had never met. Mary Morris Husband, affectionately referred to as "Mother Husband" in postwar reminiscences, was renowned for her ability to gain rare access to the battlefront, which was often denied to nurses.[10] Most famously, she served at Camp Letterman in Gettysburg, where she was offered the position of matron at the Third Corps hospital. Morris Husband was the granddaughter of founding father Robert Morris and the daughter of a member of congress and New York State assembly. Her social station was bolstered by her marriage to a "highly respectable member" of the Philadelphia bar association.[11]

Despite these advantages, Morris Husband suffered the loss of significant property in the aftermath of the war. She incurred expenses exceeding $2,000 for hospital and transportation costs, which she paid out of her own money.[12] By the time her husband died in 1880, Mary Morris Husband lived in Washington, DC, where one of her sons, a Union veteran, worked as a clerk for the US Post Office. Leveraging her connections, Husband secured a position at the pensions office, where she gained valuable insight into the intricacies of the pension application process. She eventually used her knowledge from this work to navigate the system more effectively for her own benefit.[13]

Morris Husband's pension report was passed by Congress on April 11, 1884, and she was granted a pension by a "Special Act of Congress." The process essentially resembled the passage of any other congressional bill, but this special act was specifically designed for those who were not covered under other pension legislation. Her basis for appeal rested on several important factors: her meritorious volunteer service and patriotic lineage, her current infirm state, and the precedent set by previous congressional special acts.[14] Her distinguished service as a Civil War volunteer was presented by several men who had witnessed that Morris Husband was "kind, faithful, and skillful in her management of the wounded ... relieving suffering soldiers wherever found and of whatever color, whether 'blue' or 'gray.'"[15] Additionally, she was a widow, over sixty years old, and her health had begun to decline. She had broken her hip and was thus categorized as a "confirmed cripple."[16] Finally, Morris Husband referred in her application to two previous pensions granted through a special act of Congress to Mrs. Elizabeth Leebrich and Miss Amanda Stopes, both of whom had also served the Union army as nurses.[17] Between the end of the Civil War and 1892, when the Army Nurses Pension Act was passed, Congress granted approximately 200 special acts to women based on their military service.[18]

In her appeal to Congress for a pension, Morris Husband presented over a dozen testimonies from supporting veterans and leading institutional figures, who noted how the war had taken a toll on her personal finances and health. One of the men from whom she requested an affidavit was Reverand Frederick N. Knapp, the head of the Special Relief Service of the United States Sanitary Commission (USSC). He had appointed Morris Husband to serve as a relief agent, where he attested that she had performed "arduous and valuable service, with the same devotion of spirit and rare executive ability which gave efficiency to her work for the soldiers."[19]

Mary Morris Husband's successful appeal prompted Knapp to contact Mary Bickerdyke and begin exploring a similar solution for her reward.

Knapp reached out to Bickerdyke in California from Massachusetts. He relayed the news of Morris Husband's victory and inquired about Bickerdyke's interest in pursuing a pension. Bickerdyke indignantly replied that Husband's appeal "should have opened the way for all our faithful women nurses myself among them—but it has been told us that women nurses could not get pensions." She conveyed a sense of disappointment and frustration that, despite small strides toward pensions for nurses, most women were still denied any compensation. Her sentiment highlighted the prevalent gendered discrimination and showed that women's contributions in the war were often undervalued or ignored. She recommended that several high-ranking generals could attest to her wartime service, including "[John A.] Logan, [William] Rosencrans, [William T.] Sherman." Bickerdyke reasoned that Knapp and these male wartime witnesses could use their positions to assist her in this "matter of justice" to formally gain recognition and renumeration as a nurse veteran.[20]

The long process to obtain Bickerdyke's pension revealed that it would be necessary to rely on the efforts of private organizations that were also interested in her compensation. Individual Grand Army of the Republic (GAR) posts across the country occasionally raised and sent funds to Bickerdyke for her support. For example, Western posts of the GAR took her case into their own hands and assessed themselves a small sum per capita on an annual basis.[21] Men from across the country who had received "vigilant care" under Mother Bickerdyke felt that she had, through these efforts, "thousands of adopted sons; and if adopted joint heirs." This biblical reference demonstrated the seriousness of veterans' commitment to take care of their "Mother." Part of their duty as heirs was to provide comfort and care to their aging matriarch. Ohio GAR posts raised several hundred dollars to serve as a substitute pension.[22] Other GAR posts took up occasional collections and sent them to her. Piecemeal efforts to provide for Bickerdyke communicated her worthiness and the esteem she had earned from soldiers, but they did not constitute a steady or reliable income. It was a noble gesture from her heirs of wartime mothering, but over time it became evident that "such dribblets [were] inadequate" to meet her consistent financial needs.[23] These fundraisers reflect the depth of veterans' gratitude, but their help could not match a congressional stipend and the federal government's recognition of Bickerdyke's worthy service.

The stage was set for Bickerdyke's special act to be introduced, but her advocates bemoaned their "numerical weakness," noting that it would be difficult to "move the great mass of Posts to act with any degree of unanimity upon any central front."[24] The Nineteenth National GAR Encampment held in Portland, Maine, in June 1885, helped propel a supplementary pension campaign to augment the efforts of veterans devoted to her support. The process highlighted the challenges of coordinating a unified response across a decentralized network of local posts, ultimately revealing the limitations of grassroots support to ensure the financial stability of those who had sacrificed so much for their country.

The GAR encampment was a national forum for the representation of local posts and the affiliated Woman's Relief Corps (WRC), and the gathering provided another avenue to gain support for Bickerdyke's pension. The encampment presented an opportunity to raise and pass a consolidated resolution or statement that could more visibly endorse a steady pension through a congressional special act. A message from a national entity stood a chance to influence Union veterans in positions of power.[25] A resolution on Bickerdyke's behalf reflected a larger effort on the part of the WRC to bolster fledgling attempts to set up a general relief fund for nurses in the absence of congressional support. By the time of the 1886 GAR encampment, one year later, the National Pension and Relief Committee of the WRC was overwhelmed by letters from army nurses who were under the impression that the WRC or Congress would soon be funding their pensions. The scheme on Bickerdyke's behalf was partially successful. A resolution was adopted at the June 1885 Portland encampment, which stated that "the Woman's Relief Corps, auxiliary to the Grand Army of the Republic, in national convention assembled, do most earnestly and confidently petition the Congress of the United States of America that they will by special enactment place the name of Mary A. Bickerdyke on the pension roll for the sum of $16 per month."[26] Eventually, that statement would be printed on the report delivered to Congress.

Caleb C. Davis, who knew Bickerdyke from the war as a member of the Fifty-Fifth Illinois Infantry Regiment, moved on from the convention and strategized about finding the appropriate congress members to sponsor the bill for her pension. He advised Knapp that they should try to locate the few "worker-talkers in Congress" who might oppose a nurse's pension and whip them to the majority side that wished for Bickerdyke to have her pay. It was not a heavy lift, Davis claimed, as "every intelligent Congressman in the land is well aware that her claims are just."[27] Vocal opponents to pension expansion, like President Cleveland, were concerned about exorbitant spending and welfare abuse but did not have personal qualms about Mary Bickerdyke. Davis's conversation with Knapp after the GAR convention demonstrated a shift in attitude and emphasized the states' responsibilities to provide for their Civil War heroines.

Knapp collected a cache of letters from Bickerdyke and a few interested veterans affirming her wartime service and forwarded them to a congressional representative who could introduce a bill. The laudatory correspondence included exchanges with rank-and-file men who had reached out over the years, although Bickerdyke feared that these "beautiful and appreciate letters" would have "no especial bearing" on her case.[28] Despite a large body of evidence from rank-and-file soldiers, Bickerdyke's claim needed name recognition and political persuasion to succeed. She had crossed paths with important Civil War men who rose to power after the war's conclusion, but Bickerdyke suggested that of all her references, Mary A. Livermore of Melrose, Massachusetts, "knows of my work; She can give you valuable information and is ready with her influence to help me in my pension."[29]

Mary Livermore was one of the leading women in the Chicago branch of the USSC. She leveraged her upper-class philanthropy for reform work during and after the war. Livermore's most noted contribution to the USSC effort was the organization of the wildly successful Northwestern Sanitary Fairs that raised at least $80,000.[30] After the war, Livermore became a staunch supporter of women's suffrage, establishing *The Agitator*, a paper that eventually merged into *Woman's Journal*.[31] Livermore's public-facing influence made her a powerful ally in navigating the postwar political landscape. Moreover, her advocacy for women's rights and her prominent role in the suffrage movement made her well-suited to champion Bickerdyke's pension claim, as it represented an opportunity to further the recognition of women's vital contributions during the Civil War.

Mary Livermore contacted her congressional representative and former governor, John D. Long of Massachusetts. He agreed to introduce Bickerdyke's bill and worked in tandem with his constituents, Knapp and Livermore, to organize the claim. Long had no intimate knowledge of Bickerdyke's accomplishments. Instead, he was introduced to her wartime work through an emerging genre of Civil War literature, which included an account of Bickerdyke in addition to Knapp's and Livermore's personal recommendations.[32] The collective support was convincing, and Long introduced H.R. 700—A Special Act for Mary A. Bickerdyke—to the House of Representatives on January 11, 1886.[33] The bill, along with hundreds of others submitted that day, was referred to the congressional committee on pensions.

On March 31, Senator Charles Van Wyck, a Nebraska senator on the pensions committee, submitted the report on Bickerdyke for final passage. That same day, the committee also submitted, without amendment, reports for other women's pension claims, all of which belonged to widows or dependents of soldiers.³⁴ There were other nurses who applied for special acts in the same period as Bickerdyke, and those women represented the beginning stages of testing this approach. On May 8, resolutions passed for Amelia Gill, "a volunteer nurse in the late war, at the rate of twenty-five dollars a month"; Mrs. Ellen S. Tolam, "late an Army nurse, at the rate of twenty-five dollars per month"; and Augusta M. Richards, "a volunteer nurse in the late war, and pay her the sum of twenty-five dollars per month."³⁵ The growing number of nurses applying for pensions through special acts underscored the need for a more efficient and comprehensive system that could handle the increasing demands placed on the pension bureaucracy. These pioneering women, including Bickerdyke, laid the groundwork for future reforms that would streamline the pension process and provide more equitable support for the countless individuals who had served their country during the Civil War.

Bickerdyke's final report presented to the Senate included targeted excerpts from an affidavit by Dr. A. Goslin, the medical director of the Fifteenth Army Corps, as well as from the resolution of the WRC convention. Goslin's affidavit emphasized Bickerdyke's maternal reputation: "After a day's work was done in the cooking department she would go into the wards and nurse some poor dying soldier and speak words of comfort to him of home, mother, sister. No wonder she was known in the Army and called by the endearing name of 'mother.' She was truly a mother to hundreds of sick and dying soldiers."³⁶ The report also mentioned her current employment as a laundry worker at the US Mint in San Francisco and her continued work to secure pensions for poor and needy veterans.

In preparing the report, decisions were made to exclude the testimony from several letters that Knapp and Bickerdyke had forwarded to Long. For example, James E. Yeatman, the president of the Western Sanitary Commission, noted in his affidavit that Bickerdyke was "more than a nurse; her services were more like those of a commanding officer in looking after and providing for the needs of the sick and wounded." To stress the importance of Bickerdyke's work, Yeatman coupled this marshaling ability with her willingness to give herself "wholly up to this mission of mercy."³⁷ Yeatman's testimony heavily emphasized Bickerdyke's assertive maternal characteristics, while the final report contained a more subdued recollection of her domesticity, virtue, and motherly zeal. Though Mary Bickerdyke was an intense and forceful woman, the Senate report needed to strategically dial back her martial qualities for public consumption.

After the report was presented, "Mother" Mary A. Bickerdyke was awarded $25 a month, the "usual" pension amount for these cases.³⁸ The strategic inclusion of Goslin's testimony and the WRC convention resolution in the final pension report reveals the critical role that maternal imagery and gendered expectations played in shaping the public perception of female Civil War nurses. By emphasizing Bickerdyke's nurturing and comforting presence, as well as her willingness to perform domestic tasks like cooking and laundry, the report sought to frame her wartime service within the acceptable bounds of nineteenth-century womanhood. This carefully curated representation of Bickerdyke as a maternal ideal with an ongoing commitment to veteran welfare aimed to garner sympathy and support for her pension claim while also downplaying the more controversial aspects of her assertive and unconventional behavior during the war. The selective nature of the evidence presented in the final report underscores the challenges faced by women like Bickerdyke, who had to navigate societal expectations and gender norms while advocating for recognition and compensation for their vital contributions to the war effort.

Once special acts made their way through Congress, they were passed on to President Cleveland. The only Democratic president elected between 1860 and 1913, he opposed new pensions as wasteful government spending and refused to sign bills granting pensions to six former nurses in 1886, including Bickerdyke. He claimed such requests dripped with government charity.[39] Because Congress remained in session after Cleveland's refusal, the acts became law after ten days. Bickerdyke's special act was finally certified on June 14, 1886.[40] Justice, even if partial and delayed, had been served.

Was the successful pension award for Mother Bickerdyke an antecedent toward a maternalist welfare state in America? If Mother Bickerdyke and other Union army nurses could win pensions for their labor, then their professionalism and its cultural value gained recognition. This is the Progressive Era pattern identified by Theda Skocpol: "Social circumstances and political arrangements in the turn-of-the-century United States facilitated middle-class women's consciousness and mobilization, and encouraged women to make collective and hegemonic demands."[41] More recently, Elizabeth Gardner Masarik argued that sentimentalism as a cultural movement gave language to advocates as they demanded that mothers receive protection.[42] In Mother Bickerdyke's case, maternity was central to her claim and to the widespread support from soldiers and congressional backers. Bickerdyke's successful pension claim can be seen as a precursor to the maternalist welfare state that emerged more fully in the early twentieth century. By recognizing the importance of her maternal role during the Civil War, the government set a precedent for providing support to women who performed vital care work.

This acknowledgment codified the significance of maternal labor and laid the foundation for later reforms that sought to support mothers. Moreover, the broad support for Bickerdyke's pension claim from both rank-and-file soldiers and influential political figures demonstrates the growing cultural recognition of the value of women's contributions during times of crisis. This recognition helped to legitimize women's demands for greater rights and protections, ultimately contributing to the development of a more inclusive and responsive welfare state that acknowledged the unique needs and contributions of women.

After her pension was awarded, the GAR and the WRC compiled and published a book "for the Benefit of Mother Bickerdyke."[43] The effusive biography was intended to supplement the government's "wholly insufficient" pension reward.[44] Post members could buy a copy, own a souvenir of Bickerdyke's exploits, and contribute to her continued comfort and care as she aged. This innovative method to support Bickerdyke suggested an enduring commitment to ensure the well-being deserved by their "Mother." This ongoing effort to support Bickerdyke through various private means, even after her pension was secured, highlights the limitations of the government's support and the need for grassroots efforts to fill the gaps. Ultimately, the publication of this biography served as a testament to the power of maternal sentiment in shaping the cultural and political landscape of post–Civil War America, paving the way for the emergence of a more comprehensive and inclusive welfare state.

Special acts became the stopgap measure for almost a decade before the passage of the Army Nurses Pension Act of 1892. In 1888, the WRC, the Army Nurses' Association (ANA), and Congress began a four-year struggle to reach a compromise over a more efficient and liberal pension process for women who had served as nurses.[45] Finally signed into law by Republican President Benjamin Harrison, the 1892 measure entitled all women who served as nurses in the Union army during the American Civil War to a pension of $12 per month, a woefully meager amount. The act fell short of providing adequate financial support; nevertheless, it represented a crucial step forward in acknowledging the vital contributions of these women. It took nearly three decades after the end of the Civil War for this legislation to be enacted, highlighting the deeply entrenched societal barriers that women like Mary Bickerdyke had to overcome in their pursuit of justice. Although the Army Nurses Pension Act was a belated and insufficient response to the sacrifices made by female Civil War nurses, it stands as a testament to the power of their collective advocacy and the gradual, albeit slow, progress toward a more inclusive and equitable society.

## Justice Extended: Guardianship Case Studies

After Bickerdyke navigated the complexities of the pension claim process, she became acutely aware of the gaps in the system and the hardships that claimants faced while awaiting their rewards. Pension claims could drag on for years while claimants' conditions demanded more proximate attention. While the government was still deliberating over welfare responsibilities, Bickerdyke took initiative. She applied traditional concepts of motherly care to address welfare shortfalls in claimants' local communities. The following cases illustrate how Bickerdyke skillfully navigated the institutional framework of the pension system while simultaneously employing innovative, extra-institutional methods of care to ensure that the most vulnerable claimants received the support they desperately needed.

Over the course of her long pension process, Bickerdyke reconnected with veterans, whose encouragement and kind remembrances spurred her to become a more active and official advocate for pension work. From 1884 to 1887, she transitioned from San Francisco back to Kansas, where she connected with local men and women in need of care. The state had established a precedent for probate court guardianship as a legal term for oversight and distribution of estate funds. The pension distribution system did not anticipate a parallel type of guardianship for disabled veterans, and so probate courts took up cases as they arose, which was infrequently in Kansas. For her part, Mary Bickerdyke did not detect many discernible differences between the maternal obligation to veterans and the procedural mandates of traditional probate guardianship. Her role as "Mother" during the war expanded beyond any biological limitations of motherhood. Bickerdyke helped men and women gain their rewards; more importantly, she provided maternal support as they faced illnesses, loss, destitution caused by disability, and impending death. As historians of Civil War disability and war trauma have noted, disabled veterans struggled simultaneously to assert their masculine independence and admit their real need for assistance.[46] Bickerdyke stepped into this cultural negotiation and served them as she had on the battlefield: as a steadfast guardian, unwavering in her dedication to alleviating their suffering and ensuring that their compassionate care went beyond monetary reward.

### James H. Cook

James Cook lived in the same Kansas town as Bickerdyke. She had met him during his service and recollected his bravery as a private scout.[47] Cook had been rendered disabled during wartime imprisonment, which had lasted from December 1, 1864, to April 17, 1865. When he was released, he had lost a stunning ninety-three pounds and faced a daunting physical recovery. Twenty years later, the lingering effects of that bodily trauma rendered Cook unable to dress or feed himself, let alone work for his family's provision.[48] In addition, his marriage to Eliza Cook was fraught with conflict and difficulty and was aggravated by some of his grown children taking sides and requesting portions of his monthly pension award.

Initially, a GAR comrade corresponded with Bickerdyke, representing James Cook's interests. He inquired whether she might be able to help Cook get an increase in his monthly pension, noting that the local post had determined that the $30 stipend was insufficient to attend to his growing medical needs and complicated familial responsibilities.[49] Bickerdyke obliged, and Cook's pension was eventually increased to $50 a month. Additionally, the probate court of Russell County, Kansas, appointed William Richards to be Cook's official guardian to help ensure that the stipend was spent for Cook's benefit.[50] The probate court appointed a guardian when an individual could not make or communicate responsible decisions regarding personal care. The guardian could evaluate and make assessments for the individual concerning medical treatment, residential placement, social services, and various other needs for those under conservatorship. Once appointed, guardianship was legally binding, and the recipient of the services did not have easy legal recourse to change the court's designation.

The situation appeared initially to be resolved, but Richards neglected his official duty as Cook's guardian. Over time, the Cooks registered dissatisfaction and looked to the protective comradery of the local GAR to file a petition for a different guardian. The GAR petition complained that Richards had withheld permission for basic food and household supplies because he had determined that the family was unwisely spending on unneeded items. Such actions, the petition noted, were contrary to his guardian duties and put the Cooks in "destitute circumstances."[51] The case was left unresolved for several more months because Richards refused to appear in probate court, and the pension bureau's termination of the appointment hinged on his cooperative participation. Finally, Richards was dismissed as James Cook's pension guardian.[52]

In November 1889, the GAR post reached out again to Mother Bickerdyke and pleaded with her to intervene on behalf of the Cook family. Cook's Kansas GAR post officers determined that they needed a person of moral authority for Cook's guardianship, and they were familiar with Bickerdyke's commitment "to look after the poor old comrads [sic]." After hearing Cook's need, Bickerdyke took on the role of legal guardian and organized the backlog of convoluted paperwork caused by Richards's negligence. Without Bickerdyke's intervention, the GAR's independent legal battle and advocacy on Cook's behalf would not have had the same effect.[53]

Immediately after Bickerdyke took over guardianship, James Cook was placed into the Kansas State Military Home, where agents hoped to sort out his case in alignment with the most recent pension legislation. Bickerdyke was left to settle the dozens of merchants' accounts that the Cooks had accrued and continued to stockpile.[54] Letters poured in to Bickerdyke with late-payment statements and appeals for her advice, as Mrs. Cook and her daughters continued shopping without the means to pay. One store owner told Bickerdyke that when Eliza Cook sent her daughter in for more items while still owing him almost a hundred dollars, "I informed the girl that we could not let her have any more goods until we could hear from you unless she would bring an order from you."[55] Although it was a difficult decision for neighbors and businesses in a small town to make, Bickerdyke had now been given responsibility for managing and delegating the family's financial affairs.

Managing the Cook family's financial allowance became a primary duty of Bickerdyke's guardianship and forced her to assert her moral and maternal authority. To resolve all the bills that the Cook women had racked up at various businesses since 1889, Bickerdyke made the decision to give Eliza Cook a fixed allowance of $20 a month and provisions for food and fuel.[56] This move enraged Mrs. Cook, who complained that Bickerdyke was denying her a livable income. She threatened, "If this thing goes on much longer I shall have to go to some higher power to get my rights for I know enough about pension law to know that my mony don't have to go through a dozon [sic] pair of hands before I get it."[57]

Bickerdyke, on her side, felt justified in her position and decision and stood firm in her assessments as guardian. Bickerdyke faithfully followed the instructions of the court to provide for Mrs. Cook and settle community debts by devising her own system of distribution. However, Mrs. Cook constantly opposed this arrangement and rebelled against Bickerdyke's rules. Eliza Cook moved about the region, sent her dependent children off to live with her grown children, and sought temporary employment to supplement her stipend. As a result, Bickerdyke regularly chided Mrs. Cook for her financial decisions and began to provide moral instruction regarding her maternal negligence and resistance to peaceable community social norms.

Bickerdyke regularly wrote to the schoolmaster and requested attendance reports to ensure that Eliza was sending her children to school. Bickerdyke consulted with and confirmed Mr. Cook's wishes for the girls to be properly educated and therefore took it as her mission to ensure that this happened.[58] When Eliza sent her younger children out to her older children, without supervision on the long journey and in the middle of the academic year, the mother-guardian responded in no uncertain tone. When news reached Bickerdyke, she demanded an explanation: "Now Mrs. Cook tell me what you are going to do? How came you to break up house keeping and scatter your things as you did? Why didn't you tell me what you was going to do, did you ever have a better friend then I have been, Mrs. Cook? And if you wanted to break up, why didn't you send Fannie to me? Did you know that child went across the country in that dreadful storm . . . and if she had of been frozen, who would have been responsible, Mrs. Cook?" Bickerdyke spoke firmly, placing maternal judgment, expectation, and obligation squarely on Mrs. Cook's shoulders. She offered to house and educate young Fannie if Eliza could not accept her duty as the only capable parent. She gave Mrs. Cook the ultimatum: "Answer me candidly on this question [for] Fannie's destiny hangs on yes or no, and you are responsible."[59]

For Bickerdyke, court-appointed guardianship was not limited to her duty to discharge the monthly pension as she saw fit. Her intimate involvement caused her to go beyond the intentions of the institutions that employed her. Her definition of guardianship was determined by her sense of maternal authority and the ways that culture, religion, and personal experience had instructed her to guard the moral and physical well-being of the person or persons in need. In this case, Eliza Cook had failed to meet those cultural parameters of expected maternal behavior, and Bickerdyke leveraged not only her moral authority and reputation but also the unusual authority granted to her by the probate court. Eliza continued to go to battle with Bickerdyke, constantly fighting for more of James's pension money, even after she filed for divorce in the fall of 1891.[60]

After repeated disagreements over pension distribution, a special examiner was dispatched by the US Pension Bureau to review the case.[61] The examiner unequivocally sided with Mother Bickerdyke, who chided Mrs. Cook for neglect of her children, an untimely divorce request, and a culturally improper decision to take up with another man while requesting pension funds from her invalid husband. A separate examiner confirmed Bickerdyke's maternally driven moral evaluation that Eliza Cook was living in adultery while conducting "missionary work."[62] Bickerdyke balanced the issues of the distribution of pension money to the family and Eliza's perceived moral failures against James's medical needs and costs until his death in 1894.[63]

The situation with the Cooks was tedious, confusing in its details, and convoluted, as Bickerdyke was forced to make real-time judgments about human behavior and immediate medical and welfare needs. The probate court that assigned her guardianship did not provide a handbook with a set of guidelines and potential scenarios that she might face in the position. Instead, they trusted her as one "possessed of the necessary qualifications to enable her to render clients valuable service in the presentation of their pension claims and to advise and assist them as such."[64] Her good reputation and moral standing within the community were the only qualifications that she needed to be trusted with a family's life and wellness in her care. Pension guardianship was a fitting institutional arrangement for Bickerdyke because she was given official power to exercise her private maternal training in a public professional setting with little oversight and regulation but with significant authority.

*Thomas Bolton*

Thomas Bolton was born in Ireland and immigrated to the United States with his family in May 1848 when he was nine years old.[65] He enlisted in the Twenty-Seventh Massachusetts Infantry, where he served throughout the conflict as a private. Bolton was captured by Confederate troops at the Battle of Drewry's Bluff, Virginia, and was incarcerated at the notorious Andersonville Prison on May 15, 1864.[66] He was imprisoned for at least six months and developed health problems that plagued him until his death.

Upon his release from Andersonville, he was transferred to Savannah, Georgia, where Mother Bickerdyke oversaw a temporary hospital for former prisoners of war. Upon his arrival, Bolton was near death from malnutrition and scurvy. His friends found Mary Bickerdyke and pleaded with her to help. They recounted how she "snatched him from the grave and to him she was indeed and in truth *Mother* Bickerdyke."[67] Her reputation for homelike care had preceded her, and Bickerdyke's ministrations exceeded ordinary medical attention. Her maternal style and her aid in his recovery bonded Bolton to her and created lifelong trust in matters of both life and death.

After the war and his initial recovery from the scurvy that almost took his life, Bolton moved to Santa Barbara County, California. He joined scores of other Union veterans who migrated across the country in search of a new start on their own terms.[68] Some veterans struggled to reintegrate into their old family and community routines and expectations after the war, and the West offered an opportunity to exist among other like-minded veterans who understood one another's wartime experiences.[69] He put down roots in San

Francisco, and Bolton became active in the local GAR chapter. He struggled with his health and finances and eventually became estranged from his wife and lost custody of his only daughter, who was given over to a guardianship.

Bolton's personal situation and continuous health concerns caused him to try to utilize any resources that might help him as a veteran. At the age of 51, Bolton began to actively seek out his military pension and wrote to pension attorneys in Washington, DC. His first attorney, however, collected a devastating charge that accused Bolton of "Heavy Drinking."[70] Such an accusation had disastrous effects in pension cases of this era, where individual benefits were awarded based on sympathy and moral merit rather than completed service. To counter this damning claim, Bolton wished to leverage Bickerdyke's involvement in the case to procure a positive outcome. As his health deteriorated, he knew that if he did not receive his benefit before his death, he would leave his debts for surviving friends and family.

Hoping for a positive character reference to speak on his behalf, Bolton began to search for Mother Bickerdyke's whereabouts. Bickerdyke, struck by the urgency of Bolton's situation, went to work on his behalf. She wrote several letters to Kansas lawmakers and other men of distinction to assist her California friend. When Thomas Bolton received his certification in March 1891, Bickerdyke thanked her legislative contact, Senator Preston B. Plumb, and expressed her indebtedness to him for Bolton's pension.[71] Bickerdyke recognized the crucial role that influential men in government played in expediting pension requests, but her own moral authority as a nationally respected mother, known for her virtue and sound judgment, was even more critical. By advocating for Bolton, she helped him overcome damaging accusations of alcoholism and debauchery that could have jeopardized his pension claim. After he received pension certification, Bolton appointed Bickerdyke as the official pension attorney for his case.[72] He also granted her medical power of attorney, allowing Mother Bickerdyke to make binding health care decisions on his behalf. As the end of Thomas Bolton's life was near, Bickerdyke invited him to travel across the country and stay with her until his passing. Without saying goodbye to his daughter or friends, Bolton hastily made a will and boarded a train bound for Russell County, Kansas.[73] It was an extraordinary decision, predicated on an unwavering faith in Bickerdyke's nursing ability and the maternal comfort that she embodied.

He arrived in Russell with $80 to his name and a "shabby and soiled suit," Mother Bickerdyke remarked. "Now scarcely, his soul and body hangs together."[74] Bolton took to his bed as soon as he arrived, struggling even to sit up. For a month, Bickerdyke provided the highest level of care for this now-grown soldier boy. During his suffering and through his final moments, Bickerdyke felt assured that she had "done evry [sic] thing in my power, for his comfort. I spared not pains." As a final request, Bolton asked for a new suit for his burial, a gesture that reflected his hope for a meaningful and dignified death. Bickerdyke spent $35 of his money to buy a respectable blue three-piece outfit, a burial uniform fit for a long-suffering soldier of the Union army.[75]

The GAR network, while local in its functional nature, spanned the country. The GAR post of Russell, Kansas, understood its duty to help Bolton die, even though he was not a member of the local post. After his death, Bickerdyke published a "Card of Thanks" in the *Russell Record* on behalf of herself, Bolton, and his extended family: "We wish to extend out warmest thanks to the many friends who rendered assistance and words of cheer to comrade Dr. Thomas Bolton, of Lompoc, Cal., during his last illness at our home; to the citizens and GAR Post of this city for their kindly offices at his funeral and burial."[76] Dying as a Civil War veteran afforded men a sense of community that provided recognition of their sacrifice to the nation and, perhaps more importantly, an acknowledgment of their long suffering as co-witnesses to the horrors of war.

Mother Bickerdyke arranged for Bolton to be buried in the town's small burial grounds, and the paper noted that "Mother Bickerdyke took the same care of him as she would had he been her son, and members of the GAR were always ready to do all they could."[77] Bolton's sister, removed from her brother's death by 1,600 miles, was heartened to know that he had died in the company of a substitute family and was honored by men who shared the bonds of combat duty. For years, she arranged for Bickerdyke to place flowers by Bolton's grave each Memorial Day.

Bolton's final days were a gloomy affair. Afterward, Bickerdyke called it one of the saddest deaths she had ever witnessed. Her duties, both private and publicly recognized, were borne out of an intrinsically driven lifelong dedication to attending to the men who had sacrificed during the Civil War. She felt this way about veterans and their relatives, knowing that military service extended into veterans' homes as well. Without a government system in place to address the variable health needs of aging veterans and their families, extraordinary efforts, such as those demonstrated in the case of Thomas Bolton, represented her small contribution to her steadfast belief in their entitlement to care until death.

*Lucy Nicholson*

Bickerdyke's intervention in Lucy Nicholson's case stands out as a prime example of the swift, local assistance she provided when government aid was delayed. Harmon Nicholson enlisted to serve in the Second Michigan Cavalry and was eventually promoted to the rank of Union Major.[78] After the war, Nicholson and his wife, Lucy, settled among the first emigrants in Russell, Kansas. Harmon labored as a farmer and carpenter to provide a meager income for his family.[79] Despite his industriousness, Major Nicholson suffered years of failing health from a disease he had contracted during the war. The ailment resulted in "severe affliction upon his system, increasing in intensity until it ended his life."[80] By this description, he was eligible for the revised pension qualifications under the Arrears Act of 1879, but his rapid deterioration hindered his ability to apply for assistance. Harmon Nicholson died in 1887, leaving Lucy with little money and several children in her charge.[81]

In the years following Major Nicholson's death, Lucy's situation became more difficult to manage on her own, and creditors came after the Nicholson house in the summer of 1891.[82] In desperation, Lucy reached out to Mother Bickerdyke. Bickerdyke knew that Lucy qualified for a widow's pension under the Dependent Pension Act of 1890, but she was also acutely aware of the bureaucratic hurdles involved in applying for a pension. Immediate relief was the only practical solution for Lucy Nicholson, and such measures required a local effort and response while Bickerdyke worked on a longer-term solution from the pension bureau.

Along with Kansas GAR officers, Bickerdyke issued "Special Order No. 32," calling for donations of any amount to be remitted to "Mother M. A. Bickerdyke" for distribution to Mrs. Nicholson, a widow who was in "indigent circumstances."[83] Faithfully, GAR posts across the state of Kansas sent in $1.00 donations to Bickerdyke for Nicholson's aid.[84] Mother Bickerdyke acted as Lucy Nicholson's guardian during the contribution period, tallying the money received and circulating petitions for Nicholson's relief. Bickerdyke reasoned that if every Kansas GAR post contributed a proportional amount, they could raise close to $1,000 to pay off Nicholson's accrued mortgage debt.[85] The temporary financial assistance and Bickerdyke's campaign for relief allowed time for Nicholson to finally receive her pension, which she did in June 1892. During the yearlong process, Bickerdyke navigated the pension application while also ensuring that Nicholson's family received immediate support to survive the winter.[86] Both short- and long-term solutions were needed, and as a grassroots advocate, Bickerdyke was able to integrate solutions for individual cases when the government could not meet immediate relief needs.

PENSION DISTRIBUTION WAS anything but foolproof for recipient citizens, despite the government's ongoing attempts to cast a wide and liberal net of benefits. When those oversights affected Bickerdyke's extended network, she did not hesitate to step in and advocate for more localized support. Through her actions, she expressed her belief that it was a mother's responsibility to oversee the well-being of soldiers—the sons of the nation—and their families. She saw herself in a position of civic motherhood, marshaling health resources to serve those populations until her death in 1901. These case studies exemplify the role of civic motherhood in filling the gaps left by a government that was ill-equipped to fully support its veterans. Bickerdyke's efforts were successful largely because of the influence of maternal sentiment in shaping public discourse and policy.

Bickerdyke's story sheds new light on the complex interplay between gender, activism, and social welfare in the post–Civil War period. Her ability to navigate both formal institutions and informal networks of care underscores the fluid boundaries between public and private spheres, as well as the ways in which women's maternal authority could be leveraged for political and social influence. Bickerdyke's work contributes to an understanding of how gender shaped the development of American social policy in the late nineteenth and early twentieth centuries.

Mary Bickerdyke's legacy lies not only in the countless lives she affected through her direct acts of care and advocacy but also in the impact she had on the evolution of American social policy. Her work exemplifies how maternal compassion, woven into the very fabric of her public service and medical care, pushed the boundaries of what government support could and should provide. By stepping into a role of civic motherhood, Bickerdyke illuminated a path toward a more compassionate state and a model in which maternal care and public welfare were intertwined, setting the stage for the maternalist welfare reforms of the early twentieth century. Mother Bickerdyke's pension efforts demonstrate that societal progress often begins with the unrelenting determination to infuse institutional systems with empathy and human connection, and that the cross of old age and disability was not for soldiers and nurses of the Civil War to bear alone.

CHAPTER SEVEN

# The Passing of the Mother
## Mary Bickerdyke and Constructed Remembrance

Six years after Mary Bickerdyke's death, Jenkin Lloyd Jones found himself staring at a blank page, tasked with crafting a thirteen-page memorial that would encapsulate the life and legacy of the woman known as "Mother" to countless Civil War soldiers.[1] Jones had become a prominent Unitarian minister in Chicago after he established All Souls Church in 1885. He was widely known as one of Mary Bickerdyke's "boys" and had advocated on her behalf for her pension years before. During the Civil War, he served as a private in the Sixth Independent Battery, Wisconsin Light Artillery, attached to General William Sherman's Fifteenth Corps. His path often intersected with Bickerdyke's, as both endured the horrors of war. Jones first met her in the aftermath of the Second Battle of Corinth in October 1862, when she found him "a fever-smitten patient, weak and wasted, with an unwashed body, wrapped in a coarse flannel shirt, fouled by two weeks of fever."[2] For Bickerdyke, he was a stark embodiment of the dire sanitary conditions she fought to improve. With "helpful indignation," she firmly impressed on the young soldier the importance of hygiene. Jones later recalled how she "scolded me soundly, threw me into a capacious clean nightshirt, and slapped me around generally, but kept me in mind."[3]

Jones often retold this story at veteran reunions, his humiliation recast as a humorous tribute to Bickerdyke's maternal authority.[4] At just eighteen, young "Jenk" should have been home under his own mother's watchful care. Instead, the war had thrust Bickerdyke into that role, dispensing both discipline and medical expertise to young men in need of guidance and care. Her "blessed abusiveness and irrepressible cheer" left an indelible mark on those who survived because of her care.[5]

By 1892, Bickerdyke was long removed from tending to suffering soldiers, but she remained keenly aware of how she would be remembered. That year, she wrote to Jones, asking him to help solidify her national image. "My dear neglected soldier boy," she began, before explaining that the Kansas Columbian Association was assembling materials for the upcoming Chicago World's Fair. "There is a mantle piece at the Kansas building, made of Russell County rock, and my picture is to be hung over it . . . 28 by 32," she wrote. "I didn't put any placard on it, but left that for you to do. I thought you would know what to put on it better then [sic] I could with out being extravagant. How is 'Mother Bickerdyke who battled for the boys in blue from 1861–1865'?"[6] She signed this letter with affection as "Mother B."[7] The suggestion offers a striking glimpse into how Mary Bickerdyke actively participated in the construction of her own legacy. By enlisting allies like Jenkin Lloyd Jones, she strategically crafted the narrative surrounding her wartime service, ensuring that she would be remembered not just as a nurse but as a national symbol of selfless devotion and maternal care during one of the country's greatest crises.

Remembering Mother Bickerdyke was not as simple as compiling a record that enumerated her tender ministrations, firm rebukes, and professional accomplishments. Such an account was interpreted and composed amid a swell in national sentiment related to Civil War remembrance, which gained momentum in the late 1880s and continued through the turn of the century. Surviving soldiers like Jenkin Lloyd Jones met annually at Grand Army of the Republic (GAR) encampments and, through their jolly campfire reunions, reconstructed the meaning of the Civil War for themselves and for the nation. Historians have addressed the importance of remembering for Civil War veterans toward the turn of the century, a period that Gerald Linderman referred to as the "revival" of soldiers' memories.[8] David Blight highlighted how veterans' competing memories often clashed with public memory, ultimately hindering the development of a professional historiography of the war.[9] As Civil War veterans aged, their collective acts of remembrance helped shape a historical narrative that honored their experiences and influenced how the war—and figures like Bickerdyke—would be remembered for generations to come.

The reconstruction of Mary Bickerdyke's legacy was shaped by her own efforts and those who worked alongside her, both the allies who amplified her image and those who were later erased from her story. This chapter explores these layers of remembrance: Bickerdyke's intentional shaping of her legacy, the biographical narratives that emerged late in her life, her sons' efforts to defend her memory, and the overlooked role of Lydia Foster, her longtime ghostwriter whose contributions remain largely absent from historical accounts. Unpacking these layers of mythology and purposeful reimagination reveals how perspectives, narratives, and meanings shift over time. The human experience is continually framed through filters of gender, race, class, interpretation, and memory, ultimately producing a repurposed historical narrative. This process, which Michel-Rolph Trouillot termed the power of production, underscores the ways history is constructed and reconstructed.[10] By unraveling these threads, a new generation of historians can engage with the complexities of the American past and reconsider how figures like Bickerdyke have been remembered.

## A Decade Behind Mother's Pen: Lydia S. Foster

Lydia Foster was a young, educated Black woman who served as Bickerdyke's live-in housekeeper and amanuensis during the last decade of her life. Foster played a crucial role in Bickerdyke's work as a pension attorney and advocate for Civil War veterans, yet her contributions have been largely omitted from historical narratives. This omission reflects broader patterns of racial, class, and gender exclusion in post–Civil War memory. By rendering Foster invisible, the historical narrative perpetuates the notion that Bickerdyke's accomplishments were the result of her own efforts, obscuring the critical role that Foster's labor and literacy played in enabling Bickerdyke's productivity.

Throughout her life, Bickerdyke relied on scribes and assistants for letter-writing and accounting, a practice she continued in her later years when she hired Foster. Despite Foster's significant role, Bickerdyke's biographers have barely acknowledged her, omitting details of her race and labor.[11] Ultimately, Lydia Foster's contributions to Bickerdyke's success were significant, and the exclusion of those contributions illuminates the preferential treatment given to White motherhood in the historical record. Recovering Foster's role not only challenges these historiographical silences but also offers a fuller, more nuanced understanding of Bickerdyke's legacy. By uncovering the hidden labor behind the "Mother" persona, this chapter reveals the complexities of race, gender, and power in shaping historical narratives.

After thirty years of professional struggle and frequent relocations, Bickerdyke made one final move to Kansas in 1888. Limited opportunities for women forced her to constantly seek positions suited to her skills as a palliative care nurse. The death of her stepdaughter Mollie from breast cancer in 1887 prompted her decision to "settle down" with J. R. in Russell, Kansas.[12] Reflecting on this final phase of her life, Hiram noted, "Mother was at home with Brother James longer than at any other time since 1861."[13] By the time she made it home to Kansas, she had won a long pension battle backed by the Woman's Relief Corps, and the accompanying campaign had resulted in new biographies that brought her Civil War activities back into the national conversation.

After establishing herself in her new home, the seventy-one-year-old—never one to stay idle—took on several cases as a pension attorney and guardian for Civil War veterans. This position required a considerable amount of correspondence, and Bickerdyke understood her limitations. In addition, it was during this period that she began to receive attention and renewed correspondence with former soldiers and colleagues because of the newly published biographies that featured her wartime exploits. Taken together, the load was far more than she could handle on her own, so she hired Foster to help carry the professional burden.

Mary Bickerdyke's sustained employment as a pension guardian and attorney for the US Pension Bureau was dependent on Lydia Foster's labor. Foster's indirect employment for the US Pension Bureau adds a dimension to Brandi C. Brimmer's concept of a "grassroots pension network."[14] That network, which Brimmer identified as a Southern system that grew out of the "development and maturation of black institutions and political achievements in the electoral arena during the Reconstruction era," reached northward to Kansas and other US regions as Black families migrated out of the South in the post-emancipation era. Foster's work within the extension of the grassroots pension network signals the possibility that other educated Black women may have been involved in the procurement of government pensions for both Black and White men and women in the late nineteenth century.

Very little is known about Lydia Foster outside of the few notes left behind in the Bickerdyke record and the sparse birth, marriage, and death notices. What is available implies the fascinating social dynamics of the post-emancipation American West and the nature of historical construction, wherein her labor was folded into Bickerdyke's accomplishments. Lydia's father, Wesley Foster, was a veteran of the Forty-Ninth Wisconsin Regiment of the United States Colored Infantry, and her mother, Eliza-Ousley Foster, was the White daughter of a poor Kentucky farmer.[15] Because of the slow change in state miscegenation laws, the couple was illegally married in Rock Island, Illinois, in 1872.[16] Their first child, Lydia Foster, was born a year later while they still lived in the Prairie State. The Fosters emigrated to Kansas around 1878–79, a move that coincided with the Exoduster migration from the South.[17]

Compared to Illinois, legal attitudes in Kansas toward race, including interracial marriage, were less severe, although not necessarily more progressive.[18] The 1859 Kansas Constitution opened the state to all settlers, regardless of their ethnic or racial background.[19] After the Civil War, Kansas advertised itself as a potential place for African Americans to settle, find a sense of relative freedom, and cultivate land ownership and self-employment. The recruitment campaign was successful, and between 1860 and 1870, the African American population in Kansas rose dramatically from 625 to 17,108.[20] Black settlement concentrated primarily in the eastern part of the state, particularly in Atchison, Douglas, Leavenworth, and Wyandotte counties, but the Fosters found themselves in the middle-western part of the state, in Russell County, where the total population went from 156 in 1870 to 7,351 by 1880.[21] Their move from Illinois to Kansas coincided with Benjamin "Pap" Singleton's Exoduster movement in 1879. As the Fosters came to Kansas, so too did up to 10,000 former slaves from the Deep South.[22] By 1880, Wesley Foster and his young family had established themselves with other Black farmers in the area.[23] The Fosters maintained a 200-plus acre farm that brought home $175 worth of production in 1875.[24]

Historians have investigated the literary societies of the urban North to expand the understanding of early Black literacy. Although technically free, the Northern population of Black men and women faced systemic resistance to their desire to gain and use literacy. To combat this, Black men and women sought to ensure that they would not be excluded from the benefits of education and developed literary societies in many cities across the North.[25] The significance of Black education in small communities outside the South is understudied in the post-emancipation context, particularly in its earliest forms prior to larger waves of migration.[26] In one documented case in southeastern Kansas, the ambivalent implementation of Jim Crow laws allowed for Black children to be educated in separate classrooms until the school board decided to erect a "separate but equal" facility for "Black scholars" a mile across town, literally on the other side of the railroad tracks.[27] Such an example is instructive of early educational arrangements but does not necessarily apply to the Fosters and other Black migrants before *Plessy v. Ferguson*. This court decision provided legal justification for institutionalized segregation in education. In the small hamlet of Center, Russell County, where the Fosters lived, the 1880 census reveals that approximately seven out of the 305 families were Black, and five of those families had school-age children. If they were able to attend school, they likely joined other White students in the town or county and may have been separated into another room by race, as seen in other cases. Or, Lydia Foster might have been educated alongside White boys and girls in a one-room schoolhouse because the community demographics did not provide the resources for a separate classroom and instructor.

When Lydia was hired to work for Mary Bickerdyke in 1887, she was approximately fifteen years old.[28] Her ability to compose and dictate correspondence skillfully suggests that she had received a formal education. To contextualize her schooling, a comparison with another Black family in Russell County, the Browns, is useful (see table 7.1). According to the 1880 census, Sarah Brown (age 18), Mahala Brown (age 11), and Mary A. Brown

TABLE 7.1 Comparative Black literacy in Russell County, Kansas, 1880

| Name | Age | Race | Township | County | Occupation | Cannot Read | Cannot Write |
|---|---|---|---|---|---|---|---|
| Lydia Foster | 6 | Black | Center | Russell | — | — | — |
| Sarah Brown | 18 | Black | Russell | Russell | Attending school | — | — |
| Mahala Brown | 11 | Black | Russell | Russell | Attending school | — | Yes |
| Mary A. Brown | 9 | Black | Russell | Russell | Attending school | Yes | Yes |

Data compiled from the 1880 US Census. Census Place: Center, Russell, Kansas; Roll: 395; Page: 59C; Enumeration District: 290. Tenth Census of the United States, 1880. (NARA microfilm publication T9, 1,454 rolls). Records of the Bureau of the Census, Record Group 29. National Archives, Washington, DC.

(age 9) all attended school, likely at the same or a similar institution that Lydia attended later in the decade. The census data provides insight into literacy acquisition among Black youth at these ages: Mary A. Brown had not yet gained literacy, Mahala could read but not write, and Sarah had presumably attained full literacy. This pattern suggests that between the ages of 11 and 15, young Black women in rural Kansas schools typically acquired reading and writing proficiency. The history of Black education in Reconstruction-era America demonstrates the implementation of educational reform as men and women strove for excellence and rigorous academic achievement. Black literary pursuits were built on the examples set forth by Black legacies such as James Forten, who was a vocal advocate for Black education decades before the Civil War and emancipation made widespread Black literacy a reality.[29] But like Forten before them, the Fosters and countless unheard others understood the essential nature of education for Black Americans in the contentious but liberating postwar environment.

Bickerdyke's move to employ Lydia Foster allowed her to be one of the few women engaged in pension attorney and guardian practices. During Lydia Foster's decade of employment in the Bickerdyke household she was listed officially in the census as a "servant," but it is evident from family correspondence that her role went far beyond that description.[30] Her archival record contains over 200 letters to various parties from 1891 to 1894, almost all penned by Foster and likely only a portion of the actual volume of letter-writing associated with her position.[31] After Bickerdyke's eightieth birthday in 1897, Foster kept a discreet correspondence list in the back of an autograph book created by Bickerdyke's friends as a birthday gift.[32] It shows one snapshot of the extensive secretarial work required as "Mother's" amanuensis, listing dozens of letters written each week.[33] The fact that Lydia's role was never publicly acknowledged, while Bickerdyke received all the praise for her work on behalf of Union veterans, highlights how gender, race, and class norms were being challenged—though only in private. Foster's use of literacy as a tool within this restricted sphere became her sole means of asserting public agency.

Bickerdyke's use and exploitation of Foster's literacy indicate that she recognized she needed cheap labor to achieve her professional goals as a pension agent and guardian, knowing that her own abilities could not match those of a young, educated ghostwriter. But Bickerdyke also shrewdly took advantage of Foster's Blackness, leveraging her talent to dictate correspondence, cook meals, and clean houses—presumably at a lower price than a White servant and ghostwriter would have demanded. Could Bickerdyke have achieved the same volume or impact of pension work without exploiting the social and racial dynamics that were deeply embedded by the late nineteenth century? That question cannot be answered without considering the perspectives of either Bickerdyke or Foster; however, it is crucial to acknowledge Bickerdyke's complicity in the power structure that put her White motherhood on a pedestal while Lydia Foster's personhood held its support in place.

After Bickerdyke's death in 1901, Lydia continued to keep the house clean and occupied for James's benefit. She did the work at a meager wage and was allowed only $5 a month for her efforts. Professor J. R. Bickerdyke spent most of the year at a boarding house as a superintendent of a school.[34] He encouraged Foster to collect money by selling eggs from the Bunker Hill farm. When writing to his brother in Montana, Bickerdyke expressed his obligation to Lydia's welfare, stating that "again, Lydia seems a part of my family as she took care of Mother for 10 yrs."[35] She may have been "part of" the family, but the racialized and gendered tasks assigned to Foster were folded into the work agreement.

While she was still living, Lydia Foster's literacy allowed Mary Bickerdyke to maintain her productivity well beyond her professional prime. Foster's excellence behind the pen of a revered White mother is a powerful reminder of the influence that White Americans have had in crafting a narrative about their own accomplishments that, for much of the nation's history, should rightfully be attributed to people of color. As Trouillot observed, "Any historical narrative is a particular bundle of silences, the result of a unique process, and the operation required to deconstruct these silences will vary accordingly."[36] As history has revered Mother Bickerdyke as an archetype of patriotic American motherhood, even at the turn of the twentieth century, her words were largely interpreted, dictated, and skillfully produced by a Black woman. The result is a large collection of letters that were interpreted through a "unique process" of historical construction, and Mother Bickerdyke's voice should be heard through Lydia Foster's interpretive perspective during this period. Foster's excellence behind the pen of an admired White mother is also a powerful reminder of the "thicket around the truth" that Bickerdyke's historical and memorial narrative has suggested.[37] The "bundle of silences" that surround Foster's contribution required a chance discovery to begin the process of deconstruction because contemporary voices never acknowledged Foster's contribution.[38]

The insatiable thirst for education characterized the postwar cultural environment for Black Americans who had been legally denied the dignity of literacy under slavery. In the post–Civil War South, "a whole race [was] trying to go to school. Few were too young, none too old, to make the attempt to learn," according to Booker T. Washington.[39] However, commitments to educational excellence were not new in the Black community after the Civil War's end. Historians have underscored the long lineage of learning for Black people, even in the face of unjust literacy laws and systemic oppression. Kabria Baumgartner writes about Black women dating back to the beginning of the nineteenth century who cultivated literacy as a form of "purposeful womanhood" that represented "a way to resist white supremacy and second-class citizenship while promoting black civil rights."[40] Black literary societies bloomed and flourished across the urban North as freed people sought "places of refuge for the self-improvement of their members but [also] as acts of resistance to the hostile racial climate that made the United States an uncomfortable and unequal place for all black Americans, regardless of their social or economic position."[41] Literary societies were necessary because the common school movement of the 1830s was framed around ideas of education for citizenship, which excluded Black Americans until after the passage of the Fifteenth Amendment.[42]

The juxtaposition of a historically recognized, well-regarded, and covertly uneducated White mother with her concealed, forgotten, and skilled Black laborer reveals the complexities of how Mary Bickerdyke navigated authority and respectability. Denied educational opportunities in her youth, Bickerdyke relied on amanuenses like Lydia Foster to navigate literacy challenges. However, she strategically obscured Foster's role to maintain her own image of competence and middle-class professionalism. This dynamic reflects the broader historical pattern that Jacqueline Jones Royster identifies, in which Black women's labor and intellect have been "persistently subjected to measures of value and achievement that have been set and monitored by others, who have not had their interests or potential in mind and who have been free historically to discount, ignore, and disempower them."[43] Bickerdyke's role as a "Mother" granted her the respectability and leadership often denied to women in a patriarchal society, yet it also conferred upon her the power to condescend to and control those under her charge, particularly Foster. Despite her reliance on Foster's skills, Bickerdyke's determination to cast her collaborator in the shadows demonstrates how she upheld outdated cultural norms of respectability, positioning herself as the singularly capable figure in her professional sphere.

This reveals another dimension of what "Mother" meant—one deeply embedded in the racial ideology of paternalism. Just as paternalism couched practices of hierarchy and exploitation in familial language, maternalist attitudes could do the same, legitimizing power structures under the guise of care. As Corinne Field's work illustrates, age and generation intersected with gender in ways that shaped authority and subordination, and Bickerdyke's role as a maternal guardian reinforced her dominance over Foster, despite the latter's crucial contributions.[44] In this dynamic, Foster's labor was recast as service to Bickerdyke's authority, illustrating how maternalist power depended on the subordination of others' work. The authority of adulthood—something sexism often denied to women—was conferred upon Bickerdyke through the label of "Mother," granting her both the legitimacy to lead and the power to exert control over those she deemed dependents. By examining Bickerdyke's reliance on Foster, it becomes evident that maternalist authority operated as a means of care and as a tool of racialized control, reinforcing hierarchies even within spaces of supposed female solidarity.

Switching between modes of care in public and private spaces throughout her life involved the intersectional dynamics of race, class, and education. Examples of amanuenses from Mary Bickerdyke's archival records demonstrate the complexities and intersectionality of historical construction while illuminating the community dynamics that made categories of class, race, and gender a means of competition during the late nineteenth century.[45] Examining Mary Bickerdyke's relationship with her most long-standing amanuensis, Lydia Foster, explores the cultural pressures of middle-class professionalism for women who were forging their way in the public sphere. Women's rights activists, particularly Elizabeth Cady Stanton, reconfigured emerging

164 *Chapter Seven*

sociological thought to position White women as "mothers of the race," using this construct to justify female enfranchisement.[46] Bickerdyke, striving for respectability and opportunity, seems to have internalized these ideas, adopting an approach that prioritized her own visibility at the expense of acknowledging the contributions of those who worked alongside her. From Civil War soldiers to a Black woman, those who wielded the pen for Bickerdyke offer new insight into class, race, and identity in post–Civil War America. Her engagement with middle-class respectability politics suggests that she adopted a Stanton-styled Comtean positivism, requiring the subordination of others' efforts to sustain the image of her individual success.

For Bickerdyke to be embraced as a "Mother" in American consciousness, she had to rely on the assistance of others to meet the expectations of maternal devotion and professional competency. This was difficult for several reasons, mostly because she had not completed the same levels of education or secured a comfortable income that could support her endeavors. But her strategic choices to obscure the contributions of others reflect the slow and uneven nature of social change, even for women who pushed boundaries in other ways. Her correspondence demonstrates that she continuously ran in middle-class social circles, and as such, she took measures to communicate with them in middle-class ways. Consequently, her contemporary and posthumous biographies memorialized her as a model of maternal sacrifice and patriotic devotion. However, this narrative is deceptive. A deeper examination of archival materials reveals layers of interaction and rich social dynamics that complicate the image of Bickerdyke as an independent maternal model of dogged industriousness mingled with patriotism. Looking behind the pen exposes a more intricate reality that shows how the work of others, particularly Lydia Foster, was instrumental but uncredited in shaping Bickerdyke's public legacy.

The erasure of Foster's contributions raises significant questions about how motherhood was constructed and remembered. Why did Bickerdyke, her later biographers, and even her own sons withhold recognition from Foster, who undertook a substantial portion of the labor on Bickerdyke's behalf? Whether the decision was deliberate or simply a consequence of historical context that habitually left Black contributions out, the effect was that Lydia Foster was made invisible while Mother Bickerdyke's fame was bolstered in her final years and up to the present day in historical representations. The public saw a venerable White mother hitting her professional stride in her late years while the labor and voice and intellect of a Black woman was ultimately behind her success. This follows the trend that some historians have noted: nineteenth-century White motherhood was built on the backs of

Black motherhood.[47] In this case, Bickerdyke's maternal prominence relied on Foster's invisibility.

Unless someone is carefully scouring an archive, painstakingly scraping for some nugget of discovery, these bits of information stand to be lost and erased, as "opaque winding sheets" with no sharp outline of truth to tell.[48] The process of tracing a lower-class White woman's path toward professionalism led to the discovery of the even more deeply obscured legacy of Lydia Foster. Recovering her story allows this work to reinstate a Black voice in the historical record, restoring a narrative that has long been buried. Like Charlotte Forten and other Black educators and intellectuals, Foster understood the critical role of education in the postwar era, when opportunities for Black advancement remained contested but deeply significant. Moreover, this case underscores a broader truth: Black voices were integral to constructing White histories, even when their contributions were ignored. There must be a diligence to identify the systemic structures that have buried Black influence and excellence and accomplishment in the national narrative. Without Lydia Foster, an important aspect of Mary Bickerdyke's professional development would not have reached the archive for historical discovery.

Mother Bickerdyke was a complex figure whose life defied easy classification. While she was revered in her time as a servant deserving of honor, her story is far more nuanced than a basic internet search would suggest. Her struggle with class identity and limited education compelled her to redefine traditional notions of motherhood, forging a path that was uniquely her own. Through determination and perseverance, she leveraged maternal authority to break into spaces that might otherwise have excluded her. Yet this same authority was used to obscure those who enabled her success. Her story is not only a powerful testament to the agency of individuals in shaping their legacies, but it is also a reminder of how historical memory often privileges certain narratives at the expense of others.

Bickerdyke's legacy has been celebrated, but for reasons that fail to account for the full scope of her experience. A more accurate understanding of her impact would recognize her struggles and the people she relied on to achieve success. Her failure to publicly acknowledge these individuals meant that she reinforced racial and class hierarchies rather than challenged them. The burial of contributors like Foster was not merely an oversight; it was a structural issue tied to the broader cultural elevation of White motherhood at the expense of Black women's labor and intellect. Uncovering this hidden narrative sheds light on the complexities of social and professional mobility for women in the late nineteenth century, particularly those from marginalized backgrounds. Foster's silenced voice speaks to the persistent devaluation of Black women's contributions. It underscores the need for a more inclusive and nuanced approach to history that actively works to recover the voices that shaped, but were written out of, the past.

### Preparing for Mother's Death: Communicating Life and Legacy through the Grave

Mary Bickerdyke clearly understood the power of memory and the importance of controlling her own story. Her reliance on Lydia Foster's literary skills while deliberately choosing to omit Foster's contributions suggests a woman keenly aware of how narratives shape legacy. This awareness extended beyond her lifetime, as Bickerdyke took deliberate steps to ensure that her memory would be preserved and celebrated long after her death. Her meticulous preparations for her final resting place reflect this historical consciousness. Despite the many years and miles that separated her from her husband's grave in Galesburg, Illinois, she remained steadfast in her desire to be buried beside him. In doing so, she established Galesburg as her adopted hometown and the site of her memorial.

Bickerdyke's experiences as a Civil War nurse, surrounded by death, prepared her for her own inevitable fate. Prior to the war, Mary and her young children buried Robert Bickerdyke and the couple's infant daughter at Linwood Cemetery in Galesburg. Though healthy and robust, Mary knew that her position in the war put her in harm's way. Her participation meant that she was not only exposed to battlefield combat conditions but also regularly worked in close contact with communicable diseases. Aware of these risks, Bickerdyke took steps to secure her final resting place. In September 1863, before heading deeper South for the Vicksburg campaign, she formally purchased the cemetery plot next to her husband's.[49] Without such arrangements, her remains might have been left in an unmarked battlefield grave or in a hospital cemetery. Before the government established a formal system for naming and recording the Civil War dead, Bickerdyke ensured that a permanent, identifiable burial site would be accessible to her surviving family members.[50]

The Illinois town was far from Bickerdyke's ancestral family in Ohio and her eventual home in Kansas, but Galesburg became her adopted hometown because her family was now integrated into the soil of the town. When Bickerdyke turned eighty, she wrote from her home in Bunker Hill, Kansas, to an old acquaintance from Galesburg, Sue Allen. Like Bickerdyke, Allen was a Woman's Relief Corps (WRC) member, an organization charged with publicly remembering Civil War veterans and fallen. Allen's response to Bickerdyke indicated that the gravesite needed some maintenance and preparation. The deed drafted during the war was "in bad shape," according to the secretary of Linwood Cemetery.[51] In their initial effort to remake the arrangements, the Galesburg committee struggled to find the correct plot, indicating that the Bickerdyke headstones had suffered severe neglect and damage between 1859 and 1897. Despite these challenges, Allen and the citizens of Galesburg were eager to include Bickerdyke in the process of restoring her final resting place. The renewed interest in her legacy, fueled by a resurgence of her fame in the 1880s and 1890s, conferred a sense of honor upon her. Allen emphasized this sentiment in her letter, writing that there were "not words in our vocabulary to express the esteem in which you are held and remembered by Galesburg people."[52]

For the Galesburg GAR, for Mary and J. R. Bickerdyke, and for Civil War–era Americans in general, the acceptance of and preparation for death was a community process. Bickerdyke gave the WRC committee precise directions to help them locate her husband's grave and her prospective plot. She wrote, "Enter the southeast gate. And go up the street until you come to the street turning North. It is a corner lot on the left-hand corner facing the North. There was Maple trees set out all along the streets 36 years ago. It must be quite a forest now. There were two Maple trees and two Evergreen trees on my lot. They were from 20 to 25 ft high when I last saw them."[53] Bickerdyke's vivid recollection of the spot where she buried her husband thirty-seven years earlier reflects the indelible mark left by grief.

By early 1898, members of the Galesburg GAR post made a formal offer to the Bickerdyke family to arrange and execute the aging Mother's final wishes:

> Our local Post remembering with gratitude the noble services of "*Mother*" *Bickerdyke* during the late war and . . . that this was her home before the war and recognizing the fact that sooner or later our spirits will take their flight and our bodies be committed to mother earth feel it incumbent upon them to ascertain what her wishes are as to her final resting place and for that purpose [we have] appointed a committee. And if it be her wish to be buried here by the side of her husband to offer their assistance in any way. That her wishes may be carried out.[54]

Just as Bickerdyke had guided so many through their final days, preparing their spirits for departure and ensuring their bodies were laid to rest, the people of Galesburg embraced their role in honoring her legacy. The war and its lasting presence in public memory, particularly among surviving veterans, expanded the community of care beyond the immediate Bickerdyke family.

Recognizing this, the Bickerdykes welcomed Galesburg's involvement in the planning process. Accepting the committee's offer of assistance, the family worked alongside them to carefully plan how "Mother" would be remembered at her final resting place.

Upon hearing news of her illness and just days before Bickerdyke's death, the Galesburg GAR communicated with J. R. Bickerdyke to finalize the family's wishes. The post's commander promised the son a "fine appropriate funeral," assuring him that a crowd of mourners and post members would attend the graveside services for Bickerdyke.[55] When Mary Bickerdyke died on Friday, November 8, 1901, at 3:40 p.m., Kansas mourners were poised to remember her before her body would be transported to Galesburg. Bunker Hill citizens crowded the high school assembly hall to lay memorial wreaths and hear speeches of remembrance from neighbors and friends.[56] A monthly subscription periodical for Civil War veterans, the *Western Veteran*, dispatched a special correspondent to share Bickerdyke's funeral proceedings with the nation. The publication's coverage not only memorialized Bickerdyke's passing but also openly affirmed the family's decision to inter her in Galesburg, reinforcing the town's significance in her legacy and legitimizing her final wishes within the broader public memory.[57]

For posterity, J. R. recorded the songs that were sung at the memorial, including some that his mother had chosen years before her passing.[58] The first selection, "I Would Not Live Alway," was played at Robert Bickerdyke's funeral in 1859 and therefore had obvious sentimental ties for the entire family. When Mary Bickerdyke suffered from a protracted illness in 1885 in San Francisco, she made sure to remind her son of the song's significance in her life, death, and remembrance.[59] The hymn's author drew the singer to the biblical story of Job, who suffered devastating and repeated losses as a test of his faith and trust in God's careful design and control over human activity.[60] Job was acutely aware of life's frailty, God's sovereignty, and the hope and promise of heaven's reprieve from earthly suffering. Such a message resonated deeply with Mary Bickerdyke, who had repeatedly witnessed the death and suffering of those surrounding her. To her last minute, she poured out her life as a nurse, a guardian, a mother, and an advocate so that her patients and "her boys" could live and die with the dignity of competent care. She knew and communicated through her professional and personal life the sentiments of her family's memorial hymn:

> I would not live alway: I ask not to stay
> Where storm after storm rises dark o'er the way;

The few lurid mornings that dawn on us here,
Are enough for life's woes, full enough for its cheer.[61]

As Mother Bickerdyke's body was escorted to Galesburg by the Santa Fe Railroad, the GAR and WRC posts in Galesburg prepared the entire city to receive her body as a community of mourners. They adorned buildings with flags and black crepe and opened local homes to veterans who traveled to the small town to pay tribute to "Mother" Mary Bickerdyke.[62] Mourners and well-wishers poured their condolence letters and remembrances out to J. R. Bickerdyke. After reading five different papers and the *Western Record*, one woman remarked to J. R., "I think it must be very gratifying to you to see how much she was beloved and esteemed by all who knew her I hope you will become reconsiled [sic] to the loss it is just as natural to die as to be home."[63]

For J. R. and the Galesburg community, the monumental task of remembering "Mother" was transferred to them upon her death. J. R became fiercely protective of his mother's memory and took on several tasks of remembrance in collaboration with Galesburg's various interested parties. The Galesburg WRC, for example, "started a movement" to raise money to erect a stone monument at Mary Bickerdyke's grave—a $3,000 project.[64] For the purposes of fundraising for the gravestone, the WRC created a separate Mother Bickerdyke Memorial Association to plan, organize funds, and hire the appropriate workers for the headstone.[65] Many Illinois WRC posts were interested in the endeavor, and the humble task of acquiring an appropriate headstone expanded into a broader memorial project. The headstone monument was finally installed during a "small affair" in late June 1904 while the Mother Bickerdyke Memorial Association continued making plans for a more fitting memorial.[66] Curious about its appearance, James wrote to a nephew and requested that he travel to Galesburg to ensure that all previous agreements were intact. The nephew reported back: "Well in answer to the monument yes it rests at the end of her grave and stands five feet high and 2 1/2 or 3 feet wide and about 1 1/2 ft thick its of gray marble no they did not molest your father's monument."[67] His parents, it seems, were finally at rest.

## "The Passing of the Mother": The Bickerdyke Sons' Attempt at Historical Construction

J. R. Bickerdyke embarked on a singular mission in the months and years following Mary Bickerdyke's death in 1901. He assembled, organized, and recruited willing participants who could help solidify his version and vision of his mother's legacy. He became obsessed with his family's genealogy, a hobby that his mother also shared in her later years. When he shared aspects of his own heritage, he manipulated details to attribute esteemed American heritage to the Bickerdyke name. Additionally, he used familial connections to recruit a famous poet to write a memorial poem celebrating Mother Bickerdyke. And finally, he picked battles with his mother's most recent biographer, Julia Chase, and the Kansas State Historical Society as he jealously worked to guard his mother's legacy, turning it into something of his own design. He was successful in his efforts to some extent, as some of J. R.'s derivations on the truth have made their way into twenty-first-century encyclopedic entries.[68]

Within weeks of his mother's death, J. R. wrote to Will Carleton in New York to inquire whether he might be interested in writing a poem to memorialize Mother Bickerdyke.[69] Will Carleton rose to literary prominence in the United States after the publication of "Over the Hill to the Poor House" in 1872 and subsequently became a regular contributor to *Harper's Weekly*. The piece attracted national attention for its exploration of the plight of the elderly and poor in an era of newfound social concern. The poem tells the story of a son who found independence and success in the West but used his earnings to care for his struggling and aging mother, which may have resonated with J. R. in his own life.[70] Carleton became renowned for his poetic descriptions of rural, Midwestern life. He focused his verses on the simplicity and monotony of everyday existence. Through a rustic Americana style, Carleton wrote dramas, comedies, and tragedies that depicted the complexity of the human experience through relatable scenes. J. R. may have been impressed by Carleton's 1877 Decoration Day elegy for Arlington National Cemetery titled "Converse with the Slain." The fifty-five-verse poem featured a dialogue between the living and the dead that earned him accolades, especially from those interested in preserving the memory of the Civil War, like J. R. Bickerdyke.[71]

Will Carleton's impact on the literary scene of the late nineteenth century was regional and contemporary. In 1886, the Columbus, Nebraska Lyceum organized a debate: "Who is the greater poet, Burns or Carleton?"[72] The comparison to Robert Burns reflected Carleton's Midwestern reputation as a poet of the people, whose plain, sentimental verse aimed to capture the experiences of everyday rural Americans much as Burns had memorialized the lives and dialect of Scottish farmers. Others across the country provided more critical reviews of Carleton's work. Newspapers commented on public readings performed by Carleton, observing, "Mr. Carleton doesn't seem to have any idea of expression or elocutionary effect and recites the lines in a rapid monotone, that almost fails to convey their meaning to the hearer."[73] Other literary critics insisted he was "no poet." But readers saw worth in his style enough to come to his defense. One editorialist commented, "Will Carleton is not a Shakespeare; but he has had the courage to be simply Will Carleton. The critics fight shy of him, but the common people receive him gladly."[74] Despite mixed reviews, Carleton filled high school gymnasiums, hotel halls, and county fairs across Kansas and the Midwest.

Carleton's initial correspondence back to J. R.'s cousin, George Washington Clark, indicated the popular poet's disdain for such targeted invitations of commissioned work. Despite this reluctance, he expressed admiration for Mary Bickerdyke, stating that her "noble life and character appeal both to the imagination and the heart."[75] Recognizing Carleton's interest, Clark immediately wrote to his cousin, urging J. R. to send biographical materials and books to New York without delay: "The poetic spirit is evidently moving him. I guess he will write the poem."[76] J. R. acted quickly, gathering his mother's materials and responding to Carleton's request by December 23, 1901. The documents J. R. provided shaped the narrative Carleton would craft, effectively guiding the poet's interpretation of Bickerdyke's legacy. Carleton ultimately incorporated his poem about Mother Bickerdyke into a larger collection published the following year.

Shortly thereafter, Will Carleton published *Songs of Two Centuries*, a collection of poems that included "Passing of the Mother: Mary A. Bickerdyke—War Nurse." The volume was dedicated to "the memory of the nineteenth and the success of the twentieth," signaling the collection's intention to juxtapose the nation-building experience and struggles of the past with the future possibilities of America.[77] As an anthology, *Songs of Two Centuries* was organized into several sections of poems that created a narrative arc highlighting both the natural and the societal splendor of the United States. In his typical style, Carleton celebrated common scenes, places, and occurrences to make his case for America's greatness with poetic collections that celebrated "Songs of Months and Days," "Songs of Home Life," "Songs of Pleasure and Pain," and so on. Each subsection of poems addressed ordinary subjects—"Farmer Stebbins at the Fair," for instance, or "Up in the Loft"—that describe the humble majesty of American life and the dedication of hardworking, industrious farmers and homesteaders, who provided for themselves and their communities with "plenty an' to spare."[78]

The section that included the poetic ode to Mary Bickerdyke was entitled "Songs of the Nation." The eighteen poems contained within spanned both centuries, starting with a poem called "Greater America" to the Civil War's "The March of the Volunteers," jumping to "In the Wreckage of the Maine," about the invasion of Cuba in 1898, and ending with the more prophetic and prescriptive "Liberty's Torch."[79] Meant to be a tribute to a successful American project, Carleton was preoccupied with the way that wars both tore apart and built up the American national ethos. Carleton used the warning of past grief and death to admonish present and future peace, lest Americans suffer the same personal tragedies wrought by the wars of the nineteenth century. "Do not forget the wounded," he warned. "Study the past: my words have all been said."[80] National messages were communicated through the individual stories of patriotic but tragic loss.

"The Passing of the Mother" was the four-page result of Carleton's "poetic spirit," with Bickerdyke as his muse. The poem depicted an imagined scene of her entering heaven at the end of her long life, where she was welcomed by "swift-footed legions" of veterans who honored her above any king, queen, or millionaire to have passed through the pearly gates before her.[81] In the poem, she was as insistent in her death as in her life on maintaining humility, and Bickerdyke responded to the effusive praise accordingly: "My heroes, 'tis done: Rise to your feet, every one. Naught in my work was of grandeur or beauty: Love was my countersign—Help was my duty."[82] The poem then shifted perspectives, as one by one, soldiers recounted how she had saved them from a bitter death or eased their suffering through her battlefield care. Notably, these characters framed her legacy around her success in palliative care and her particular caregiving approach—simultaneously motherly and medical, displaying the "Heart of a Christian and nerves of a Stoic" who "Charged with her might on the cohorts of Grief—Gave every suf'ring relief."[83] This idealized portrayal reinforced the mythology surrounding Bickerdyke, celebrating her as a singular force whose compassion and resilience transcended traditional boundaries of gender and professional identity.

One of the three soldiers in the poem assumed the voice of the Fort Donelson soldier whom Bickerdyke found after she heard his moaning, determined to carry out her midnight mission after detecting life in the frozen scene.[84] Each of the three soldiers echoed the tales that had been repeated for decades. Understandably, Carleton chose those anecdotes that promised the most literary flair for the purposes of the poem. His aim and accomplishment were to capture the essence of the widespread esteem for Bickerdyke. It was a sentiment that superseded reality, but that was the crux of Carleton's interpretation. Where Bickerdyke felt she was simply performing a duty assigned to her, the impact of her actions extended beyond earthly expression.

The fourth and final visitor in Carleton's vision of heaven was none other than Jesus, "the Christ of Humanity."[85] His climactic exchange between Bickerdyke and Jesus Christ served as the culmination of her celestial orientation and Carleton's poetic interpretation of her character. The Son of Man presented Bickerdyke with a crown, symbolizing her Christian inheritance and the culmination of a life dedicated to service. Yet, true to form, Bickerdyke refused to accept the reward without protest, responding:

> Then said the woman, "O Master of Mission!
> Hear thee, I pray thee, a humble petition
> Let me work on, my vocation pursuing:
> Nought have I done to what yet needs the doing.
> Stow this sweet gift in some worthier place,
> While I still toil for my race!"[86]

Her response, marked by a distinct nineteenth-century hubris cloaked in humility, reflected her tireless devotion to duty. Here stood an aged, "wrinkled and weary and old" eighty-four-year-old woman who, even in death, rejected divine reward in favor of continued labor.[87] To a turn-of-the-century audience, her refusal may have appeared admirable; it was a testament to her unyielding dedication to others and her country. No one who knew Bickerdyke's story would question the volume or impact of her work or her propensity to rebuke idleness. Carleton's ending subtly suggested that no amount of reassurance, no declaration of a life well lived, could satisfy her restless spirit. Even in the afterlife, Bickerdyke was unwilling to embrace the finality of rest.

Carleton's "The Passing of the Mother" served as a tribute and an instructive model, reinforcing patriotic ideals of labor and sacrifice within the larger collection of poems. Through Bickerdyke's example, Carleton urged Americans to commit to productive work that would contribute to national development. Bickerdyke's dutiful help, accomplished through love of men and country, saved the nation from division and allowed for the perpetuation of liberty. In this vision, individual freedom required the willing sacrifice of all citizens in the performance of their assigned duties across gender, class, and race.

The narrative arc of Carleton's "Songs of the Nation" reflects the exceptionalist imperialism common in turn-of-the-century American thought. Carleton did not hide his pride for his country—"Grandest of nations earth ever has known!"—while mourning the harrowing journey and cost of the trek toward inevitable greatness.[88] Bickerdyke's presence in the collection also underscored the gendered nature of care-switching, the fluid movement between public and private caregiving roles that enabled women's professionalization. She embodied a cultural transition as she shifted between domestic maternal care and battlefield medical work, ultimately transforming both into a patriotic duty. By positioning her as a model for women's labor in the nation-building project, Carleton reinforced the idea that professional caregiving was not just a skill but a moral and national obligation.

The lukewarm reception of Carleton's "The Passing of the Mother" and its eventual obscurity underscore the complexities of historical construction and the limits of controlled legacy-making. Despite J. R.'s efforts to enshrine his mother's memory through poetry and Carleton's literary reputation, the poem failed to secure a lasting place in the national consciousness. This outcome reveals the unstable nature of public memory, where even well-intentioned commemorations are subject to shifting cultural priorities and competing narratives. Carleton's attempt to frame Bickerdyke's life within the patriotic and moralistic framework by placing her memorial poem in the "Songs of the Nation" section of the volume reflected a broader effort to position women's professionalization within the rhetoric of national service. However, the poem's idealized portrayal of Bickerdyke ultimately reduced her to a symbol, detached from the material realities of her labor and the gendered and racialized systems that shaped her work.

## The Straight of It: Controversy over Mother's Legacy

The most significant and accurate biography of Mary Bickerdyke was written in 1896 by Julia Chase. By then nearing eighty, Bickerdyke worked closely with Chase, providing details and clarifying omissions or embellishments found in earlier biographical accounts. The two women shared a genuine friendship during Bickerdyke's years in Kansas, collaborating on several projects for the Kansas WRC. Chase's deep connection with Bickerdyke informed her yearslong effort to produce the most definitive work of Mother Bickerdyke to date.[89]

Chase's goal was twofold: to write the book as a dictated firsthand account of Bickerdyke's life and to fundraise for the WRC.[90] Her job, as she understood it, was to abide by the wishes of the Kansas WRC and Mary Bickerdyke to write an authentic biography of Bickerdyke's life.[91] Released in time for Bickerdyke's eightieth birthday, the Kansas GAR sent out resolutions and general orders that every local post should procure "one or more copies of the admirable book on the life and services of Mother Bickerdyke," securing a welcomed reception for the book and guaranteed revenue.[92] The work ultimately cost the WRC more money than it made.⁹³ Chase titled the biography, *Mary A. Bickerdyke, "Mother": The Life Story of One Who, as Wife, Mother, Army Nurse, Pension Agent and City Missionary, Has Touched the Heights and Depths of Human Life*. After its publication, Bickerdyke took great pride in this version of her life's events and advertised the book to veterans who contacted her, asking for a $1.00 contribution to WRC funds.

In January 1902, just months after Bickerdyke's passing, Chase presented her book's findings in a paper to the Kansas State Historical Society, aiming to document and memorialize the major events of Bickerdyke's life. However, the public reading of this personal history unexpectedly sparked a minor local controversy, exposing tensions in contemporary historical practice and the competing claims over how Bickerdyke's legacy should be remembered. Some citizens of Saline County, Kansas, contended that Chase's portrayal of the facts conflicted with their own recollections of events. Aware of the influence of the historical record, they were determined to challenge her account and contribute their own perspectives. Dan Wagstaff, the main editorialist in the controversy, took umbrage with Chase's account of events and publicly stated in the local newspaper that her reports of the 1868 "Indian raids" were false. In an article titled "The Straight of It," he claimed that many "old timers" of the town were asked about their memories of the raids, and they reportedly contradicted Chase. Wagstaff confirmed that "all testify to the inaccuracy of Mrs. Chase's contribution to the history of this county."⁹⁴ Chase's credibility as Bickerdyke's primary historian was publicly called into question. Facing direct challenges to her work, she turned to the Bickerdyke sons and the Kansas State Historical Society, seeking their support in determining how to respond.

The situation frustrated Chase and mortified J. R. Bickerdyke, both of whom felt responsible for representing Bickerdyke's legacy. The dispute centered on fewer than two pages of Chase's 145-page book, specifically minor details regarding the location of the raid, the participants, and the nature of the injuries sustained by White settlers.⁹⁵ However, Chase's focus was not on the raids themselves but on Bickerdyke's response and her efforts to mobilize resources to alleviate suffering in the aftermath. Letters from Bickerdyke's archive documented her appeals for rations and clothing to aid the "extreme suffering and destitution of these Setters [*sic*]."⁹⁶ Despite documentary evidence of Bickerdyke's involvement, the historical discipline at the time lacked standardized norms for resolving such disputes. In the end, as was often the case, the prevailing interpretation was determined not by factual accuracy but by those with the most societal power.

Chase clapped back in her own defense, using the same public forum as the editorialists. In the *Salina Daily Republican-Journal,* Chase disagreed with the editorialist's corrections, citing her distrust of Dan Wagstaff as a trustworthy source.[97] While she was writing the book, Chase had access to the letters kept in the Bickerdyke house but was unprepared when the integrity of her documentation and interpretation was called into question several years after its initial publication. She hoped to obtain a statement from J. R. and Hiram, who were teenagers at the time of the raids and likely had some memories of the events as well as knowledge of their mother's involvement.[98]

Because the book claimed to be an authoritative biography, supervised by Bickerdyke herself, the falsification of a single event might unravel the validity of the whole book. Chase and the Kansas State Historical Society were more concerned with the validity of the project and were unwilling to squabble over details with the Salina objectors. As a result, Chase decided to "eliminate the portion of her paper about which there is controversy."[99] The secretary of the Kansas State Historical Society, George W. Martin, weighed in on Chase's decision and explained to J. R., "I think this is wise, because your mother's main reputation as an army nurse is beyond question, and it should not be effected by a controversy of this character."[100]

Chase did not realize how fraught the act of historical construction would be when she took on the Bickerdyke project. In defense of her work, she explained her methods and sources as transparently as possible. She responded to the accusations in a letter to the *Salina Daily Republican-Journal*:

> [Bickerdyke] gave me the Indian raid story, as I have it in the book. I copied from the book for this part of my sketch for the Historical Society. I also copied from the "History of Kansas" compiled by A. L. Andreas, and published in 1883. I found there, on page 210, the statement regarding the extent of the raid and the action of Gov. Crawford, which seemed to corroborate what Mother Bickerdyke had told me, and in these years since the book was published, this is the first time, so far as I know, that the account has been called into question.[101]

Chase defended her efforts to faithfully construct a historical narrative. She received the assault on her book and her integrity with humility and humor but showed obvious frustration that the work would come into question so long after its publication and after Bickerdyke's death, forfeiting the possibility that she could defend her own story.

This controversy highlights fundamental questions about historical construction: Whose account should be believed—Mother Bickerdyke's or Dan

Wagstaff's? Which details mattered, and did they alter the broader interpretation of events? The dispute between Chase and Wagstaff reflected a larger shift in the historical discipline, transitioning from a predominantly literary genre to a social scientific field.[102] It also underscored an enduring challenge for historians who navigate "the shifting theoretical ground we all now seem to occupy."[103]

While the specifics of the raid were significant to those who had lived through it, they were peripheral to Chase's purpose. She intended to narrate the ways that Bickerdyke had "touched the heights and depths of human life," as her title advertised. She had the instincts of a historical thinker: argumentation built on available evidence. Upon a more detailed investigation of her claims, it became clear that while Chase and Mother Bickerdyke did not falsify their accounts, Bickerdyke misremembered a couple of details about the attacks.[104] Hiram sent J. R. several clippings and documentary evidence that corroborated the narrative written by Chase, but J. R. was too overwhelmed by the whole affair to publish those findings.[105] The newspaper debacle, which questioned her integrity, did not deter Chase from her archival work.[106] Instead, she incisively thanked the detractors for "the thoughtful warning of the coming thunderbolt" but sardonically reassured any readers: "I'll survive the shock. . . . I am in no danger of having to resign my position as housekeeper."[107] Julia Chase was not pretending to be a leading authority on the Salina Indian raids of 1868. The controversy sparked by "The Straight of It" revealed the limitations of adjudicating historical disputes in the early twentieth century and foreshadowed the ongoing reinterpretation of Bickerdyke's legacy long after her death.

J. R., however, did not emerge from the controversy with the same resilience. He jealously guarded his mother's legacy after her death but struggled with the weight of her absence. Immersing himself in schoolwork, he left his Bunker Hill home in the care of his mother's housekeeper, Lydia Foster, finding it "lonely and forsaken since dear Mother has gone."[108] Over the next year, he seriously considered leaving the home he had lived in for over thirty years to reunite with his younger brother Hiram and his family in Montana. Though he claimed to be in "excellent" health, his lifelong battle with chronic illness made such periods of wellness fleeting. On December 25, 1904, at the age of 55, James Robert Bickerdyke passed away before his brother could respond or reach his bedside.[109]

J. R.'s death disrupted Mother Bickerdyke's estate, which included her documents, artifacts, and possessions. With no surviving relatives in Kansas to oversee the materials, questions arose about inheritance. A trunk of goods was sent to Hiram in Montana, while some letters were donated to the Kansas State Historical Society for research. However, others felt entitled to portions of Bickerdyke's legacy, particularly those that J. R. had kept. Julia Chase believed she had been unfairly denied items that had been promised to her and felt mistreated by J. R. in the process. After dedicating herself to Mother Bickerdyke's memorial, Chase worried that all that work might be destroyed when the estate was dissolved after his death. She had hoped that J. R.'s death would create an opportunity to recover the work and other promised mementos from Bickerdyke's possessions.[110] She complained to a local friend, "[J. R.] never so much as thanked me or reimbursed a penny of the expense I incurred. Now I presume he never even published it, and if this manuscript is among his papers I feel it properly belongs to me. Don't you?"[111] Chase contacted Hiram with the grievance as well, citing her care for "Mother" on her deathbed and her care for James in the weeks after their mother's death. She requested a few copies of any surviving memorial booklets as promised compensation for her work on the project and "some little remembrance . . . a book, or cane," of Mother's.[112]

The principles of mourning dictated that Chase's proximity to Bickerdyke at the end of her life afforded her some physical artifacts to properly remember her. In Chase's mind, J. R.'s refusal to let go of his mother's things or his decision to ignore her was an unwarranted snub. Hiram responded kindly to the "very frank letter" from Chase.[113] He offered an apology for his brother's ill-treatment and told her that he did not think that J. R. ever published the booklet, partially due to financial constraints. His letter insinuated that the larger issue was that his brother was influenced by the "statements made by the Papers Published at Saline disputing the *truthfulness* of Mother's statements on facts and incidents concerning the Indian Raids of 1868."[114] The public indictment on his mother's story and Chase's interpretation made J. R. "most hopeless" and "much depressed."[115] The incident only exacerbated the nervousness that had overcome the elder brother after his mother's death. After J. R.'s passing, Hiram assumed charge of his mother's papers and used professional resources in Kansas to try to determine the best course of action for preserving her documents or keeping them in the state archive. He kept some for himself, donated some to the state archive, and told Chase, "As to the book you speak of you shall have it. As to a memento or any thing you desire of Mothers in remembrance, you are entitled to it. *Name it.*"[116]

These episodes give insight into the acts of historical construction that subtly shifted Mother Bickerdyke's legacy after her death. Multiple parties believed that the "true" history had yet to be fully extracted, weaving different versions into their own interpretations. As the historical discipline transitioned into a professionalized social science, facts became paramount, and the flowery prose of the nineteenth century was increasingly dismissed as unreliable. Salina's residents rejected Chase's account in favor of their own, despite documentary evidence that could have proven otherwise. In his correspondence with Chase, Hiram Bickerdyke insisted that he could provide records to set the record straight regarding the Indian raid. However, he recognized his limited authority, especially if George Martin, a key player in Kansas historical preservation, sided with the Saline County citizens who wished "the whole matter cut out."[117] Resigned, Hiram admitted, "If this be so I have no desire to intrude, or push any documents contrary to the feelings of any citizens of the State of Kansas."[118] It seemed improbable to Hiram Bickerdyke that he could change the minds of those who firmly subscribed to their version of events, and it was a fool's errand to make the attempt.

George Martin stated soon after that he would gladly receive any papers that Hiram was willing to furnish, believing that "history will finally rest on documents and not on opinions."[119] Martin clearly explained his theory on history, trusting that the documentary evidence could produce the cold, hard facts to clear up any doubts about the chronological record of events. He viewed professionalized history as a shift toward objective data collection rather than interpretive storytelling.[120] Data gathering became paramount to the discipline, employing archivists like Martin to collect and organize the facts that could eventually produce the type of historical synthesis envisioned by the leaders of the discipline.[121] In Martin's estimation, Chase was part of a previous generation of historical works, and she provided too much opinion and interpretation of Bickerdyke's life and legacy. Martin, though, was not a professional historian. His understanding of the developing philosophies of historical research ultimately undermined Chase's influence and reflected local antiquarians who were obsessed with details that mattered only to them. Sadly, Chase's interpretation, a valuable resource that focused on her subject's substantial contribution to nursing and the palliative care process, fell victim to the judgments of the men who claimed authority with their new scientific methods. As a result, subsequent interpretations of Bickerdyke's legacy continued to misrepresent her contributions, shaped by those who wielded authority over accounts of the past.

As I Knew Her

When Florence Shaw Kellogg initially contacted him in 1905, Hiram Bickerdyke was skeptical of her inquiry to use Mother Bickerdyke's personal papers and manuscripts to start yet another book project.[122] Unfamiliar with his mother's friends and with few connections in the community since his brother's passing, Hiram—who had not lived in or visited Kansas since he was young—knew he needed help to find someone who could honorably capture his mother's legacy. He turned to Julia Chase, believing that she knew more about Bickerdyke's local relationships. "What do you know about her?" he asked. "My opinion is that [Kellogg], without Mother's presence, cannot compile the story as you did ... and do the subject justice."[123] Eventually, with Chase's blessing, he decided to give Kellogg permission to pursue the writing project.

Kellogg, working under the direction of Unitarian minister Jenkin Lloyd Jones through the Abraham Lincoln Center in Chicago, produced *Mother Bickerdyke, As I Knew Her*. Though the title suggested a close friendship, Kellogg and Bickerdyke were likely only casual acquaintances, living in the same Kansas town during Bickerdyke's later years.[124] Kellogg's account mentioned occasional visits until illness prevented her from leaving home in 1895, after which she received encouraging letters from Bickerdyke.[125] Their relationship was sparsely detailed in Kellogg's book, appearing only 126 pages into the narrative, and is largely absent from archival records.

Kellogg was not a professional historian, and much of her book was a near duplication of Chase's earlier biography, incorporating entire excerpts from Chase's work and Mary Livermore's *Story of the War*. Notably, Kellogg was the only Bickerdyke biographer to mention Lydia Foster, describing her as a "maid servant" whom Bickerdyke treated "more like that of a daughter ... than of one who worked for the weekly wage," but she omitted Foster's race and role as Bickerdyke's amanuensis.[126]

Since *As I Knew Her* was produced under Jones's supervision, its content reflected his interests as a Unitarian minister. For example, an entire chapter on Bickerdyke's religious life was the first of its kind in any biographies of her life. The book claimed that Bickerdyke was "not creed-bound in any way," a truly Universalist sentiment.[127] The chapter afforded Kellogg space to include conversations she had with Bickerdyke that indicated the impetus for her creedless faith. Kellogg's conclusion was that Bickerdyke had been "consecrated by sorrow."[128] Kellogg argued that Bickerdyke's deep faith and ministry of palliative care were born from the multiple personal tragedies that she had faced. Kellogg recalled a conversation wherein Bickerdyke shared that in the years prior to the war "God had taken seventeen of those I loved best from me—among them my husband.... By my sorrow I was taught sympathy for others' sorrows, by my suffering I learned how to lessen the sufferings of others."[129] Kellogg argued that Bickerdyke was led to palliative care during the Civil War because she had an acute understanding of sorrow and felt that a divine power consecrated her for the work. Her understanding of death and its processes prepared her for the work on the battlefield attending to the Civil War dead:

> Tenderly as his own mother might have done, she listened to the last, low-spoken words of the dying soldier, soothingly she sang his "Swan Song," as death came nearer and nearer, and his soul, upborne by her singing, by the thoughts of love and home and Heaven, of which she sang—floated bravely out into the silence—God's silence. Tenderly then she gathered up the little keepsakes he had cherished and wrote the letter to send with them to those who waited at home. . . . Think how many times she did this through those dreadful years. What but mother love could have prompted it? What but God's love could have sustained and strengthened her for it all?[130]

Decades after the war had concluded, these persistent thoughts and conversations continued to occupy Bickerdyke, highlighting the importance of her life's most defining work. Unfortunately, these significant memories of the war and her reasons for pursuing palliative care, even with their religious implications, were obscured by the repetitiveness of the first half of Kellogg's narrative. Such analytic treasures rewarded persistent readers, but the tropes and repeated anecdotes found more influence in popular memory.

The other significant contribution of *As I Knew Her* was its introduction, which was the promised memorial to Mother Bickerdyke by Reverend Jenkin Lloyd Jones. As the editor of the book, Jones had creative and financial oversight over the biography.[131] His introduction, filled with emotional and proselytizing rhetoric, framed Bickerdyke's contributions in a cosmic moral context. A Civil War veteran turned pacifist, Jones used the opportunity to argue for an end to war: "For war is to cease, not because it becomes too expensive, too terrible, or so triumphant that none dare challenge it, but because human nature will become too noble; men will grow too wise and women too influential to resort to such coarse, cruel and wasteful settlements of disputes."[132]

Jones also misrepresented Bickerdyke's origins, elevating her lineage without documentary proof. His assertions were far more questionable than the small historical errors in Chase's Salina stories, but no one cared to set the record straight. Jones presented Bickerdyke family lore as though it were gospel truth, asserting that Bickerdyke's compassionate patriotism stemmed from a lineage that coursed through the family's veins. He claimed that Bickerdyke's "best blood" connected her to the *Mayflower* and that her grandfather had assisted George Washington during the crossing of the Delaware, later receiving socks from Martha Washington in return. Jones further claimed, without evidence, that "the blood of her paternal grandfather mingled with that of Mary Ball, the mother of Washington."[133] Future historians seeking to retell Bickerdyke's story inherited an additional layer of myth to unravel. Jones's fabrications became deeply embedded in public memory, as later writers trusted his account as a firsthand source on Bickerdyke and regarded him as a respected spiritual leader. His perceived credibility led others to repeat and reinforce his claims, further entrenching the false history.[134]

The construction of Bickerdyke's legacy was complex: shaped by the efforts of her sons, the selective narratives of her biographers, and the broader forces of historical memory and forgetting. Ultimately, the enduring power of Mary Bickerdyke's example lies in her individual achievements and in the collective impact of the countless women who became professionals after the Civil War. From the nurses and widows who found solace and support through pension claims to those inspired by her courage and determination, Bickerdyke's legacy endures as a testament to the transformative power of compassion, dedication, and an unshakable belief in the dignity and worth of human life.

# Epilogue
## What Did Mother Mean?

In 1897, the Woman's Relief Corps (WRC) of Kansas opened a facility that they named the Mother Bickerdyke Home and Hospital. The home was established by the WRC as a gendered annex to the state soldiers' home. The main facility was dotted with small cabins to house aging Civil War nurses or soldiers' widows and their dependent children. The WRC was keenly aware of Bickerdyke's commitment to the lives and deaths of veterans, and the facility's name represented that acknowledgment. At the dedication, Bickerdyke joined them to clearly articulate her decades-long mission: "No widow or orphan, of those gallant heros [sic] who have passed away, must be neglected. And there is no such thing as fail. Little by little things are done in this world."[1] The WRC envisioned the facility as "a monument" to her work, ensuring that nursing care and relief remained available to those who had sacrificed during the war.[2] As she and the other nurses of the war aged, the facility signaled a gesture of state-sponsored health care and relief.

After Bickerdyke's death, the Mother Bickerdyke Home and Hospital continued to be a sanctuary for the elderly women, nurses, and widows and their families who had served and sacrificed in the Civil War. The WRC continued its annual tours of the facility for several years, even after its financial management was transferred to the state in 1901. The organization felt a lasting sense of duty to honor Bickerdyke's legacy. After one of these tours, Alice Long of the WRC reflected on this enduring tribute, describing how Bickerdyke's presence "smiled at us from above the entrance, bidding us a motherly welcome to the home that she loved so well."[3] She continued in her report:

> We were also shown over the Home and were all pleased to note the evidence of the generosity of the various corps all over the state, in the comfortable, even elegant, furnishings. It made us proud of our womanhood and of our order to see the generous provisions for these near and dear the brave men who saved our union, and who, though "non-combatants," fought the hardest battle of the war. The little family who have here found refuge looked so comfortable and showed such evidence of the good care they receive that I could not help thinking that if ever the hand of misfortune should be laid heavily upon me and I, poor and bereft, a soldier's

widow, should be compelled to seek shelter in a Home, that I could wish for no more homelike a retreat than could be found at the Mother Bickerdyke Home.[4]

Long's description of the home as a dignified and comforting refuge underscored how deeply the values of care and service shaped its mission. In many ways, the facility reflected the evolution of Bickerdyke's own career, bridging the personal and institutional aspects of caregiving.

Over the course of her more than forty-year nursing career, Bickerdyke had transitioned from institutional to private care nursing, navigating the professional barriers placed on women in medicine. The Mother Bickerdyke Home and Hospital transformed her personal efforts back into an institutionalized and sanctioned model of care, illustrating how the profession had come to recognize women as competent medical authorities. It also affirmed the growing acceptance of structured, "homelike" environments for end-of-life care. Far from "doing nothing" in the face of death, Bickerdyke anticipated and responded to the values of her generation as they aged and neared life's end.

The Mother Bickerdyke Memorial Cemetery lies on a hill overlooking Ellsworth, Kansas. The small cemetery is the final resting place for thirty-two women who were Civil War nurses, widows, or daughters of Civil War veterans. They were "Mothers" in their own right, each one known for her maternal abilities and competencies to heal and help, both during the war and afterward. The women interred in the small country plot died between 1902 and 1919 and were residents of the nearby Mother Bickerdyke Home, connected to the war by service or by the death of their loved ones. Their names, less recognized than Bickerdyke's, are the incomplete remnants of the Civil War era of women who knew enough of death and dying to feel themselves capable nurses and proto-professionals to the men of the Union army. They inherited the fruits of Bickerdyke's lifelong labor to provide peaceful and dignified deaths. Even after she was gone, Bickerdyke was able, through this institution in her name, to give proper and honorable deaths to the Civil War participants to whom she dedicated her life's work.

Mary Bickerdyke's multiple motherhoods, both ordinary and extraordinary, both simple and intricate, give an incisive and alternative perspective into the changing United States from before the Civil War until the turn of the twentieth century. Bickerdyke's personal and professional lives during and after the war complicate broader historical narratives of how White women's primary roles as mothers intersected, interfered, or otherwise affected their attempts to work outside the home. Despite many scholarly attempts by notable historians, a persistent tale of domesticity pervades the popular consciousness of this period of American history. Bickerdyke's professionalism over the course of several decades is just one more story in the attempt to shift the view toward women's consistent and constructive workplace contributions in the wake of the Civil War.

This book provides an example of a woman whose participation in that shift toward maternal professionalism did not come from progressive ideologies or determinations of women's right to work. Instead, Mary Bickerdyke was committed to traditional ways of home care, and in many ways, her methods were anathema to the changes in the medical profession that were happening around her. She preferred and professed medical techniques, particularly in the arena of palliative care, that reflected more traditional norms and customs surrounding the "good death." In other areas of care, she relied on home remedies but was also not opposed to the intervention of medical professionals in cases that required specialized knowledge, as was seen in her stepdaughter's cancer case. Over time, Bickerdyke deftly blended old and new medical approaches and therapeutics in a way that put those under her care at ease as Americans slowly started to rely on doctors and hospitals for their health care. Her trusted position as a mother was a critical component in that process.

Cultural ideas of motherhood shifted across class and geography in the second half of the nineteenth century as women, like Bickerdyke, asserted their maternal identities for various purposes and in different settings. It should be telling, for example, that the woman who is historically known as Mother Bickerdyke existed primarily in lower-class contexts, rather than the middling ethos that has dominated the understanding of nineteenth-century White mothers. Where Catharine Beecher, Sarah Josepha Hale, and other cultural contributors shared stories of and instructions for mothers, Bickerdyke exemplified how one's motherhood could be shared beyond domestic spaces. As she neared the end of her life and continued to advocate for women's pensions in the wake of their husbands' deaths, Bickerdyke's interactions with these women show a changing attitude of the national government toward women that would eventually culminate in more sweeping protections and reforms in the early twentieth century.

Public performances of femininity and motherhood during the Civil War era influenced popular ideas and conversations about mothers for the rest of the century and into the present. Without Bickerdyke's persistent and notable actions during the Civil War and the stream of biographical literature that followed, she would not have had the same grassroots impact that she did. Many veterans and their families could rely on Bickerdyke's public performances during and then after the war as reassurance that their continued care mattered and should matter to the state. In this instance, Bickerdyke's maternity signaled a lasting commitment to veteran care that emboldened old soldiers to seek help and assistance as they aged.

Of course, this work is not conclusive. There still could be, and likely will be, future interpretations of Bickerdyke's efforts. Even more likely are the ways that parts of her archival collection will be used by historians to make any number of observations about the nature of motherhood or mothers' work during the Civil War period. The richness of further research lies in the exploration of women's roles in institutional development in the western United States. Bickerdyke's ventures into private nursing in Nevada and California reveal how rudimentary the medical structures of the far West were in comparison to their eastern counterparts.

The results of this research demonstrate the intricacies of a singular life, left behind in fragments and remembered in diverging ways. It reveals the beautifully complicated task of the historian and the endless possibilities that historical inquiries have to offer. There were moments during the research process when some intimate knowledge and deep understanding of Mary Bickerdyke and what her motherhood meant felt within reach. One such moment emerged with the discovery of a short sample of handwriting included in a letter from Hiram and James Bickerdyke to their mother (see figure E.1).

The letter begins with a set of symbols drawn by Hiram, which, according to his brother, were arranged in a hieroglyphic-like form meant for their mother to interpret. The image captures a moment of childhood playfulness—Hiram's cryptic script reflecting youthful mischief while his older brother's commentary suggests both amusement and exasperation at the use of valuable paper. Their fraternal dynamic is evident in this undated note buried deep in Bickerdyke's papers. Like the symbols on the page, the emotions behind them remain layered with meaning. It is easy to imagine the smile that must have crossed Mother Bickerdyke's face as she opened the letter, followed by a bittersweet ache and an acute awareness of the distance that separated her from her sons' daily lives, their developing personalities, and the private jokes she could only partially decipher from such a distance. She had made decisions that reflected her own desires and the pressures of her long-term economic situation. She wanted what was best for her children, for herself, and then for the men and women who would become her adopted children under her care. Moments like these revealed the competing emotions of fulfillment and heart-

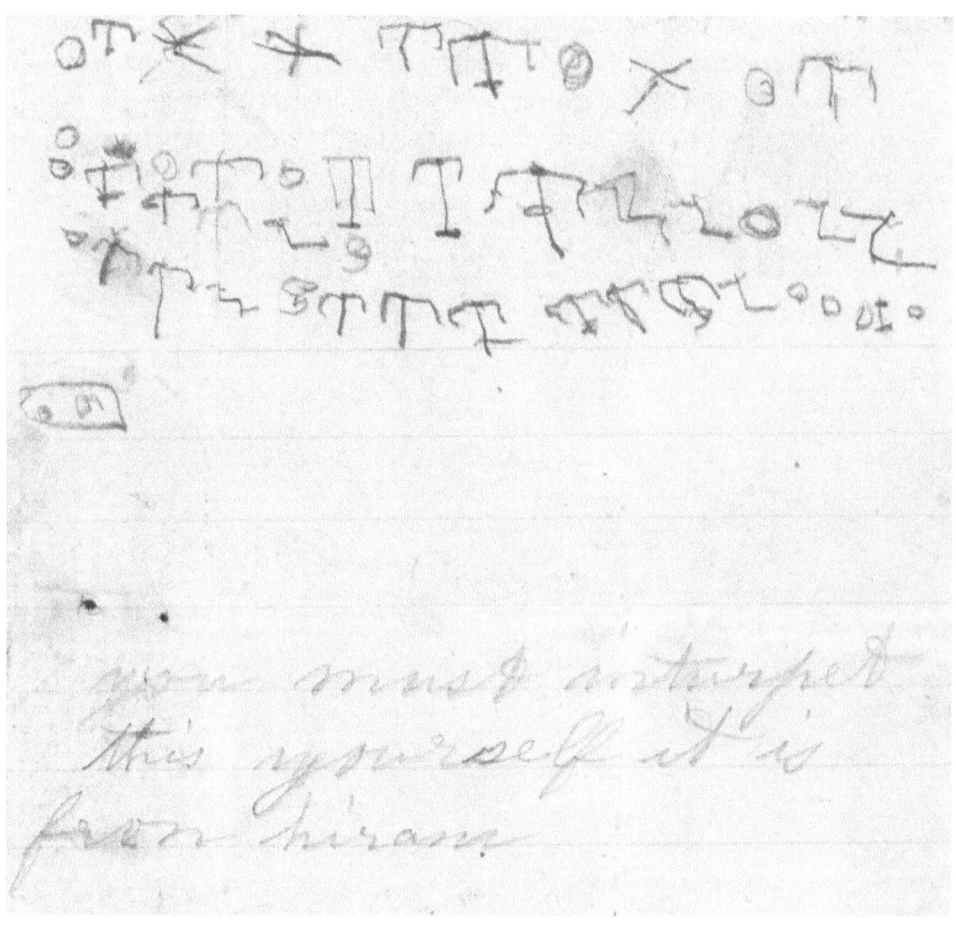

FIGURE E.1  Hiram's hieroglyphs and James Bickerdyke's "interpretation."
Courtesy of the Library of Congress.

ache that filled her everyday decisions. As she assumed each maternal role, she did so with the acknowledgment that both fulfillment and heartache accompanied each move that she made. And yet still, she continued to move.

The Civil War and its aftermath proved that motherhood was no longer a role that could be limited to the private spaces of the home; Bickerdyke's example demonstrates the utility of maternal professionalism and actions in public spaces. There was an imperative to care for and relieve soldiers, veterans, and a multitude of citizens across the country, which the growing medical institutions were still not equipped to address. Mary Bickerdyke's methods for treating patients and her trusted position as "Mother" proved instrumental in addressing that need.

Motherhood, in many ways, is a language unto itself. It is fluid, multifaceted, and ever-changing. It is both intuitive and learned, assumed and performed, deeply personal yet inherently collective. Like Hiram's hieroglyphics, its meaning is not always immediately clear, and "you must interpret this yourself."[5]

# Notes

*Abbreviations*

| | |
|---|---|
| FNK Collection | Federick N. Knapp Collection, 1862–86, MS 0209, Kiplinger Research Library, DC History Center, Washington, DC |
| IHC | Indian History Collection #590, Depredations, subfolder Indian Depredations, 1868, Kansas State Historical Society, Topeka, KS |
| KCSC | Knox College Special Collections and Archives, Manuscripts Collection, Galesburg, IL |
| MAB Collection | Mary Ann Bickerdyke Collection, 1862–1908, Kansas State Historical Society, Topeka, KS |
| MAB Papers | Mary Ann Bickerdyke Papers, Manuscript Division, Library of Congress, Washington, DC |
| NARA | National Archives and Records Administration, Washington, DC |
| USSC | United States Sanitary Commission Records, Western Department Archives, Manuscripts and Archives Division, New York Public Library |

*Preface*

1. Rubie Loring to James Bickerdyke, December 16, 1901, MssCol 19224, box 1, folder 15, images 142–45, MAB Papers.

2. Phillip W. Magness, "What the Data Say about Civil War Monuments," June 23, 2020, American Institute for Economic Research, https://www.aier.org/article/what-the-data-say-about-civil-war-monuments/.

3. Mother Bickerdyke Memorial Association to James Bickerdyke, June 27, 1904, box 1, folder 15, image 189, MAB Papers.

4. "Monument to Mother Bickerdyke Unveiled at Illinois Encampment with Ceremonies," *Champaign Daily News*, May 23, 1906; "Outranked General Sherman: Mother Bickerdyke, War Nurse, Gets a Monument," *Butte Daily Post*, November 15, 1906; "'Mother' Bickerdyke Monument Will be Erected at Galesburg, Ill," *Inquirer* (Lancaster, PA), April 28, 1906.

5. "Outranked General Sherman," *Butte Daily Post*, November 15, 1906.

6. "Encampment at Galesburg: Fittingly Opened with Dedication of Statue to Mother Bickerdyke, the War Nurse," *Rock Island Argus*, May 23, 1906.

7. "Monument to Mother Bickerdyke Unveiled," *Champaign Daily News*, May 23, 1906.

8. "Monument to Mother Bickerdyke Unveiled."

9. Ken Burns, *The Civil War: A Film by Ken Burns*, episode 5, "The Universe of Battle (1863): 'She Ranks Me,'" aired September 5, 1990, PBS, segment beginning at 52:14, quote from 56:00–56:32.

10. The 1,800-item collection is now digitized and freely accessible to researchers through the Library of Congress.

## Introduction

1. Ferber, *Mother Knows Best: A Fiction Book*. Ferber's 1927 novel consists of a series of short stories and was eventually adapted into a screenplay. The phrase then became more ubiquitous and continues to be used to this day. Although this common phrase has origins embedded in American popular culture of the 1920s, maternal knowledge and authority extend much farther back in history.

2. Schultz, *Women at the Front*.

3. Culpepper and Adams, "Nursing in the Civil War," 982.

4. Jacoby, *Strange Career of William Ellis*; Young, *Shoemaker and the Tea Party*; Young, "George Roberts Twelves Hewes." For this type of construction in historical writing, see the excellent work of Alfred Young and Karl Jacoby, cited here.

5. The first medical schools that allowed women to be trained as doctors were in cities in the East. Pragmatically, this excluded women without the means to travel, pay for relocation and education, or live away from their homes during medical training.

6. Ginzberg, *Women and the Work of Benevolence*, 144; Schultz, *Women at the Front*, 63–64, 119; Cutter, *Domestic Devils, Battlefield Angels*, 189; Marten, *Children for the Union*, 87–88.

7. Silber, *Daughters of the Union*, 212.

8. Apple and Golden, "Introduction: Mothers, Motherhood, and Historians," xiii.

9. Giesberg, *Army at Home*, 10.

10. Faust, *Mothers of Invention*, 5.

11. Valenčius, *Health of the Country*; Abel, *Hearts of Wisdom*, Beier, *A Matter of Life and Death*. Beier's work provides a more localized study of health care in the Midwestern region and the slow development of medical practice prior to the Civil War, whereas the other books are more regional in scope.

12. Humphreys, *Marrow of Tragedy*; Brooks and Hallett, *One Hundred Years of Wartime Nursing Practices*; Giesberg, *Civil War Sisterhood*; Hall, *Women on the Civil War Battlefront*; Attie, *Patriotic Toil*.

13. Sklar, *Catharine Beecher*; Sklar, *Florence Kelley and the Nation's Work*; Fischer, Nackenoff, and Chmielewski, *Jane Addams and the Practice of Democracy*; Oates, *A Woman of Valor*; M. M. Jones, *American Red Cross from Clara Barton to the New Deal*; Ginzberg, *Elizabeth Cady Stanton*; Gardner, "When Service Is Not Enough." These life histories and examinations of prominent nineteenth-century women provide a view of White women in different socioeconomic contexts than Mary Bickerdyke.

14. Skocpol, *Protecting Mothers and Soldiers*; Abramovitz, *Regulating the Lives of Women and Politics of Domesticity*; Michel and Koven, *Mothers of a New World*. An examination of Bickerdyke's involvement in local, state, and national institutions adds to this body of scholarship.

15. Hodes, *Sea Captain's Wife*, 18.

16. N. Doyle, *Maternal Bodies*, 148; Hulbert, *Raising America*; Masarik, *Sentimental State*; Vandenberg-Daves, *Modern Motherhood*.

17. McCurry, *Women's War*, 10.

18. McCurry, *Women's War*, 10.

19. Marten, *Children's Civil War*; Clement, *Growing Pains*; Mintz, *Huck's Raft*.

20. Tetrault, *Myth of Seneca Falls*; Fahs and Waugh, *Memory of the Civil War in American Culture*; Janney, *Remembering the Civil War*; Blight, *Race and Reunion*.

21. Lepore, "Historians Who Love Too Much," 130.

22. Levi, "On Microhistory," in *New Perspectives on Historical Writing*, 107; Ginsburg, "Microhistory," 203; Lüdtke, *History of Everyday Life*; Szijártó, *What Is Microhistory?*, 28. Examples include Giovanni Levi, Carlo Ginsburg, Emmanuel Le Roy Ladurie, and Alf Lüdtke, who all pioneered and articulated microhistorical approaches.

23. Ware, "The Book I Couldn't Write," 13.

24. Digital paleography refers to the use of digital tools and computational methods to analyze handwriting and script. These tools allow researchers to compare, identify, and classify scripts across documents. More than simply digitizing manuscripts, digital paleography allows for pattern recognition and stylistic comparison through image analysis and data processing. In the case of Lydia Foster, whose own voice and records are largely absent from the archival record, I employed a hybrid methodology that combined traditional archival research with digital handwriting analysis. Using open-access software to analyze targeted letters from Mary Bickerdyke's professional correspondence in the 1890s, I was able to group amanuenses by task and compare handwriting features. This process generated similarity scores that confirmed Foster's consistent authorship of letters during Bickerdyke's pension work in the 1890s, thereby revealing her unacknowledged role as Bickerdyke's amanuensis. It was corroborated by census data that placed Lydia Foster as a servant in the Bickerdyke home during that same period, as well as letters written between the Bickerdyke brothers after Mary Bickerdyke's death.

25. Schultz, *Women at the Front*, 64.

26. Giesberg, *Civil War Sisterhood*.

*Chapter One*

1. "Population Schedule [Knox County, Ohio]," 1820 United States Federal Census database, Ancestry.com, https://www.ancestry.com/search/collections/7734/?residence=_knox-ohio-usa_1630; "Population Schedule [Knox County, Ohio]," 1860 United States Federal Census database, Ancestry.com, https://www.ancestry.com/search/collections/7667/?residence=_knox-ohio-usa_1630; "Population Schedule [Hamilton County, Ohio]," 1820 United States Federal Census database, Ancestry.com, https://www.ancestry.com/search/collections/7734/?residence=_Cincinnati; "Population Schedule [Hamilton County, Ohio]," 1860 United States Federal Census database, Ancestry.com, https://www.ancestry.com/search/collections/7667/?residence=_cincinnati-hamilton-ohio-usa_51335.

2. Lauck, *Good Country*, 3.

3. Cayton and Gray, "The Story of the Midwest," 13.

4. Welter, "The Cult of True Womanhood," 152.

5. Welter, *Dimity Convictions*.

6. Hoganson, *Heartland*, xxii.

7. Jalland, *Death in the Victorian Family*, 230–50.

8. Litvin, *Young Mary*, 29. Martin Litvin's work is important in Bickerdyke scholarship because of Litvin's personal and direct access to Bickerdyke's trunk, maintained by her grandchildren. In his research for this book, which vehemently denies any claim of neglect or wrongdoing on Bickerdyke's part, Litvin became close friends with many of Bickerdyke's descendants.

9. Pope, "Adult Mortality in America before 1900," in *Strategic Factors in Nineteenth-Century American Economic History*, 271.

10. Mary Bickerdyke to George W. Clark, MssCol 19224, box 1, folder 25, MAB Papers. Mary Bickerdyke became fascinated with her family genealogy in the final years of her life. She spoke of her family lineage with a sense of pride and belonging, despite her displacement from her father's household after her mother's death. She also participated in the Ball family reunions as late as 1898, indicating her self-identification as part of the family. See her correspondence with a cousin, George Clark, cited here.

11. Litvin, *Young Mary*, 29.

12. Sam Starkweather to Mary Bickerdyke, March 25, 1863, MssCol 19224, box 2, folder 4, images 5–7, MAB Papers.

13. Abel, *Hearts of Wisdom*, 37.

14. Litvin, *Young Mary*, 44–45.

15. Robert Bickerdyke to Mary Bickerdyke, July 9, 1847, MssCol 19224, box 1, folder 21, images 2–3, MAB Papers.

16. *Daily Cincinnati Commercial*, February 28, 1848.

17. *Daily Cincinnati Commercial*, February 28, 1848. The report stated that "preparation is being made for a complimentary concert at the Assembly Rooms, to Mr. Robert Bickerdyke, who apart from the heavy losses sustained by the recent flood, has strong claims upon the patronage of the community, both as an accomplished musician and a gentleman."

18. Chase, *Mary A. Bickerdyke, "Mother,"* 8.

19. D. H. Doyle, *Social Order of a Frontier Community*, 62.

20. T. R. Mahoney, *From Hometown to Battlefield in the Civil War Era*, 7.

21. "Sudden Death," *Weekly Hawk-Eye and Telegraph* (Burlington, IA), April 12, 1859.

22. "Sudden Death."

23. Abel, *Living in Death's Shadow*, 5.

24. Abel, *Inevitable Hour*, 15.

25. "Galesburg Academy of Music Resolution and Condolence to Mary Bickerdyke," April 18, 1859, MssCol 19224, box 2, folder 2, image 3, MAB Papers.

26. Litvin, *Young Mary*, 45.

27. Halttunen, *Confidence Men and Painted Women*, 136.

28. Abel, *Hearts of Wisdom*, 37.

29. Josephine Dexter to Professor Irving, January 14, 1875, MssCol 19224, box 2, folder 13, images 2–3, MAB Papers.

30. "Mary A. Bickerdyke [Knox County, Illinois]," 1860 United States Federal Census database, Ancestry.com, https://ancestry.com/search/collections/7667/records/37731588; "Root's Galesburg Directory, 1861," box 4, Local History Series, KCSC.

31. Flannery, "The Early Botanical Medical Movement."

32. Haller, *People's Doctors*, 241.

33. Flannery, "Early Botanical Medical Movement," 448.

34. Valenčius, *Health of the Country*, 54; Haller, *Medical Protestants*; Dinger, "The Doctors in This Region Don't Know Much"; Hudson, "The Indian Doctress in the Nineteenth-Century United States."

35. Starr, *Social Transformation of American Medicine*, 30–60.

36. Warner, *Against the Spirit of System*, 223–53; Ulrich, *A Midwife's Tale*. These works offer a more nuanced investigation on American antebellum ideas on the increased professionalization, organization, and distribution of medical practitioners.

37. Starr, *Social Transformation of American Medicine*, 51.

38. Flannery, "Early Botanical Medical Movement," 450.

39. Chase, *Mary A. Bickerdyke, "Mother,"* 8.

40. Kirschmann, *A Vital Force*, 30.

41. "Mary A. Bickerdyke [Knox County, Illinois]," 1860 United States Federal Census database, Ancestry.com; "Root's Galesburg Directory, 1861," box 4, Local History Series, KCSC.

42. Perry, *History of Knox County*, 242–43.

43. Muelder, "Galesburg: Hot-Bed of Abolitionism," 216.

44. Norman, "The Other Lincoln-Douglas Debate," 5–6.

45. Guelzo, *Lincoln and Douglas*, 231.

46. McDonald, "Edward Beecher and the Anti-Slavery Movement in Illinois," 9.

47. Meredith, *Politics of the Universe*, 107.

48. McDonald, "Edward Beecher and the Anti-Slavery Movement in Illinois," 30.

49. "The Illinois Congregationalists on the War," *Chicago Tribune*, May 29, 1861.

50. Woodward, "Mother Bickerdyke: One of the Grandest Women of the War," 99.

51. Rosenberg, *Care of Strangers*, 18, 217.

52. Humphreys, *Marrow of Tragedy*, 2; Beier, *Health Culture in the Heartland*, 11.

53. Devine, *Learning from the Wounded*, 271.

54. Woodward, "Mother Bickerdyke: One of the Grandest Women of the War," 100.

55. Baker, *Cyclone in Calico*, 6.

56. Baker, *Cyclone in Calico*, 11.

57. Baker, *Cyclone in Calico*, 11, 15.

58. Chase, *Mary A. Bickerdyke, "Mother,"* 5; Litvin, *Young Mary*, 29–32.

59. Hogeland, "Coeducation of the Sexes at Oberlin College," in *Education*, 134.

60. Fairchild, *Co-education of the Sexes as Pursued in Oberlin College*, 18.

61. Even the Library of Congress website on Bickerdyke perpetuates the myth that Bickerdyke studied "herbal medicine" at Oberlin in the 1840s. Martin Litvin, in his meticulously researched book on Bickerdyke's younger years, consulted with enrollments at Oberlin to determine that she never attended the school. For more on the methodology employed in his research, see Litvin, *Young Mary, 1817–1861*.

62. Chase, *Mary A. Bickerdyke, "Mother,"* 6; Juettner, *Daniel Drake and His Followers*, 167. When recounting her life to Julia Chase, Bickerdyke made some key claims to education and religion that, when checked with the historical record, do not align.

63. Lafayette Sherwood to Mary Bickerdyke, August 25, 1864, MssCol 19224, box 2, folder 5, images 82–83, MAB Papers. There are several examples of soldiers who wrote to Bickerdyke during the war, expressing these sentiments and thoughts. Lafayette Sherwood's letter to Bickerdyke in 1864 complains about his new nurse since Bickerdyke was relocated to another Union position.

64. Hoge, *Boys in Blue*, 117.

65. Woodward, "Mother Bickerdike: One of the Grandest Women of the War," 98; Chase, *Mary A. Bickerdyke, "Mother,"* 4.

66. Cutter, *Domestic Devils, Battlefield Angels*, 188–91; Silber, *Daughters of the Union*, 203–12.
67. Schultz, *Women at the Front*, 64.
68. Reverby, *Ordered to Care*.
69. Hoge, *Boys in Blue*, 120.
70. Woodward, "Mother Bickerdike: One of the Grandest Women of the War," 99.
71. James Bickerdyke to Mary Bickerdyke, MssCol 19224, box 1, folder 16, MAB Papers. This folder contains a partial collection of letters from James to his mother.
72. James Bickerdyke to Mary Bickerdyke, January 7, 1864, MssCol 19224, box 1, folder 16, images 7–8, MAB Papers.
73. Mary Bickerdyke to Hiram Bickerdyke, June 13, 1869, MssCol 19224, box 1, folder 15, images 21–22, MAB Papers.
74. Mary Bickerdyke to James Bickerdyke, August 8, 1875, MssCol 19224, box 1, folder 14, images 31–33, MAB Papers.
75. James Bickerdyke to Mary Bickerdyke, April 22, 1864, MssCol 19224, box 1, folder 16, images 9–10, MAB Papers.
76. James Bickerdyke to Mary Bickerdyke, March 20, 1865, MssCol 19224, box 1, folder 16, images 14–16, MAB Papers.
77. Buhle, *Women and American Socialism*, 50.
78. Brockett and Vaughan, *Woman's Work in the Civil War*, 172.
79. Woodward, "Mother Bickerdike: One of the Grandest Women of the War," 98.
80. Martin Litvin, "Sister Colton and Sister Bickerdyke," booklet, box 4, file 3, Mary Bickerdyke Papers, KCSC.
81. Vandenberg-Daves, *Modern Motherhood*; Clement, *Growing Pains*.
82. Illick, *American Childhoods*, 12.
83. Marten, *Children's Civil War*, 3; Mary Bickerdyke to Hiram Bickerdyke, June 9, 1864, MssCol 19224, box 1, folder 14, images 2–3, MAB Papers.
84. Mintz, *Huck's Raft*, 132.
85. Hodes, *Sea Captain's Wife*, 224.
86. "The Happy Family," *The Mother's Magazine*, May 1839, 111; Lewis, "Mother's Love," in *Mothers & Motherhood*, 57; Fass, *End of American Childhood*, 80.
87. Holt, *Children of the Western Plains*, 12; West, *Growing Up with the Country*, xix; Fass, *End of American Childhood*, 80.
88. Marten, *Children's Civil War*.
89. Mary Bickerdyke to Hiram Bickerdyke, July 28, 1864, MssCol 19224, box 1, folder 12, images 4–5, MAB Papers.
90. Mary Bickerdyke to James and Hiram Bickerdyke, April 7, 1874, MssCol 19224, box 1, folder 14, images 27–28, MAB Papers.
91. Mary Bickerdyke to James and Hiram Bickerdyke, April 7, 1874, MssCol 19224, box 1, folder 14, images 27–28, MAB Papers.

*Chapter Two*

1. Hoge, *Boys in Blue*, 116.
2. Intisar K. Hamidullah, "The Impact of Disease on the Civil War," *Yale National Initiative*, January 29, 2015, http://teachers.yale.edu/curriculum/viewer/initiative_10.06.02_u.

3. Hoge, *Boys in Blue*, 117.
4. "Attention Girls!" *Janesville Weekly Gazette* (Janesville, WI), August 12, 1863.
5. Eliza C. Porter, "Report of the North-Western Commission for Jan. and Feb., 1864," *Niles Democrat* (Niles, IL), March 19, 1864.
6. "A Long Journey," *Brooklyn Union*, August 12, 1865.
7. Schultz, *Women at the Front*, 63–64, 119.
8. Silber, *Daughters of the Union*, 212.
9. Giesberg, *Civil War Sisterhood*.
10. Humphreys, *Marrow of Tragedy*, 132.
11. Humphreys, *Marrow of Tragedy*, 132.
12. The most direct and plausible account comes from Benjamin Woodward's own recollection. He solicited Bickerdyke's assistance through a plea to the Congregational Church in Galesburg, Illinois, which took up a collection. Bickerdyke left her children in the hands of community members and her older stepchildren and took the donations down to Cairo.
13. Brinton, *Personal Memoirs of John H. Brinton*.
14. Lemuel Adams, "Lemuel Adams Memoirs, 1831–1893," 86, Lemuel Adams Papers, Abraham Lincoln Presidential Library, Manuscripts Collection. The first recorded instance of the use of the "Mother" honorific came after the Battle of Belmont on November 7, 1861.
15. Women could not obtain official nursing positions until 1862, after Dorothea Dix's appointment as "Superintendent of Female Nurses in the Army," which mobilized women throughout the nation. Even then, Dix's professional norms and values for female nurses imposed age limits on official nurses. Mary Safford remained a volunteer nurse, constrained by her age.
16. Hoge, *Boys in Blue*, 68.
17. Livermore, *My Story of the War*, 207.
18. L. H. Fischer, "Cairo's Civil War Angel, Mary Jane Safford," 241.
19. Beier, *A Matter of Life and Death*, 11.
20. Cairo's strategic importance outweighed practical concerns about environmental threats, leading to the construction of a levy in the 1850s to hold back the rivers and allowing for modest development of transportation systems. The Civil War created a set of circumstances that superseded concerns about sickness or natural hazards.
21. "II. Cairo, Memoir," n.d., MssCol 19224, box 3, folder 9, image 12, MAB Papers.
22. "II. Cairo, Memoir," image 12.
23. Newberry, *US Sanitary Commission in the Valley of the Mississippi*, 36. Henry Bellows was the chief planner and president of the United States Sanitary Commission based out of New York; Frederick Law Olmsted was the executive secretary. John Strong Newberry toured Cairo with Bellows as a commissioned army surgeon who would become the secretary of the USSC Western Department. In this position, Newberry supervised all the work of the commission in the Mississippi Valley, with his headquarters in Louisville, Kentucky.
24. Ralph N. Isham and William Weston Patton, "Report on the Conditions of Camps and Hospitals at Cairo and Vicinity, Paducah and St. Louis," Documents of the United States Sanitary Commission, no. 38, Chicago History Museum, Manuscripts Collection.
25. "An Account of the Executive Organization," November 17, 1862, Documents of the United States Sanitary Commission, no. 60, 54, Chicago History Museum, Manuscripts Collection.

26. "An Account of the Executive Organization," 54.
27. This is an impulse that I describe as "competitive benevolence."
28. "II. Cairo, Memoir," n.d., MssCol 19224, box 3, folder 9, image 14, MAB Papers.
29. C. Baker to Mrs. Bickerdyke, April 1, 1862, MssCol 19224, box 2, folder 3, images 2–3, MAB Papers; Mary C. Brayton to Mrs. Bickerdyke, April 28, 1862, MssCol 19224, box 2, folder 3, image 4, MAB Papers. These represent individual donations provided to Bickerdyke before she was added to the USSC payroll.
30. Adams, "Lemuel Adams Memoirs," 86. Emphasis in original.
31. Adams, "Lemuel Adams Memoirs," 86.
32. Cooling, *Fort Donelson's Legacy*, 5.
33. This assumption is based on tactical maps from Forts Henry and Donelson as well as Bickerdyke's personal account in her unpublished memoir.
34. Tucker, *Unconditional Surrender*, 80.
35. "II. Cairo, Memoir," n.d., MssCol 19224, box 3, folder 9, image 33, MAB Papers.
36. "II. Cairo, Memoir," n.d., MssCol 19224, box 3, folder 9, image 35, MAB Papers.
37. "II. Cairo, Memoir," image 35.
38. "II. Cairo, Memoir," image 35.
39. "II. Cairo, Memoir," image 35.
40. Faust, *This Republic of Suffering*, 144.
41. Faust, *This Republic of Suffering*, 9.
42. Neff, *Honoring the Civil War Dead*, 11.
43. Faust, *This Republic of Suffering*, 31.
44. "II. Cairo, Memoir," n.d., MssCol 19224, box 3, folder 9, image 14, MAB Papers. This part of the event is recorded in her personal papers and unpublished memoir and, as a result, should be taken as an account adjusted for accuracy after subsequent retellings.
45. "II. Cairo, Memoir," n.d., MssCol 19224, box 3, folder 9, images 36–37, MAB Papers. Hot milk punch would have been a milk-based brandy or bourbon beverage that also contained sugar and vanilla, if available. The drink, in this context, would have been a warming liquid, with flavors that might revive or comfort a person.
46. "II. Cairo, Memoir," n.d., MssCol 19224, box 3, folder 9, image 37, MAB Papers.
47. "II. Cairo, Memoir," image 37.
48. Chase, *Mary A. Bickerdyke, "Mother,"* 14.
49. Hoge, *Boys in Blue*; Henshaw, *Our Branch and Its Tributaries*; Newberry, *US Sanitary Commission in the Valley of the Mississippi*.
50. Henshaw, "Prefatory Statement," *Our Branch and Its Tributaries*.
51. Henshaw, *Our Branch and Its Tributaries*, 50.
52. "The Great Victory," *Chicago Tribune*, February 18, 1862.
53. Henshaw, *Our Branch and Its Tributaries*, 22.
54. Henshaw, *Our Branch and Its Tributaries*, 54.
55. Newberry, *US Sanitary Commission in the Valley of the Mississippi*, 31.
56. H. A. Warriner and C. W. Christy, ed., "Draft: Fort Donelson and Shiloh to Corinth, Warriner's Volume," 1866, MssCol 22263, box 95, folder 13, Historical Bureau Archives, United States Sanitary Commission Records, Manuscripts and Archives Division, New York Public Library.
57. Warriner, "Draft: Fort Donelson and Shiloh to Corinth," 24–25.

58. Henshaw, *Our Branch and Its Tributaries*, 32.

59. Warriner, "Draft: Fort Donelson and Shiloh to Corinth," 21.

60. "To the Honorable Senate and House of Representatives Convened in General Assembly for the State of Illinois," n.d., MssCol 19224, box 3, folder 8, images 3–6, MAB Papers; Hoge, *Boys in Blue*, 95.

61. Hoge, *Boys in Blue*, 111.

62. Hoge, *Boys in Blue*, 121; "II. Cairo, Memoir," n.d., MssCol 19224, box 3, folder 9, image 38, MAB Papers.

63. Hoge, *Boys in Blue*, 157–58.

64. Hoge, *Boys in Blue*, 69.

65. Hoge, *Boys in Blue*, 111.

66. Hoge, *Boys in Blue*, 121.

67. By the end of the war, the USSC had taken the rudimentary practices of early experimentation on hospital steamers and began to outfit ships expressly for the purpose of hospital transportation. The ships, such as the *D. A. January*, were engineered according to sanitary principles, with proper ventilation, adequate space for patients, and fully furnished kitchens and laundries.

68. Whelan, *Nursing the Nation*, 8.

69. Reverby, *Ordered to Care*, 76.

70. Bickerdyke was paid for her work for the USSC, but it was notably less than her male counterparts were paid, and many of the documented anecdotes, like the midnight mission, were initiated outside of her assigned duty.

71. D'Antonio, *American Nursing*, 14; Abel, *Hearts of Wisdom*, 4.

72. Nightingale, *Notes on Nursing*, 6.

73. Monteiro, "On Separate Roads: Florence Nightingale and Elizabeth Blackwell," 523.

74. Downs, *Maladies of Empire*, 89.

75. Downs, *Maladies of Empire*, 91.

76. Longfellow, "Santa Filomena," *The Atlantic Monthly*, November 1857.

77. Longfellow, "Santa Filomena."

78. Devine, *Learning from the Wounded*.

79. US War Department, *War of the Rebellion*, ser. 3, vol. I: 107.

80. Brown, *Dorothea Dix*, 274.

81. "Mortality and Sickness of the US Volunteer Forces, 1861–1862," Documents of the Sanitary Commission, no. 46, Chicago History Museum, Manuscripts Collection.

82. Burton, *Woman Who Battled for the Boys in Blue*, x.

83. Burton, *Woman Who Battled for the Boys in Blue*, ix.

84. US Congress, "Fifty-Second Congress. Sess. I, August 5, 1892," *Report of Committees of the Senate of the United States for the First Session of the Fifty-Second Congress*, 348.

85. Burton, *Woman Who Battled for the Boys in Blue*, 44–45.

86. Nightingale, *Notes on Nursing*, 165.

87. Torreno, "The Art and Politics of Chicago's Sanitary Fairs"; Greene, "Nothing Daunts Chicago," 71–97.

88. Livermore, *My Story of the War*, 476.

89. Livermore, *My Story of the War*, 9.

90. Anna Webb-Peck, "A Sketch of Hospital Life and Work," 1862–1897, Kansas State Historical Society, 11, accessed August 20, 2025, http://www.kansasmemory.gov/item/219263.

91. Many accounts explain the creative ways that Bickerdyke recycled resources from wounded or deceased soldiers, gained help from "contrabands" or refugees from slavery, and restored hygiene and cleanliness to camps, steamers, and hospitals.

92. Woodworth, "Introduction," in *The Shiloh Campaign*, 1.

93. Webb-Peck, "Sketch of Hospital Life and Work," 11–12.

94. Hoge, *Boys in Blue*, 124; Henshaw, *Our Branch and Its Tributaries*, 70; "Record of Mrs. M. R. M'Coll as Hospital Nurse and Matron in US Military Hospitals, from 1863 to 1866," 1897, MssCol 19224, box 5, folder 4, images 94–99, MAB Papers.

95. Chicago Sanitary Commission, "Appointment as Sanitary Commission Nurse," box 4, file 3, Book Selections, Mary Bickerdyke Papers, KCSC.

96. George W. Weeks to James and Hiram Bickerdyke, February 19, 1863, MssCol 19224, box 3, folder 7, image 125, MAB Papers.

97. Faust, *This Republic of Suffering*, 85.

98. Hoge, *Boys in Blue*, 339.

99. Faust, *This Republic of Suffering*, 87.

100. George W. Weeks to Mrs. Abbott, February 19, 1863, MssCol 19224, box 3, folder 7, image 126, MAB Papers.

101. Mrs. Abbott's Drawing of Sherman Abbott Grave Location, n.d., MssCol 19224, box 3, folder 11, image 35, MAB Papers.

102. "Battle Unit Details: Union Illinois Volunteers, 26th Regiment, Illinois Infantry," n.d., National Park Service, https://www.nps.gov/civilwar/search-battle-units-detail.htm?battleUnitCode=UIL0026RI.

103. "List of Hospital and Sanitary Goods Transferred to Mrs. Bickerdyke by Capt. J. G. Klinck Hamburg Tenn," August 29, 1862, MssCol 19224, box 3, folder 12, image 2, MAB Papers. Mary Bickerdyke was in Hamburg, Tennessee, for an unknown amount of time but did receive hospital and sanitary goods there in late August 1862.

*Chapter Three*

1. "II. Cairo, Memoir," n.d., MssCol 19224, box 3, folder 9, images 20–22, MAB Papers.

2. Webb-Peck, "Sketch of Hospital Life and Work," box 1, image 11, MAB Collection.

3. Livermore, *My Story of the War*, 487.

4. Livermore, *My Story of the War*, 488.

5. Schultz, *Women at the Front*, 22.

6. Livermore, *My Story of the War*, 487.

7. Livermore, *My Story of the War*, 488.

8. Taylor, *Embattled Freedom*, 127.

9. LaPointe, "Military Hospitals in Memphis, 1861–1865," 332.

10. Henshaw, *Our Branch and Its Tributaries*, 114.

11. Henshaw, *Our Branch and Its Tributaries*, 114–15.

12. Henshaw, *Our Branch and Its Tributaries*, 114–15.

13. Hoge, *Boys in Blue*, 125.

14. Hoge, *Boys in Blue*, 263, 264.

15. Livermore, *My Story of the War*, 503–4.

16. Thomas Hannah Jr. to Elizabeth Hannah, January 31, 1863, Hannah Family Papers as shared with "Historic-Memphis," accessed March 10, 2024, https://www.historic-memphis.com.

17. Livermore, *My Story of the War*, 505.

18. Henshaw, *Our Branch and Its Tributaries*, 138; Livermore, *My Story of the War*, 502.

19. Livermore, *My Story of the War*, 503.

20. Livermore, *My Story of the War*, 507.

21. Livermore, *My Story of the War*, 509.

22. Schultz, "Seldom Thanked, Never Praised, and Scarcely Recognized."

23. Morantz-Sanchez, *Sympathy and Science*, 27; Reverby, *Ordered to Care*, 2; Beier, *Health Culture in the Heartland*, 11.

24. Brockett and Vaughan, *Woman's Work in the Civil War*, 21.

25. Brockett and Vaughan, *Woman's Work in the Civil War*, 23. As previously stated, Mary Livermore visited Memphis in March 1863 with a contingent of Chicago Sanitary Commission representatives. Along with Jane Hoge and Henrietta Colt, Livermore interacted and worked alongside Mary Bickerdyke during her time in Memphis.

26. Livermore, *My Story of the War*, 510.

27. Livermore, *My Story of the War*, 510.

28. Livermore, *My Story of the War*, 510. Bickerdyke would have been forty-five years old at the time of this incident.

29. Brockett and Vaughan, *Woman's Work in the Civil War*.

30. Sherman, *Memoirs of General William T. Sherman*, 280.

31. N. B. Hood to Mother Bickerdyke, December 9, 1895, MssCol 19224, box 2, folder 24, image 22, MAB Papers; John Gerdes to Mother Bickerdyke, January 11, 1898, MssCol 19224, box 3, folder 3, images 4–5, MAB Papers. It is most likely that neither of these men witnessed the "she ranks me" moment but were instead former patients or "boys" of Mother Bickerdyke and assimilated their memory of Civil War events with other stories that they read in later years.

32. "Wanted—One Hundred Cows!" *Chicago Tribune*, July 21, 1863; "A Plan for Supplying the Memphis Hospital with Milk," *Cleveland Daily Leader*, September 5, 1863.

33. Brockett and Vaughan, *Woman's Work in the Civil War*, 177.

34. "A Noble Enterprise," *Wisconsin State Journal*, August 4, 1863.

35. "An Opportunity to Do Good," *Daily Illinois State Journal*, July 22, 1863.

36. Bender, "Old Boss Devil," 80.

37. Wittenmyer, *Under the Guns*, 83; Mary Livermore, *My Story of the War*, 521; Chase, *Mary A. Bickerdyke, "Mother,"* 94.

38. James Yeatman to "Sir," June 6, 1863, MssCol 19224, box 2, folder 4, image 10, MAB Papers.

39. Mary A. Livermore to Mary A. Bickerdyke, August 13, 1863, MssCol 19224, box 4, folder 2, image 2, MAB Papers.

40. "A Noble Enterprise," *Wisconsin State Journal*, August 4, 1863; "Special Dispatch to the Chicago Tribune: From Springfield," *Chicago Tribune*, August 1, 1863.

41. Emily J. Bancroft to Mary Bickerdyke, August 4, 1863, box 2, folder 4, image 12, MAB Papers; James E. Yeatman to Mrs. M.A. Bickerdyke, August 13, 1863, box 2, folder 4, image 16, MAB Papers; Mary A. Livermore to Mary A. Bickerdyke, August 13, 1863, MssCol 19224,

box 4, folder 2, image 2, MAB Papers; John Williams to Thomas Harrison, September 2, 1863, MssCol 19224, box 4, folder 2, images 17–18, MAB Papers.

42. John Williams to Thomas Harrison, September 2, 1863, MssCol 19224, box 4, folder 2, images 17–18, MAB Papers; "A Noble Enterprise"; "Special Dispatch to the Chicago Tribune: From Springfield."

43. Brockett and Vaughan, *Woman's Work in the Civil War*, 177; Hoge, *Boys in Blue*, 126; Henshaw, *Our Branch and Its Tributaries*, 179.

44. Livermore, *My Story of the War*, 531.

45. Brace, "Consecrated by Sorrow," 80. Susan Brace posited that "perhaps repeated and early losses of consistent mothering left Bickerdyke without an appreciation or a capacity for mothering her own children with a continuous maternal presence." Death was an absence in a wholly different sense than an obligation to work away from the home.

46. Michel, "The Limits of Maternalism," in *Mothers of a New World*, 294.

47. Hoge, *Boys in Blue*, 68.

48. Bickerdyke's direct superiors, Mary Livermore and Jane Hoge, had secondary education at Charlestown Female Seminary and the Young Ladies' College of Philadelphia, respectively.

49. Henshaw, *Our Branch and Its Tributaries*, 254.

50. Henshaw, *Our Branch and Its Tributaries*, 254.

51. Chicago Sanitary Commission, "Appointment as Sanitary Commission Nurse," box 4, file 3, Book Selections, Mary Bickerdyke Papers, KCSC. This starting salary was increased by the end of the war when she received $50.

52. US Sanitary Commission, Washington, DC, to Mrs. Bickerdyke, May 18, 1865, MssCol 19224, box 2, folder 6, image 44, MAB Papers.

53. Senese, "Sarah Josepha Hale and Ladies' Magazine," 67.

54. D. M. Mahoney, "'More Than an Accomplishment.'"

55. Graff, "The Literacy Myth," 18.

56. Mary Livermore to Mrs. Bickerdyke, March 21, 1864, MssCol 19224, box 2, folder 1, image 9, MAB Papers.

57. Halttunen, *Confidence Men and Painted Women*, 96.

58. Mary Livermore to Mrs. Bickerdyke, March 21, 1864, MssCol 19224, box 2, folder 1, image 11, MAB Papers.

59. "Population Schedule, 1860 United States Federal Census," NARA microfilm publication M653, 1,438 rolls, National Archives and Records Administration.

60. Henshaw, *Our Branch and Its Tributaries*, 72.

61. Hoge, *Boys in Blue*, 117.

62. Brockett and Vaughan, *Woman's Work in the Civil War*, 74.

63. J. R. Bickerdyke, "A Partial History of Mary Bickerdyke," n.d., MssCol 19224, box 3, folder 7, images 18–20, MAB Papers; Mary Bickerdyke to Hiram Bickerdyke, March 11, 1867, MssCol 19224, box 1, folder 12, images 12–13, MAB Papers; Mary Bickerdyke from San Francisco to James and Hiram Bickerdyke, February 10, 1878, MssCol 19224, box 1, folder 15, images 50–51, MAB Papers.

64. James Bickerdyke to Mary Bickerdyke, September 14, 1866, MssCol 19224, box 1, folder 16, images 34–35, MAB Papers.

65. Birk, *Fostering on the Farm*, 3.

66. James Bickerdyke to Mary Bickerdyke, September 6, 1865, MssCol 19224, box 1, folder 14, images 21–23, MAB Papers. James's request for new boots and coats was repeated on at least a yearly basis between 1865 and 1868.

67. James Bickerdyke to Mary Bickerdyke, December 17, 1866, MssCol 19224, box 1, folder 14, images 42–43, MAB Papers.

68. Mary Bickerdyke to James Bickerdyke, January 20, 1867, MssCol 19224, box 1, folder 14, images 18–19, MAB Papers.

69. Mary Bickerdyke to "My dear Sons," March 10, 1864, MssCol 19224, box 1, folder 14, image 3, MAB Papers.

70. Downs, *Sick from Freedom*; Humphreys, *Intensely Human*.

71. Mary Bickerdyke to "My dear Sons," March 10, 1864, MssCol 19244, box 1, folder 14, image 4, MAB Papers.

72. Marten, *Children's Civil War*, 70; Mintz, *Huck's Raft*, 170.

73. Sherman, *Memoirs of General William T. Sherman*, 372–90; Marszalek, *Sherman: A Soldier's Passion for Order*, 237–42; General Orders, No. 2, HQ, Military Division of the Mississippi, October 19, 1863, in US War Department, *War of the Rebellion: A Compilation of the Official Records of the Union and Confederate Armies*, series 1, vol. 30, part 4, 476.

74. Mary Bickerdyke to "the Proper Authorities," December 24, 1863, MssCol 19224, box 2, folder 4, image 45, MAB Papers.

75. Foote, *Gentlemen and the Roughs*; Mary Bickerdyke to "the Proper Authorities," December 24, 1863, MssCol 19224, box 2, folder 4, image 45, MAB Papers. The scholarship on punishment within the Union army is robust and speaks more to the reasoning behind such techniques, but it tends to be overly focused on desertion. For a valuable discussion on the roles of gender in Union army punishment, Foote's work is an excellent social history on violence in the Union army.

76. Mary Bickerdyke to "the Proper Authorities," December 24, 1863, MssCol 19224, box 2, folder 4, image 45, MAB Papers.

77. Devine, *Learning from the Wounded*, 8.

78. Charles Woodward Stearns to Bickerdyke, 1864, MssCol 19224, box 2, folder 5, images 14–17, MAB Papers; Woodward, "Mother Bickerdike," 98.

79. "Special Order No. 21" to Mrs. Bickerdyke and Mrs. Porter, January 23, 1864, MssCol 19224, box 2, folder 5, image 5, MAB Papers.

80. "Report of E. B. McCagg and E. W. Blatchford," *Bulletin of the United States Sanitary Commission* 2, no. 20 (August 24, 1864): 610.

81. Humphreys, *Marrow of Tragedy*; Giesberg, *Civil War Sisterhood*. These works provide more thorough information on the US Sanitary Commission and its ideologies of organizational efficiency and scientific bureaucracy.

82. List of the Commands at Pulaski, Tennessee, April 25, 1864, MssCol 19224, box 3, folder 12, images 8–12, MAB Papers.

83. "Western Sanitary Commission: What It Does with Its Funds and Why It Should Be Aided in Its Work," *Missouri Democrat*, March 16, 1864.

84. Mary Livermore to Mrs. Bickerdyke, March 21, 1864, MssCol 19224, box 2, folder 1, image 10, MAB Papers.

85. A. M. Read to Bickerdyke from Huntsville, April 10, 1864, MssCol 19224, box 2, folder 4, images 24–26, MAB Papers.

202  Notes to Chapter Four

86. W. H. Marsh to L. H. Everts, April 11, 1864, MssCol 19224, box 2, folder 5, image 28, MAB Papers.

87. E. C. Porter to United States Christian Commission, April 18, 1864, MssCol 19224, box 2, folder 5, image 46, MAB Papers.

88. Petition from 16th Army Surgeons of Pulaski, Tennessee, April 11, 1864, MssCol 19224, box 3, folder 10, images 15–17, MAB Papers.

89. E. C. Porter to United States Christian Commission, April 18, 1864, MssCol 19224, box 2, folder 5, image 46, MAB Papers.

90. E. C. Porter, US Christian Commission, April 29, 1864, MssCol 19224, box 2, folder 5, images 38–45, MAB Papers.

91. Porter, US Christian Commission, April 29, 1864, image 38.

92. Porter, US Christian Commission, April 29, 1864, image 39.

93. E. B. McCagg to Mary Bickerdyke, May 3, 1864, MssCol 19224, box 2, folder 5, images 74–75, MAB Papers.

94. McCagg to Bickerdyke, May 3, 1864.

95. E. B. McCagg to John Strong Newberry, March 9, 1865, MssCol 18779, box 15, folder 13, item 3, USSC, Western Department Archive.

96. McCagg to Newberry, March 9, 1865.

97. Resolution, Northwestern Sanitary Commission, Chicago Branch, February 28, 1865, MssCol 19224, box 4, folder 4, images 2–3, MAB Papers.

98. John V. Farrell, B. Jacobs, Robert Patterson, to Nathan Bishop, December 24, 1864, MssCol 19224, box 2, folder 5, image 94, MAB Papers.

99. D. L. Dix, Certificate for Mary Bickerdyke, April 1, 1865, MssCol 19224, box 3, folder 10, image 21, MAB Papers.

100. Hoge, *Boys in Blue*, 117.

101. W. A. Laurence to Mary Bickerdyke, June 29, 1865, MssCol 19224, box 2, folder 6, image 56, MAB Papers.

102. Laurence to Bickerdyke, June 29, 1865.

103. "Dear Mother Bickerdyke" / "Stories of the Beautiful Career which has just ended" / "The Idol of the Boys in Blue from the Opening to the Close of the Civil War—The High Authority She Bore," *Topeka Daily Herald*, November 11, 1901; MssCol 19224, box 4, folder 7, image 4, MAB Papers.

104. Brockett and Vaughan, *Woman's Work in the Civil War*, 173.

*Chapter Four*

1. "Report of the Board of Managers," *Chicago Tribune*, January 16, 1866.

2. Individual records and board meeting notes for the Home for the Friendless, which include the years from its conception to the time of Bickerdyke's employment (1863–1871), were likely destroyed in the Great Chicago Fire.

3. "Contract of Indenture," May 22, 1867, MssCol 19224, box 3, folder 8, image 2, MAB Papers.

4. "Contract of Indenture."

5. "Contract of Indenture."

6. Schmidt, *Industrial Violence and the Legal Origins of Child Labor*, 122–24; Ross, "Families without Paradigms."
7. "Report of the Board of Managers," *Chicago Tribune*, January 16, 1866.
8. "Report of the Board of Managers," emphasis added.
9. Skocpol, *Protecting Soldiers and Mothers*; Mink, *Wages of Motherhood*; Chappell, "Protecting Soldiers and Mothers Twenty-Five Years Later."
10. Michel and Koven, *Mothers of a New World*; Ladd-Taylor, *Mother-Work*.
11. Novak, "The Myth of the 'Weak' American State." Bickerdyke's work with orphans, mothers, and veterans through institutional interventions reinforces William Novak's "Myth of the 'Weak' American State" and shows that there were, in fact, systems in place before the turn of the century. This terminology originated with Skocpol, *Protecting Soldiers and Mothers*.
12. Prior to the Progressive Era reforms that vastly expanded the US government's role in promoting the welfare of America's children and youth, guardianships for youth were easily awarded to willing applicants. The social dislocations of the late nineteenth century eventually led to social reform movements in the 1890s that were solidified after the turn of the century with broader protective legislation. The 1909 White House Conference on the Care of Dependent Children, for example, established a national foster care system and provided mothers' pensions to assist poor families facing potential separation because of an inability to financially provide for their children's basic needs.
13. Simultaneously, there was an increased imperative to solve class issues of endemic poverty and delinquency. State institutions for orphan children hoped to serve both needs.
14. Mintz, *Huck's Raft*, 76.
15. *Daily Illinois State Journal* (Springfield), March 14, 1866.
16. Giesberg, "Orphans and Indians." In *Children and Youth during the Civil War Era*.
17. Cordelia Harvey, a state sanitary agent and wife of a former governor, advocated for a soldiers' orphans' home in Wisconsin in early 1865 upon her return from the front. In Iowa, state sanitary agent Annie Wittenmyer spearheaded efforts to create a centralized home for orphans and half-orphans of the war. Such processes in the Midwestern states mirrored Illinois's journey.
18. Illinois Soldiers' and Sailors' Children's School (ISSCS) Collection, McLean County Museum of History. After World War I, the institution was renamed the Illinois Soldiers' and Sailors' Children's Home and School.
19. "Recommendations for Tax for Destitute Families of Soldiers, Schools for Soldiers' Orphans, and a State Sanitary Bureau," *Journal of the House of Representatives of the Twenty-Fourth General Assembly of the State of Illinois*, 58.
20. "Recommendations for Tax for Destitute Families of Soldiers," 58.
21. Koerner, "The Illinois Soldiers' Orphans' Home," in *Reports Made to the General Assembly of Illinois*, 334.
22. The phrase "competitive benevolence is taken from H. A. Warriner's contemporary and unpublished history of the USSC. Henry A. Warriner and C. W. Christy, eds., "Draft: Fort Donelson and Shiloh to Corinth, Warriner's Volume," 1866, MssCol 22263, box 95, folder 13, images 73–75, Historical Bureau Archives, United States Sanitary Commission, Manuscripts and Archives Division, New York Public Library.

23. E. B. McCagg to John Strong Newberry, March 9, 1865, MssCol 18779, box 15, folder 13, item 3, USSC, Western Dept. Archive.

24. McCagg to Newberry, March 9, 1865.

25. McCagg to Newberry, March 9, 1865.

26. Preeminent examples include Annie Wittenmyer in Iowa and Cordelia Harvey in Wisconsin.

27. *Daily Illinois State Journal* (Springfield), September 2, 1865.

28. Richard J. Oglesby to Edwin Stanton, October 27, 1865, MssCol 19224, box 2, folder 6, image 81, MAB Papers.

29. Bickerdyke used an amanuensis, or ghostwriter, whenever she had longer documents to send. She was self-conscious about her apparent social "deficiencies" due to her class and lack of formal schooling.

30. Mary Bickerdyke in Washington, DC, to Maj. General M. Meigs, November 27, 1865, MssCol 19224, box 2, folder 6, image 87, MAB Papers; Mary Bickerdyke to Surgeon General Joseph Barnes, November 27, 1865, MssCol 19224, box 2, folder 6, image 88, MAB Papers.

31. Koerner, "Illinois Soldiers' Orphans' Home," in the *Seventh Biennial Report of the Superintendent of Public Instruction of the State of Illinois, 1867–1868* (Springfield, IL), 175. A generous land donation from David Davis, a Supreme Court justice and Bloomington-Normal native, allowed for building to begin. Two years after the home was incorporated, the Illinois General Assembly supplemented incoming donations and finally appropriated resources from a "deserter's fund" to maintain the project's longevity.

32. Virginia C. Ohr, "Matron's Report," *Reports Made to the General Assembly of Illinois at Its Twenty-Sixth Session, Volume 1, 1869* (Springfield: Illinois State Printing Services), 342. Virginia Ohr's narrative is the only remaining account of the home's early days. All the official orders and rules for the governance of the Illinois Soldiers' Orphans' Home were "destroyed by fire in Springfield" when they were sent to the state binder for rebinding, according to a report from John M. Snyder, Secretary of the Board to Col. M. Beardsley, President Board of Trustees, Soldiers Orphans Home, February 25, 1871. The beginnings of the Illinois Soldiers' Orphans' Home and its daily operations will, unfortunately, never be fully known.

33. F. G. Ensign to Mrs. M. A. Bickerdyke, April 3, 1866, MssCol 19224, box 2, folder 6, image 15, MAB Papers.

34. Holt, *Orphan Trains*, 5.

35. Crenson, *Building the Invisible Orphanage*, 221.

36. "Contract of Indenture," May 22, 1867, MssCol 19224, box 3, folder 8, image 2, MAB Papers; Sarah Cleveland to Mrs. Bickerdyke, June 2, 1867, MssCol 19224, box 2, folder 8, images 11–15, MAB Papers; D. F. Wharland to Mrs. Bickerdyke, June 13, 1867, MssCol 19224, box 2, folder 8, images 16–17, MAB Papers.

37. "Salina—As It Was, and Is," *Salina Herald*, February 16, 1867.

38. Peterson, "Home-Builders," 36.

39. Kansas State Historical Society, *Transactions of the Kansas State Historical Society, 1901–1902*, 192.

40. [Kansas Soldier Applicant, no signature] to Mary Bickerdyke, December 19, 1869, MssCol 19224, box 2, folder 10, image 28, MAB Papers.

41. [Kansas Soldier Applicant, no signature] to Mary Bickerdyke, December 19, 1869, MssCol 19224, image 29, MAB Papers.

42. James Bickerdyke to Mary Bickerdyke, December 17, 1866, MssCol 19224, box 1, folder 16, images 42–43, MAB Papers.

43. Laura A. Hayward to Mary Bickerdyke, January 1, 1867, MssCol 19224, box 1, folder 16, images 46–48, MAB Papers.

44. Laura A. Hayward to Mary Bickerdyke, January 1, 1867, MssCol 19224, box 1, folder 16, images 46–48, MAB Papers.

45. James Bickerdyke to Mary Bickerdyke, December 5, 1867, MssCol 19224, box 1, folder 16, images 30–32, MAB Papers.

46. L. A. Hayward to Mary Bickerdyke, 1867, MssCol 19224, box 1, folder 16, images 61–62, MAB Papers.

47. *Transactions of the Kansas State Historical Society*, 192; "Population Schedule [Salina, Saline County, Kansas], 1870 United States Federal Census," NARA microfilm publication M593, 1,761 rolls. The 1870 census suggests that the number was much closer to fifty veterans and their families.

48. M. S. Finegan to Mary Bickerdyke, April 15, 1868, MssCol 19224, box 2, folder 9, image 11, MAB Papers.

49. R. W. Hall to J. H. Knight, July 16, 1867, MssCol 19224, box 2, folder 8, image 22, MAB Papers.

50. Susan B. Anthony to Mary Bickerdyke, July 7, 1897, Mary Ann Bickerdyke Collection #276, Kansas State Historical Society.

51. Rev. G. S. F. Savage to Mary Bickerdyke, October 31, 1868, MssCol 19224, box 2, folder 9, image 24, MAB Papers.

52. Hiram Bickerdyke to James Bickerdyke, February 26, 1902, box 1, correspondence, 1898–1908 and undated, Mary Ann Bickerdyke Collection #276, Kansas State Historical Society, https://www.kansasmemory.gov/item/219272.

53. Hiram Bickerdyke to James R. Bickerdyke, March 21, 1901, box 1, correspondence 1898–1908, Mary Ann Bickerdyke Collection #276, Kansas State Historical Society, https://www.kansasmemory.gov/item/219282.

54. Hiram Bickerdyke to James R. Bickerdyke, February 11, 1902, box 1, item 219281, Mary Ann Bickerdyke Collection #276, Kansas State Historical Society, https://www.kansasmemory.gov/item/219281.

55. Frank Scott to Mary Bickerdyke, July 22, 1897, folder 5, correspondence, July–Sept, 1897, Mary Ann Bickerdyke Collection #276, Kansas State Historical Society.

56. *Junction City Weekly Union* (Junction City, Kansas), January 16, 1869.

57. *Agitator* (Chicago, Illinois), March 13, 1869.

58. Venet, "The Emergence of a Suffragist," 161.

59. Mary Livermore, "A Heroine of the Hospitals: Mother Bickerdyke's New Year's Eve, 1864," *Springfield Daily Republican*, October 23, 1869.

60. Cox, "The Grasshopper Plague, 1874–1878, and Social Welfare," in *The Struggle for Equality*, 172.

61. Mary F. Brown, "My Experiences with the Grasshoppers in 1866–67," December 5, 1908, folder 1—Hist. Grasshoppers, Grasshoppers History Collection, Kansas State Historical Society.

62. Brown, "My Experiences with the Grasshoppers in 1866–67."

63. Brown, "My Experiences with the Grasshoppers in 1866–67."

64. Kansas State Historical Society, *Transactions of the Kansas State Historical Society, 1901–1902*, 195.

65. "Philanthropy Personified," *Great Bend Register* (Great Bend, KS), December 10, 1874.

66. "Southwest," *Weekly-News Democrat* (St. Louis, MO), December 25, 1874.

67. "An Appeal!," November 18, 1874, MssCol 19224, box 13, folder 15, image 3, MAB Papers.

68. Box 2, folder 12, and box 3, folder 15, MAB Papers. These folders hold various bills of lading, letters of introduction, and donation estimates.

*Chapter Five*

1. George Duffield, Jr. to Mrs. M.A. Bickerdyke, July 30, 1867, MssCol 19224, box 2, folder 8, image 24, MAB Papers; M. S. Finegan to Mrs. Bickerdyke, April 15, 1868, MssCol 19224, box 2, folder 9, image 11, MAB Papers.

2. This less well-known instance of her aid work is discussed more thoroughly in chapter 4.

3. "Employment for Women," *Burlington Free Press* (Burlington, VT), February 12, 1868.

4. The letter from Bickerdyke to Bellows does not exist in the Massachusetts Historical Society archive where Bellows's papers reside.

5. Henry W. Bellows to Mary Bickerdyke, November 23, 1870, MssCol 19224, box 2, folder 11, image 2, MAB Papers.

6. Henry W. Bellows to Mary Bickerdyke, November 23, 1870, MssCol 19224, box 2, folder 11, image 3, MAB Papers.

7. Henry W. Bellows to Mary Bickerdyke, November 23, 1870, MssCol 19224, box 2, folder 11, image 3, MAB Papers.

8. Henry W. Bellows to Mary Bickerdyke, November 23, 1870, MssCol 19224, box 2, folder 11, image 4, MAB Papers.

9. Wittenmyer, *Under the Guns*, 83; Livermore, *My Story of the War*, 251; Chase, *Mary A. Bickerdyke, "Mother,"* 94. These are only a sample of the copious stories in the secondary literature from Civil War histories of women in the war that mention Bickerdyke's propensity to "cut red tape."

10. Schultz, "The Inhospitable Hospital," 365.

11. Johnson, *Funding Feminism*; McCarthy, *Lady Bountiful Revisited*; Green, "Humanitarianism in Nineteenth-Century Context"; Ginzberg, *Women and the Work of Benevolence*. These pieces provide a more thorough treatment of the scientific philanthropy movement that encouraged wealthy women to donate to charitable causes and fund charitable organizations.

12. George Duffield, Jr. to Mrs. M.A. Bickerdyke, July 30, 1867, MssCol 19224, box 2, folder 8, image 24, MAB Papers.

13. Maggie Trynne to Mrs. Bickerdyke, August 5, 1867, MssCol 19224, box 2, folder 8, image 25, MAB Papers.

14. Trynne to Bickerdyke, August 5, 1867.

15. *Junction City Weekly Union*, November 21, 1868.

16. Hiram Bickerdyke to Florence Shaw Kellogg, December 3, 1905, box 4, Local History Series, KCSC; Mary Bickerdyke to General Sherman, Friday, February 5, 1869, MssCol

19224, box 2, folder 1, images 14–16, MAB Papers. The first document is a letter reprinted in the *Galesburg Post* by Martin Litvin. The second document shows Hiram's easily discernable handwriting.

17. Mary Bickerdyke to "Sir," March 5, 1875, MssCol 19224, box 2, folder 13, images 18–19, MAB Papers; Mary Bickerdyke to "Sir," March 6, 1876, MssCol 19224, box 2, folder 13, images 20–21, MAB Papers.

18. Mrs. M. A. Bickerdyke to "Sir," March 5, 1875, MssCol 19224, box 2, folder 13, images 18–19. I begin referring to James as "J. R." from this point on, which is how he preferred to be addressed as a professional in adulthood.

19. Mary Bickerdyke to "Sir," March 6, 1876, MssCol 19224, box 2, folder 13, image 21, MAB Papers.

20. Mary Bickerdyke to "Sir," March 6, 1876, MssCol 19224, box 2, folder 13, image 21, MAB Papers.

21. Rosenberg, *Care of Strangers*; Morantz-Sanchez, *Sympathy and Science*; Reverby, *Ordered to Care*; D'Antonio, *American Nursing*.

22. Hilde, "Worth a Dozen Men," 110.

23. Fairman and D'Antonio, "Reimagining Nursing's Place in the History of Clinical Practice," 439; Pace and Lunsford, "The Evolution of Palliative Care Nursing Education," S9.

24. "She Wanted Pickles," *Russell Kansas Journal*, January 14, 1892.

25. Schultz, "The Inhospitable Hospital," 375.

26. Fairman and Lynaugh, *Critical Care Nursing*, 3.

27. Reverby, *Ordered to Care*, 77.

28. "She Wanted Pickles," *Russell Kansas Journal*, January 14, 1892.

29. Schultz, "The Inhospitable Hospital," 390.

30. Valenčius, *Health of the Country*, 57; Ulrich, *A Midwife's Tale*, 53.

31. Rosenberg, *Care of Strangers*, 14.

32. Rosenberg, *Care of Strangers*, 217.

33. D'Antonio, *American Nursing*, 14.

34. Buhler-Wilkerson, *No Place Like Home*, 53.

35. "Battle Unit Details, Union Wisconsin Volunteers, 2nd Regiment, Wisconsin Cavalry," National Park Service, accessed March 1, 2025, https://www.nps.gov/civilwar/search-battle-units-detail.htm?battleUnitCode=UWI0002RC; Ruth S. Eastman to Mary Bickerdyke, July 15, 1897, MssCol 19226, box 3, folder 2, image 27, MAB Papers.

36. Charlotte went by the name Ruth according to the letter that she wrote to Bickerdyke.

37. "Died," *Reno Gazette-Journal*, November 9, 1879.

38. Ruth S. Eastman to Mary Bickerdyke, July 15, 1897, MssCol 19226, box 3, folder 2, image 27, MAB Papers.

39. Ruth S. Eastman to Mary Bickerdyke, July 15, 1897, MssCol 19226, box 3, folder 2, image 27, MAB Papers.

40. Mary Bickerdyke to James Bickerdyke, May 16, 1880, MssCol 19224, box 1, folder 14, images 43–44, MAB Papers; census details are taken from "Population Schedule [Carson City, Ormsby, Nevada], 1880 United States Federal Census," NARA microfilm publication M593, Enumeration District 038, roll 759, page 46C.

41. "Soldier Details: Magee, William J.," Civil War Soldiers database, National Park Service, n.d., https://www.nps.gov/civilwar/search-soldiers-detail.htm?soldierId=E17F22B5-DC7A-DF11-BF36-B8AC6F5D926A.

42. Mary Bickerdyke to James Bickerdyke, May 16, 1880, MssCol 19224, box 1, folder 14, images 43–44, MAB Papers.

43. Fairman and D'Antonio, "Reimagining Nursing's Place in the History of Clinical Practice," 440.

44. Mary Bickerdyke to Mr. J. R. Bickerdyke, December 12, 1881, MssCol 19224, box 1, folder 14, image 47, MAB Papers.

45. Mary Bickerdyke to J. R. Bickerdyke, February 26, 1882, MssCol 19224, box 1, folder 14, image 50, MAB Papers.

46. Harbour, *Organizing Freedom*, 104.

47. Hackemer, "Civil War Veteran Colonies on the Western Frontier," in *The War Went On*, 61. Hackemer's work has more details on the prevalence of veterans' communities in the western United States.

48. For ease of understanding in this explanation of the story, I will be using Mollie.

49. Mary Bickerdyke to J. R. Bickerdyke, February 26, 1882, MssCol 19224, box 1, folder 14, image 49, MAB Papers.

50. Mollie Bickerdyke to Mary Bickerdyke, July 11, 1886, MssCol 19224, box 1, folder 20, image 26, MAB Papers.

51. Mollie Bickerdyke to Mary Bickerdyke, February 16, 1887, MssCol 19224, box 1, folder 20, images 29–30, MAB Papers.

52. Maria L. Gibson to Mary Bickerdyke, February 27, 1887, MssCol 19244, box 1, folder 20, images 31–33, MAB Papers.

53. Maria L. Gibson to Mary Bickerdyke, February 27, 1887, MssCol 19244, box 1, folder 20, images 31–33, MAB Papers.

54. Maria L. Gibson to Mary Bickerdyke, February 27, 1887, MssCol 19244, box 1, folder 20, images 31–33, MAB Papers.

55. Devine, *Learning from the Wounded*, 132.

56. Halsted, "The Results of Operations for the Cure of Cancer of the Breast Performed at the Johns Hopkins Hospital from June, 1899, to January, 1894," 297.

57. J. R. Bickerdyke to Mollie Bickerdyke, April 22, 1887, MssCol 19224, box 1, folder 15, image 83, MAB Papers.

58. "Epithelioma! Or Skin Cancer," *American Israelite* (Cincinnati, OH), July 30, 1886.

59. Fett, *Working Cures*.

60. Starr, *Social Transformation of American Medicine*, 17.

61. Maria L. Gibson to Mary Bickerdyke, February 27, 1887, MssCol 19244, box 1, folder 20, images 31–33, MAB Papers.

62. "Temmen, Mrs. J. H., 69 Dudley" of Cincinnati is listed as a physician in the city directory on a yearly basis. "Physicians, [Cincinnati City Directory, 1888]," *US, City Directories, 1822–1995*, Ancestry.com, ancestry.com/search/collections/2469/records/1101216652.

63. Details are taken from "Population Schedule [Cincinnati Ward 18, Hamilton, Ohio], 1870 United States Federal Census," NARA microfilm publication M593, roll M593_1216, page 434A.

64. Albisetti, "The Fight for Female Physicians in Imperial Germany," 101.
65. Cohn, "Nativism and the End of the Mass Migration of the 1840s and 1850s."
66. Mary Bickerdyke to James Bickerdyke, May 13, 1887, MssCol 19224, box 1, folder 14, images 35–36, MAB Papers.
67. "In Memoriam: Miss Mary E. Bickerdyke," box 1, folder 20, image 53, MAB Papers.
68. Mary Bickerdyke to James Bickerdyke, May 13, 1887, box 1, folder 14, image 37, MAB Papers.
69. Mollie Bickerdyke to Mary Bickerdyke, n.d., MssCol 19224, box 1, folder 20, image 65, MAB Papers.
70. Mollie Bickerdyke to Mary Bickerdyke, n.d., MssCol 19224, box 1, folder 20, image 66, MAB Papers.
71. "In Memoriam: Miss Mary E. Bickerdyke," n.d., box 1, folder 20, image 53, MAB Papers.
72. Vanderpool, *Palliative Care*.
73. "Deaths," *Cincinnati Enquirer*, July 28, 1887.
74. "In Memoriam: Miss Mary E. Bickerdyke," n.d., box 1, folder 20, image 53, MAB Papers.
75. "In Memoriam: Miss Mary E. Bickerdyke," n.d., box 1, folder 20, image 53, MAB Papers.
76. "In Memoriam: Miss Mary E. Bickerdyke," n.d., box 1, folder 20, image 53, MAB Papers.
77. Mary Bickerdyke to James Bickerdyke, May 13, 1887, box 1, folder 15, image 37, MAB Papers.

*Chapter Six*

1. Skocpol, *Protecting Soldiers and Mothers*; Kelly, *Creating a National Home*.
2. Ladd-Taylor, *Mother-Work*; Masarik, *Sentimental State*.
3. Edwards, *Angels in the Machinery*.
4. "Must Jesus Bear the Cross Alone?" Mss19224, box 4, folder 12, image 43, MAB Papers.
5. Noll, *Scandal of the Evangelical Mind*, 149.
6. Glasson, *Federal Military Pensions in the United States*, 125. In 1818, 1832, and 1836, Congress progressively extended and expanded pensions to veterans of the US War of Independence and their widows. The earliest legislation required veterans to demonstrate "dire poverty," but by 1836, the United States had liberalized its pension distribution to include widows of all rank-and-file soldiers and veterans, regardless of proven financial need.
7. McClintock, "Civil War Pensions and the Reconstruction of Union Families," 465.
8. "Would Not Sign the Bill: The President Refuses to Approve the New Pension Measure," *Chicago Tribune*, February 12, 1887.
9. This eventually came to include old age, explicitly stated in the 1906 amendment of this law.
10. "'Mother' Husband Dying," *Canton Independent-Sentinel*, February 6, 1894.

11. Elizabeth Lindqwister, "Mary Morris Husband," Library of Congress Research Guides, n.d., https://guides.loc.gov/civil-war-soldiers/mary-morris-husband#s-lib-ctab-24729930-1.

12. Lindqwister, "Mary Morris Husband."

13. Mary M. Husband to F. N. Knapp, January 6, 1885, container 1, folder 9, FNK Collection.

14. Courtland Cushing Matson, "Report No. 1136 to Accompany Bill H.R. 5894: Mary Morris Husband," April 11, 1884, 48th Cong., 1st sess., House of Representatives, 3.

15. John A. Douglass, M. D., to Mary Morris Husband, March 11, 1884, Civil War and Later Pension Files, 1861–1942 (Civil War Files), Records of the Department of Veterans Affairs, Record Group 15, NARA.

16. Matson, "Report No. 1136: Mary Morris Husband," 3; Mary Morris Husband to F. N. Knapp, March 22, 1884, container 1, folder 7, FNK Collection.

17. Matson, "Report No. 1136: Mary Morris Husband," 3.

18. Metheny, "'For a Woman,'" 4.

19. Matson, "Report No. 1136: Mary Morris Husband," 2.

20. Mary Bickerdyke to F. N. Knapp, December 18, 1884, container 1, folder 7, FNK Collection.

21. Mary Livermore to F. N. Knapp, February 25, 1885, container 1, folder 7, FNK Collection.

22. Tommy Sweet to Mary Bickerdyke, May 22, 1885, container 1, folder 9, FNK Collection.

23. C. C. Davis to F. N. Knapp, June 14, 1885, container 1, folder 7, FNK Collection.

24. C. C. Davis to F. N. Knapp, October 5, 1885, container 1, folder 5, FNK Collection.

25. C. C. Davis to F. N. Knapp, June 14, 1885, container 1, folder 7, FNK Collection.

26. US Congress, Senate, Report No. 351 to Accompany Bill H.R. 700, 49th Cong., 1st sess., March 31, 1886. Facsimile of the report found in container 1, folder 7, FNK Collection.

27. C. C. Davis to F. N. Knapp, October 5, 1885, container 1, folder 5, FNK Collection.

28. Mary Bickerdyke to F. N. Knapp, November 17, 1885, container 1, folder 7, FNK Collection.

29. Mary Bickerdyke to F. N. Knapp, October 19, 1885, container 1, folder 8, FNK Collection.

30. Torreno, "The Art and Politics of Chicago's Sanitary Fairs"; Greene, "Nothing Daunts Chicago," 71–97.

31. Massey, *Women in the Civil War*.

32. Mary Bickerdyke to James Bickerdyke, August 15, 1885, MssCol 19224, box 1, folder 14, images 67–68, MAB Papers; John D. Long to F. N. Knapp, November 7, 1885, container 1, folder 8, FNK Collection. For the Civil War memorial literature that includes Bickerdyke, see Brockett and Vaughan, *Woman's Work in the Civil War*; Hoge, *Boys in Blue*; Henshaw, *Our Branch and Its Tributaries*; Newberry, *US Sanitary Commission in the Valley of the Mississippi*.

33. John D. Long to F. N. Knapp, January 12, 1886, container 1, folder 5, FNK Collection.

34. US Congress, Senate, Report No. 351 to Accompany Bill H.R. 700, 49th Cong., 1st sess., March 31, 1886, container 1, folder 7, FNK Collection; Senator Charles Van Wyck

and Henry W. Blair, Speaking on the Reports of the Committee on Pensions, March 31, 1886, 49th Cong., 1st sess., S 2939.

35. Private Acts and Resolutions, Acts of the Forty-Ninth Congress of the United States, Statutes I, US Statutes at Large 24 (1886), 706–50.

36. US Congress, Senate, Report No. 351 to Accompany Bill H.R. 700.

37. James E. Yeatman to F. N. Knapp, December 3, 1885, container 1, folder 9, FNK Collection.

38. US Congress, Senate, Report No. 351 to Accompany Bill H.R. 700.

39. Grover Cleveland to Senate, July 5, 1888, in *The Public Papers of Grover Cleveland, Twenty-Second President of the United States: March 4, 1885 to March 4, 1889* (Washington, DC, 1889), 351–52.

40. Mary Bickerdyke Pension Certificate, June 14, 1886, MssCol 19224, box 4, folder 1, image 3, MAB Papers.

41. Skocpol, *Protecting Soldiers and Mothers*, 319.

42. Masarik, *Sentimental State*, 13.

43. Burton, *A New Book of Thrilling Interest*.

44. Burton, *Woman Who Battled for the Boys in Blue*, x.

45. Metheny, "'For a Woman.'"

46. Hadley-Cousins, *Bodies in Blue*, 4.

47. Mary Bickerdyke to Dr. Eastman, July 9, 1891, MssCol 19224, box 3, folder 13, images 55–57, MAB Papers.

48. James H. Cook to Mary Bickerdyke, San Francisco, November 18, 1885, MssCol 19224, box 2, folder 15, images 25–27, MAB Papers.

49. James H. Cook to Mary Bickerdyke, December 9, 1885, MssCol 19224, box 2, folder 15, image 28, MAB Papers.

50. Headquarters Motor Post to 478 GAR, Codell, Kansas, August 24, 1889, MssCol 19224, box 2, folder 18, image 8, MAB Papers; "Notice of Appointment—Guardian," *Russell Record*, June 20, 1889. The adjustment to Cook's pension amount could have been made any time after the Arrears Act.

51. Joel E. Cadry Jr. to Whom It May Concern, October 30, 1889, MssCol 19224, box 2, folder 18, images 12–16, MAB Papers.

52. "City Officers," *(Russell, KS) Journal*, September 11, 1889. Although William Richards had disappointed GAR members with his handling of the Cook case, he maintained an upstanding reputation in the small community of Russell, where he held elected positions as police judge and clerk.

53. Joel E. Cadry Jr. to Mary Bickerdyke, November 7, 1889, MssCol 19224, box 2, folder 18, images 17–18, MAB Papers.

54. Nichols to Mary Bickerdyke, December 29, 1889, MssCol 19224, box 2, folder 18, images 30–31, MAB Papers.

55. J. B. Ross and Son to Mary Bickerdyke, May 26, 1890, MssCol 19224, box 2, folder 19, image 7, MAB Papers.

56. Mary Bickerdyke to Mrs. E. C. Cook, June 8, 1891, MssCol 19224, box 3, folder 13, image 46, MAB Papers.

57. James or Eliza Cook to Mr. Ross, May 1, 1891, MssCol 19224, box 2, folder 19, image 18, MAB Papers.

58. Dr. B. D. Eastman to J. B. Ross, May 25, 1891, MssCol 19224, box 2, folder 20, images 39–40, MAB Papers.

59. Joel E. Cadry Jr. to Mary Bickerdyke, November 7, 1889, MssCol 19224, box 2, folder 18, images 17–18, MAB Papers.

60. Dr. B. D. Eastman to J. B. Ross, May 25, 1891, MssCol 19224, box 2, folder 20, images 39–40, MAB Papers.

61. Rodney Chipp, Department of the Interior, Bureau of Pensions, Denver, to Commissioner of Pensions, May 1, 1893, James H. Cook Civil War Pension File, T288, NARA.

62. Harkness Godard to Holland, February 23, 1892, James H. Cook Civil War Pension File, T288, NARA.

63. "Receipt, Mr. James H. Cook, Estate," September 21, 1894, MssCol 19224, box 3, folder 13, image 138, MAB Papers; W. W. Denison to Mrs. Bickerdyke, September 23, 1894, MssCol 19224, box 2, folder 13, image 140, MAB Papers.

64. I. W. G. Eastland, Probate Court, April 16, 1892, MssCol 19224, box 3, folder 13, image 71, MAB Papers.

65. Passenger Lists of Vessels Arriving at Boston, Massachusetts, 1820–1891, Records of the US Customs Service, Record Group 36, series M277, roll 024, NARA.

66. "Prisoner Details," Civil War Soldiers and Sailors System, National Park Service, n.d., https://www.nps.gov/civilwar/search-prisoners.htm#sort=score+desc&q=Bolton,+Thomas.

67. "A Stranger's Burial," *Russell Record*, May 21, 1891.

68. Hackemer, "Civil War Veteran Colonies on the Western Frontier," 64.

69. Eli, Salisbury, and Shertzer, "Ideology and Migration after the American Civil War," 823.

70. Tom Bolton to Mary Bickerdyke, September 7, 1890, MssCol 19224, box 2, folder 19, image 23, MAB Papers; Gardner, "When Service Is Not Enough," 43.

71. Mary Bickerdyke to P. B. Plumb, April 4, 1891, MssCol 19224, box 2, folder 20, image 6, MAB Papers.

72. Mary Bickerdyke, Pension Attorney, March 9, 1891, MssCol 19224, box 4, folder 3, images 14–17, MAB Papers.

73. C. H. Blinn to Mary Bickerdyke, May 12, 1891, MssCol 19224, box 2, folder 20, images 25–26, MAB Papers; Anna Young to Mary Bickerdyke, May 17, 1891, MssCol 19224, box 2, folder 20, image 28, MAB Papers.

74. Mary Bickerdyke to P. B. Plumb, April 24, 1891, MssCol 19224, box 2, folder 20, image 14, MAB Papers; Mary Bickerdyke to Charles H. Blinn, May 18, 1891, MssCol 19224, box 2, folder 20, images 31–32, MAB Papers.

75. Charles H. Blinn, May 18, 1891, MssCol 19224, box 2, folder 20, images 31–32, MAB Papers.

76. Mary and J. R. Bickerdyke, "Card of Thanks," *Russell Record*, May 21, 1891.

77. "A Stranger's Burial," *Russell Record*, May 21, 1891.

78. Illinois State Marriage Records, Online Index, Illinois State Public Record Offices, Records of the Office of the Quartermaster General, Record Group 92, series M1845, NARA.

79. Tenth US Census, 1880, Center Township, Russell, Kansas, roll 395, page 66A; 1885 Kansas Territory Census, Topeka, Kansas, roll KS1885_120, line 6, Kansas State Historical Society.

80. "Obituary," *Russell Record*, December 15, 1887.

81. Tenth US Census, 1880, Center Township, Russell, Kansas, roll 395, page 66A.
82. "Special Order No. 32, Department of Kansas, G.A.R.," October 21, 1891, folder 2, Correspondence 1862–June 1897, MAB Collection.
83. "Special Order No. 32, Department of Kansas, G.A.R.," October 21, 1891, folder 2, Correspondence 1862–June 1897, MAB Collection.
84. See over fifty individual responses and receipts from Kansas GAR posts to the aid of Lucy Nicholson, folder 2, Correspondence 1862–June 1897, MAB Collection.
85. "Relief of Lucy Nicholson," December 23, 1891, and "Update from Larrabee Post on Lucy Nicholson," April 9, 1892, folder 2, correspondence 1862–June 1897, MAB Collection.
86. US Civil War Pension Index, General Index to Pension Files, 1861–1934, NAI no. T288, Records of the Department of Veterans Affairs, 1773–2007, Record Group 15, roll 349; List of Claim Numbers and Soldiers/Widows, box 4, folder 3, image 25, MAB Papers.

*Chapter Seven*

1. Jenkin Lloyd Jones to James Bickerdyke, December 11, 1901, MssCol 19224, box 1, folder 12, MAB Papers.
2. Jenkin Lloyd Jones, "Introduction," in Kellogg, *Mother Bickerdyke, As I Knew Her*, 15.
3. J. L. Jones, "Introduction," 16.
4. N. B. Hood to Mary Bickerdyke, August 29, 1897, MssCol 19224, box 2, folder 15, image 48, MAB Papers.
5. J. L. Jones, "Introduction," 16.
6. Mary Bickerdyke to Jenkin Lloyd Jones, February 15, 1892, box 1, folder 14, Jenkin Lloyd Jones Papers, 1861–1932, University of Chicago Special Collections Research Center.
7. Bickerdyke to Jenkin Lloyd Jones, February 15, 1892.
8. Linderman, *Embattled Courage*, 267; Blight, *Race and Reunion*; Fahs and Waugh, *Memory of the Civil War in American Culture*; Janney, *Remembering the Civil War*; Jordan and Rothera, *War Went On*. The full book titles cited here provide a more complete treatment of soldier memory in Civil War historical construction.
9. Blight, *Race and Reunion*, 2.
10. Trouillot, *Silencing the Past*, 27.
11. Kellogg, *Mother Bickerdyke, As I Knew Her*, 111.
12. "Hiram Bickerdyke to Florence Shaw Kellogg, December 3, 1905," in Kellogg, *Mother Bickerdyke, As I Knew Her*, 36–38.
13. "Hiram Bickerdyke to Florence Shaw Kellogg, December 3, 1905."
14. Brimmer, *Claiming Union Widowhood*, 5.
15. "The Civil War: Soldier Details. Foster, Wesley," National Park Service, n.d., https://www.nps.gov/civilwar/search-soldiers-detail.htm?soldierId=77AA429E-DC7A-DF11-BF36-B8AC6F5D926A.
16. Illinois, US, County Marriage Records, 1800–1940; Illinois State Archives, *The Revised Laws of Illinois*, "An Act respecting free Negroes and Mulattoes, Servants, and Slaves, Section 3" (Vandalia: Printed by Greiner & Sherman, 1833), 473. The 1833 Illinois law stated: "No person of color, negro, or mulatto, of either sex, shall be joined in marriage with any white person, male or female, in this state, and all marriages or contracts entered into between such colored person and white person, shall be null and void in law; and any person

214  Notes to Chapter Seven

so offending shall be liable to pay a fine, whipped in not exceeding thirty-nine lashes, and be imprisoned not less than one year." This law was not overturned until 1874, two years after their forbidden marriage.

17. Painter, *Exodusters*. Nell Irvin Painter's counters the monolithic narrative the Exoduster movement.

18. Hodes, *Sea Captain's Wife*; Pascoe, *What Comes Naturally*; Monahan, "Interracial Marriage and Divorce in Kansas and the Question of Instability of Mixed Marriages," 109; Campney, "'Light Is Bursting upon the World!'" Brent Campney's article provides an excellent analysis that counters other historians' claims to more racial equity in Reconstruction Kansas.

19. "Wyandotte Constitution," 1859, Kansas State Historical Society, accessed March 13, 2025, https://www.kansasmemory.org/item/90272.

20. "African American Residents in Kansas," Kansas State Historical Society, accessed March 13, 2025, https://www.kansashistory.gov/kansapedia/african-american-residents-in-kansas/17878.

21. "Russell County, Kansas," Kansas State Historical Society, accessed March 13, 2025, https://www.kansashistory.gov/kansapedia/russell-county-kansas/15338.

22. Painter, *Exodusters*.

23. "Tenth Census of the United States [Center, Russell, Kansas], 1880, United States Federal Census," NARA microfilm publication M593, roll 395, page 59C, Enumeration District, 290.

24. US Census Bureau, Population Schedule (Russell, KS), "Productions of Agriculture in Center Township in the County of Russell, State of Kansas," enumerated by George Shearer, June 6–7, 1880.

25. McHenry, *Forgotten Readers*, 3.

26. Edwards and Friefeld, *The First Migrants*. This book provides more examples of the establishment of Black schools in Kansas, particularly after the turn of the twentieth century.

27. Patterson et al., "Educating for Success," 308.

28. Arthur, T. C. McGavic and Co to Mary Bickerdyke, December 23, 1897, MssCol 19224, box 2, folder 2, image 141, MAB Papers. This letter gives the first discernable archival mention of Lydia's employment in the Bickerdyke household.

29. Forten, *Minutes and Proceedings of the First Annual Meeting of the American Moral Reform Society*; Muhammad, "The Literacy Development and Practices within African American Literary Societies." James Forten's force and sentiment is best seen by the educational frameworks proposed and implemented by Dr. Gholnecsar Muhammad, who advocates for a modern and equitable educational framework that is inspired by nineteenth-century Black literary societies.

30. "Twelfth Census of the United States [Center, Russell, Kansas], 1900, United States Federal Census," NARA FHL microfilm 1240498, page 2, Enumeration District 0149; Blake, "'First in the Path of the Firemen.'" Most of the original schedules of the 1890 census from Kansas were destroyed in a 1921 fire in Washington, DC. For more information on this tragic erasure of American history, Kellee Blake's article provides the narrative.

31. This corpus of letters was run through the Handwriting Analysis Tool (HAT) from the University of Hamburg's Centre for the Study of Manuscript Cultures. This tool em-

ployed digital paleography to produce similarity scores and positively confirmed Lydia Foster's consistent letter-writing as Bickerdyke's amanuensis.

32. "Mary Bickerdyke's Eightieth Birthday Autograph Book," folder 3, MAB Collection, 1862–1908.

33. Lydia Foster did not sign this list, but it was run through the Handwriting Analysis Tool to confirm its authorship.

34. James Bickerdyke to Hiram Bickerdyke, July 4, 1904, MssCol 19224, box 1, folder 12, images 59–60, MAB Papers; James Bickerdyke to Hiram Bickerdyke, November 21, 1903, MssCol 19224, box 1, folder 12, images 53–54, MAB Papers.

35. James Bickerdyke to Hiram Bickerdyke, July 4, 1903, MssCol 19224, box 1, folder 12, images 42–43, MAB Papers.

36. Trouillot, *Silencing the Past*, 27.

37. May, "Ghost Writing and History," 461.

38. Trouillot, *Silencing the Past*, 27.

39. DuBois, *Black Reconstruction in America*, 641.

40. Baumgartner, *In Pursuit of Knowledge*, 107.

41. McHenry, *Forgotten Readers*, 17.

42. Moss, *Schooling Citizens*, 4.

43. Royster, *Traces of a Stream*, 4.

44. Field, *Struggle for Equal Adulthood*, 3.

45. Field, *Struggle for Equal Adulthood*, 129.

46. Elizabeth Cady Stanton, "Advice to the Strong-Minded," *Revolution* (New York, NY), January 29, 1868.

47. Faust, *Mothers of Invention*; K. S. Smith, *We Have Raised All of You*; White, *Too Heavy a Load*.

48. May, "Ghost Writing and History," 465.

49. Mary Bickerdyke, "Cemetery Plot Deed, September 1, 1863," MssCol 19224, box 4, folder 11, images 7–8, MAB Papers.

50. Faust, *This Republic of Suffering*. The United States government did not successfully put a cemetery system in place until after the war's conclusion.

51. Sue Allen to Mary Bickerdyke, April 28, 1897, MssCol 19224, box 2, folder 2, image 16, MAB Papers.

52. Allen to Bickerdyke, April 28, 1897, MssCol 19224, box 2, folder 2, image 17, MAB Papers.

53. Mary Bickerdyke to Sue Allen, May 14, 1897, box 1, file 2, Mary Bickerdyke Papers, KCSC.

54. H. A. Allen to Professor J. R. Bickerdyke, January 12, 1898, box 1, file 3, Mary Bickerdyke Papers, KCSC.

55. E. J. Harris to J. R. Bickerdyke, November 5, 1901, MssCol 19224, box 1, folder 15, images 104–5, MAB Papers.

56. "Wished Burial Here," *Western Veteran* (Topeka, KS), November 1901.

57. James Bickerdyke to Hiram Bickerdyke, November 10, 1901, MssCol 19224, box 1, folder 12, images 35–36, MAB Papers; "Back to Her Old Home," *Western Veteran* (Topeka, KS), November 1901.

58. "Songs Used at My Mother's Funeral," MssCol 19224, box 4, folder 12, image 11, MAB Papers. James Bickerdyke compiled this list in a letter written to his brother Hiram.

216  Notes to Chapter Seven

59. Mary Bickerdyke to James Bickerdyke, August 15, 1885, MssCol 19224, box 1, folder 14, images 67–68, MAB Papers.

60. Muhlenberg, *"I Would Not Live Alway,"* 1860, 9.

61. Muhlenberg, *"I Would Not Live Alway,"* 1860, 9–11. The hymn was written in 1824 and revised by the author in 1859.

62. "Services at the Grave," *Western Veteran* (Topeka, KS), November 1901.

63. Mary Wainwright to James Bickerdyke, December 22, 1901, MssCol 19224, box 1, folder 31, images 21–22, MAB Papers.

64. "Mother Bickerdyke Monument," *Western Veteran* (Topeka, KS), November 1901.

65. Mother Bickerdyke Memorial Association to James Bickerdyke, May 2, 1902, MssCol 19224, box 1, folder 15, images 156–57, MAB Papers.

66. Mother Bickerdyke Memorial Association to James Bickerdyke, June 27, 1904, MssCol 19224, box 1, folder 15, image 189–90, MAB Papers.

67. C. R. Bickerdyke to James Bickerdyke, August 28, 1904, MssCol 19224, box 1, folder 15, images 201–2, MAB Papers.

68. Harper, *Women during the Civil War*, 34–36.

69. J. R. made the inquiry through his cousin George Washington Clark, who knew Carleton personally and wrote to the poet on J. R.'s behalf.

70. Carleton, "Over the Hill to the Poor House."

71. Carleton, "The Festival of Memory; or, Converse with the Slain," 154.

72. "Columbus Lyceum: December 10," *Columbus Journal* (Columbus, NE), November 24, 1886.

73. "Will Carleton: A Good Poet Whose Forte Is Not Recitation," *Topeka State Journal*, April 26, 1892.

74. "Will Carleton," *Oberlin Herald*, May 29, 1890.

75. Will Carleton to Mr. G. W. Clark, December 18, 1901, MssCol 19224, box 2, folder 6, image 44, MAB Papers.

76. G. W. Clark to J. R. Bickerdyke, December 20, 1901, MssCol 19224, box 2, folder 6, image 45, MAB Papers.

77. Carleton, "Preface," *Songs of Two Centuries*, 3.

78. Carleton, "Farmer Stebbins at the Fair," in *Songs of Two Centuries*, 35.

79. Carleton, *Songs of Two Centuries*, 9.

80. Carleton, "Do Not Forget the Wounded," in *Songs of Two Centuries*, 105; Carleton, "A Man Has Died," in *Songs of Two Centuries*, 124.

81. Carleton, "The Passing of the Mother," in *Songs of Two Centuries*, 106.

82. Carleton, "The Passing of the Mother," 107, lines 29–32.

83. Carleton, "The Passing of the Mother," 107, lines 81–82.

84. Carleton, "The Passing of the Mother," 107, lines 39–45.

85. Carleton, "The Passing of the Mother," 107, line 111.

86. Carleton, "The Passing of the Mother," 107, lines 117–22.

87. Carleton, "The Passing of the Mother," 107, line 14.

88. Carleton, "Greater America," in *Songs of Two Centuries*, 97.

89. Hiram Bickerdyke to Julia Chase, January 12, 1905, images 1–7, MAB Collection. In this letter, Hiram acknowledged his mother's close friendship with Julia Chase.

90. Department of Kansas WRC to Mary Bickerdyke, February 15, 1896, MssCol 19224, box 4, folder 6, image 31, MAB Papers; *Salina Daily Republican-Journal*, December 17, 1895.

91. "Mrs. Chase's Reply," *Salina Daily Republican-Journal*, February 8, 1902.

92. "General Order No. 4, Mother Bickerdyke Day General Orders Booklet," GAR and WRC Kansas Resolutions, folder 2, MAB Collection.

93. Emma B. Alrich to Mary Bickerdyke, June 1896, MssCol 19224, box 3, folder 1, images 20–22, MAB Papers.

94. "The Straight of It," *Salina Daily Republican-Journal*, January 27, 1902.

95. "The Straight of It," *Salina Daily Republican-Journal*, January 27, 1902.

96. Mary Bickerdyke to General Sherman, February 5, 1869, MssCol 19224, box 2, folder 1, image 14, MAB Papers.

97. "Mrs. Chase's Reply," *Salina Daily Republican-Journal*, February 8, 1902.

98. Mrs. Julia A. Chase to Mr. George W. Martin, February 13, 1902, MAB Collection.

99. George W. Martin to James R. Bickerdyke, February 19, 1902, MAB Collection.

100. Martin to James R. Bickerdyke, February 19, 1902.

101. "Mrs. Chase's Reply," *Salina Daily Republican-Journal*, February 8, 1902.

102. Hamerow, "The Professionalization of Historical Learning," 319.

103. Cronon, "A Place for Stories," 1349; Roberts, "Reversible Social Processes, Historical Memory, and the Production of History"; Crane, *Nothing Happened*.

104. Hiram Bickerdyke to James R. Bickerdyke, February 26, 1902, box 1, MAB Collection.

105. Hiram Bickerdyke to Julia Chase, January 12, 1905, box 1, image 1, IHC.

106. Julia A. Chase to A. H. Thomas, January 9, 1905, MssCol 19224, box 3, folder 6, images 50–53, MAB Papers.

107. "Mrs. Chase's Reply," *Salina Daily Republican-Journal*, February 8, 1902.

108. J. R. Bickerdyke to Hiram Bickerdyke, May 26, 1902, MssCol 19224, box 1, folder 12, image 39, MAB Papers.

109. Lydia S. Foster to Hiram Bickerdyke, December 24, 1904, MssCol 19224, box 1, folder 15, images 204–6, MAB Papers; "James R. Bickerdyke Dead," *Great Bend Register*, December 29, 1904.

110. Julia A. Chase to A. H. Thomas, January 9, 1905, MssCol 19224, box 3, folder 6, image 50, MAB Papers.

111. Julia A. Chase to A. H. Thomas, January 9, 1905, MssCol 19224, box 3, folder 6, image 50, MAB Papers.

112. Julia A. Chase to Hiram Bickerdyke, January 5, 1905, MssCol 19224, box 1, folder 12, image 86, MAB Papers.

113. Hiram Bickerdyke to Julia Chase, January 12, 1905, box 1, image 1, IHC.

114. Hiram Bickerdyke to Julia Chase, January 12, 1905, box 1, image 2, IHC, italics in original.

115. Hiram Bickerdyke to Julia Chase, January 12, 1905, box 1, image 4, IHC.

116. Hiram Bickerdyke to Julia Chase, January 12, 1905, box 1, image 7, IHC, italics in original.

117. Hiram Bickerdyke to Julia Chase, February 27, 1905, box 1, image 9, IHC.

118. Hiram Bickerdyke to Julia Chase, February 27, 1905, box 1, image 2, IHC.

119. George W. Martin to Julia Chase, March 10, 1905, box 1, image 14, IHC.

218  *Notes to Epilogue*

120. Hamerow, "Professionalization of Historical Learning," 323.

121. Wilson, "The Variety and Unity of History." This September 20, 1904, speech was given at the Universal Exposition at St. Louis. Wilson charged, "We have seen the dawn and the early morning hours of a new age in the writing of history, and the morning is now broadening about us into day. When that day is full we shall see that minute research and broad synthesis are not hostile but friendly methods, cooperating toward a common end which neither can reach alone."

122. Hiram Bickerdyke to Julia A. Chase, March 25, 1905, box 1, images 4–5, IHC.

123. Hiram Bickerdyke to Julia A. Chase, March 25, 1905, image 5.

124. Record of Appointment of Postmasters, 1832–September 30, 1971, roll 43, Archive Publication M841, NARA. Kellogg was appointed postmaster as early as 1883 in Fay, Kansas, in Russell County, where Bickerdyke also lived in her final years.

125. Kellogg, *Mother Bickerdyke, As I Knew Her*, 126. The letters that Kellogg refers to in this passage do not exist in any public archive.

126. Kellogg, *Mother Bickerdyke, As I Knew Her*, 111.

127. Kellogg, *Mother Bickerdyke, As I Knew Her*, 129.

128. Kellogg, *Mother Bickerdyke, As I Knew Her*, 130.

129. Kellogg, *Mother Bickerdyke, As I Knew Her*, 130–31.

130. Kellogg, *Mother Bickerdyke, As I Knew Her*, 131–32.

131. Jenkin Lloyd Jones to J. R. Bickerdyke, December 11, 1901, MssCol 19224, box 1, folder 12, image 37, MAB Papers; Kellogg, *Mother Bickerdyke*, 152.

132. J. L. Jones, "Introduction," in Kellogg, *Mother Bickerdyke*, 8.

133. J. L. Jones, "Introduction," 10.

134. Baker, *Cyclone in Calico*, 14. Jones's genealogical claims can be found in Nina Brown Baker's book published for a young audience.

*Epilogue*

1. Mary Bickerdyke to Comrad Bonquet, April 20, 1892, MssCol 19224, box 2, folder 21, image 21, MAB Papers.

2. Louis H. Hendricks to Julia A. Chase, November 19, 1901, MssCol 19224, box 3, folder 6, images 37–39, MAB Papers.

3. Alice B. Long, "Regular Meeting of the WRC," n.d., MssCol 19224, box 4, folder 6, image 110, MAB Papers.

4. Long, "Regular Meeting of the WRC," n.d., MssCol 19224, box 4, folder 6, image 110, MAB Papers.

5. "Hiram's Hieroglyphics," MssCol 19224, box 4, folder 11, image 106, MAB Papers.

# Bibliography

*Primary Sources*

ARCHIVES

Bloomington, IL
  McLean County Museum of History
    Illinois Soldiers' and Sailors' Children's School (ISSCS) Collection
Chicago, IL
  Chicago History Museum, Manuscripts Collection
    The Allen C. Fuller Papers
    Chicago Home for the Friendless Records, 1858–1960, bulk 1858–1937
    Documents of the United States Sanitary Commission
    Mark Skinner Collection
    Report of Transactions of the Illinois State Sanitary Bureau (1862–63)
    Report of the Illinois State Sanitary Commission (1863–64)
  Newberry Library, Manuscripts and Ephemera
    The E. W. Blatchford Papers
    The Lloyd Lewis Papers
  University of Chicago Special Collections Research Center
    Jenkin Lloyd Jones Papers, 1861–1932
Galesburg, IL
  Knox College Special Collections
    Local History Series
    Mary Bickerdyke Papers
New York, NY
  New York Public Library, Manuscripts and Archives Division
    United States Sanitary Commission, Historical Bureau Archives
    United States Sanitary Commission, New York Archives
    United States Sanitary Commission, Western Department Archives
Philadelphia, PA
  Library Company of Philadelphia
    The Frank H. Taylor Illustration Collection
Springfield, IL
  Abraham Lincoln Presidential Library and Museum
    The David and Sarah Gregg Manuscript Collection
    The Isham Nicholas Haynie Papers, 1848–98
    The John A. McClernand Papers
    The Lemuel Adams Papers
    The Richard J. Oglesby Papers

Illinois State Archives
  Journal of the House of Representatives of the Twenty-Fourth General Assembly of the State of Illinois, at Their Regular Session, Begun and Held at Springfield, Illinois, January 2, 1865. Springfield, IL: Baker and Phillips, Printers, 1865.
  Reports Made to the General Assembly of Illinois, at Its Twenty-Sixth Session, Convened January 4, 1869. Springfield, IL: Illinois Journal Printing Office, 1869.
  Revised Laws of Illinois, "An Act respecting free Negroes and Mulattoes, Servants, and Slaves, Section 3." Vandalia, IL: Printed by Greiner & Sherman, 1833.
Topeka, KS
  Kansas State Historical Society
    Grasshoppers History Collection
    Indian History Collection
    Mary Ann Bickerdyke Collection
    Transactions of the Kansas State Historical Society, 1901–1902; Together with Addresses at Annual Meetings, Memorials, and Miscellaneous Papers, Volume 7, edited by George W. Martin. Topeka: Kansas Publishing House, 1902.
Washington, DC
  Kiplinger Research Library, DC History Center
    Frederick N. Knapp Collection
  Library of Congress, Manuscripts Division
    The Mary Bickerdyke Papers
  National Archives and Records Administration, Washington, DC
    Record of Appointment of Postmasters, 1832–Sept. 30, 1971
    Records of the Department of Veteran Affairs
    Records of the Office of the Quartermaster General
    Records of the US Customs Service
    US Civil War Pension Index

BOOKS AND MAGAZINES

Baker, Nina Brown. *Cyclone in Calico: The Story of Mary Ann Bickerdyke*. Boston: Little, Brown, 1952.

Beecher, Catharine Esther. *A Treatise on Domestic Economy, for the Use of Young Ladies at Home, and at School*, Rev. ed. Boston: T. H. Webb, 1843.

Brinton, John H. *Personal Memoirs of John H. Brinton: Civil War Surgeon, 1861–1865*. Carbondale: Southern Illinois University Press, 1996.

Brockett, L. P., and Mary Vaughan. *Woman's Work in the Civil War: A Record of Heroism, Patriotism and Patience*. Boston: R. H. Curran, 1867.

Brooks, Jane, and Christine E. Hallett. *One Hundred Years of Wartime Nursing Practices, 1854–1953*. Manchester, UK: Manchester University Press, 2015.

Burton, Margaret Davis. *A New Book of Thrilling Interest, Mother Bickerdyke: The Woman Who Battled for the Boys*. San Francisco: A.T. Dewey, 1886.

———. *The Woman Who Battled for the Boys in Blue: Mother Bickerdyke; Her Life and Labors for the Relief of Our Soldiers. Sketches of Battle Scenes and Incidents of the Sanitary Service*. San Francisco: A.T. Dewey, 1886.

Carleton, Will. "The Festival of Memory; Or, Converse with the Slain." In *Farm Festivals*. New York: Harper and Brothers, 1882.

———. "Over the Hill to the Poor House." In *Over the Hill to the Poor-House and Other Poems*. New York: Harper and Brothers, 1872.
———. *Songs of Two Centuries*. New York: Harper and Brothers, 1902.
Chase, Julia A. Houghton. *Mary A. Bickerdyke, "Mother": The Life Story of One Who, as Wife, Mother, Army Nurse, Pension Agent and City Missionary, Has Touched the Heights and Depths of Human Life*. Lawrence: Women's Relief Corps, 1896.
Cleveland, Grover. *The Public Papers of Grover Cleveland, Twenty-Second President of the United States: March 4, 1885 to March 4, 1889*. Washington, DC: Government Printing Office, 1889.
Ferber, Edna. *Mother Knows Best: A Fiction Book*. Garden City, NY: Doubleday, 1927.
Forten, James. *Minutes and Proceedings of the First Annual Meeting of the American Moral Reform Society*. Philadelphia: AMRS, 1837.
Halsted, William S. "The Results of Operations for the Cure of Cancer of the Breast Performed at the Johns Hopkins Hospital from June, 1889, to January, 1894." *Johns Hopkins Hospital Reports* 4 (1894).
Henshaw, Mrs. Sarah Edwards. *Our Branch and Its Tributaries: Being a History of the Work of the Northwestern Sanitary Commission and Its Auxiliaries during the War of the Rebellion*. Chicago: Alfred L. Sewell, 1868.
Hoge, Jane Currie Blaikie. *The Boys in Blue: Or, Heroes of the "Rank and File." Comprising Incidents and Reminiscences from Camp, Battle-field, and Hospital, with Narratives of the Sacrifice, Suffering, and Triumphs of the Soldiers of the Republic*. Chicago: C. W. Lilley, 1867.
Jones, Jenkin Lloyd. *An Artillery Man's Diary*. The Wisconsin History Commission, 1914.
———. "Introduction." In *Mother Bickerdyke, As I Knew Her*. Chicago: Unity Pub. Co., 1907.
Juettner, Otto. *Daniel Drake and His Followers: Historical and Biographical Sketches*. Cincinnati, OH: Harvey Publishing, 1909.
Kellogg, Florence Shaw. *Mother Bickerdyke, As I Knew Her*. Chicago: Unity Pub. Co., 1907.
Livermore, Mary. *My Story of the War*. Hartford, CT: A. D. Worthington, 1871.
Longfellow, Henry Wadsworth. "Santa Filomena." *The Atlantic Monthly*, November 1857. https://www.theatlantic.com/magazine/toc/1857/11/.
Muhlenberg, William Augustus. *"I Would Not Live Alway," Evangelized by Its Author*. Smithtown, NY: T. Whittaker, 1871.
———. *"I Would Not Live Alway," and Other Pieces in Verse by the Same Author*. New York: Robert Craighead, Printer, 1860.
Newberry, John Strong. *The US Sanitary Commission in the Valley of the Mississippi, during the War of the Rebellion, 1861–1866. Final Report of Dr. J. S. Newberry, Secretary Western Department*. Cleveland, OH: Fairbanks, Benedict, 1871.
Nightingale, Florence. *Notes on Nursing: What It Is, and What It Is Not*. London: Harrison Publishers, 1859.
Owen, Albert. *Integral Cooperation at Work*. New York: John W. Lovell, 1884.
Perry, Albert J. *History of Knox County*. Chicago: Clarke Publishing, 1912.
Porter, Mary H. *Eliza Chappell Porter: A Memoir*. Chicago: Fleming H. Revell, 1892.
*Report of Committees of the Senate of the United States for the First Session of the Fifty-Second Congress, 1891–1892*. Washington, DC: Government Printing Office, 1892.
*Seventh Biennial Report of the Superintendent of Public Instruction of the State of Illinois, 1867–1868*. Springfield, IL, 1868.
Sherman, William T. *Memoirs of General William T. Sherman, Volume 1*. New York: D. Appleton, 1889.

US War Department. *The War of the Rebellion: A Compilation of the Official Records of the Union and Confederate Armies*, 128 vols. Washington, DC: Government Printing Office, 1880–1890.

Wilson, Woodrow. "The Variety and Unity of History." Speech, St. Louis Exposition, September 20, 1904.

Wittenmyer, Annie. *Under the Guns: A Woman's Reminiscences of the Civil War*. Boston: E. B. Stillings, 1895.

Woodward, Benjamin. "Mother Bickerdike: One of the Grandest Women of the War." In *Camp-fire Sketches and Battle-field Echoes of 61–5*. Springfield, MA: King, Richardson, 1886.

DATABASES

Ancestry.com
   1820 United States Federal Census
   1860 United States Federal Census
   1870 United States Federal Census
   1880 United States Federal Census
   US, City Directories, 1822–1995
   US, Civil War Soldiers, 1861–1865

National Park Service
   Civil War Soldiers and Sailors

NEWSPAPERS

*Agitator*
*American Israelite*
*Brooklyn Union*
*Burlington Free Press* (Burlington, VT)
*Butte Daily Post*
*Canton Independent-Sentinel*
*Chicago Tribune*
*Cincinnati Enquirer*
*Cleveland Daily Leader*
*Columbus Journal* (Columbus, NE)
*Credit Foncier of Sinaloa*
*Daily Cincinnati Commercial*
*Daily Illinois State Journal* (Springfield)
*Galesburg Register-Mail*
*Great Bend Register*
*Inquirer* (Lancaster, PA)
*Janesville Weekly Gazette*
*Junction City Weekly Union*
*Missouri Democrat*
*Niles Democrat*
*Oberlin Herald*
*Reno Gazette-Journal*
*Revolution*
*Rock Island Argus*
*Russell Kansas Journal*
*Russell Record*
*Salina Daily Republican-Journal*
*Salina Herald*
*Sanitary Bulletin*
*South Bend Tribune*
*Springfield Daily Republican*
*Topeka State Journal*
*Weekly Hawk-Eye and Telegraph* (Burlington, IA)
*Weekly-News Democrat* (St. Louis, MO)
*Western Veteran*
*Wisconsin State Journal*
*Zephyr*

*Secondary Sources*

BOOKS

Abel, Emily K. *Hearts of Wisdom: American Women Caring for Kin, 1850–1940*. Cambridge, MA: Harvard University Press, 2002.

———. *The Inevitable Hour: A History of Caring for Dying Patients in America*. Baltimore: Johns Hopkins University Press, 2013.

———. *Living in Death's Shadow: Family Experiences of Terminal Care and Irreplaceable Loss*. Baltimore: Johns Hopkins University Press, 2017.

Abramovitz, Mimi. *Regulating the Lives of Women: Social Welfare Policy from Colonial Times to the Present*. Boston: South End Press, 1988.

Anderson, Paul Christopher. *A Short History of the American Civil War*. London: Bloomsbury, 2020.

Apple, Rima D., and Janet Golden. "Introduction: Mothers, Motherhood, and Historians." In *Mothers & Motherhood: Readings in American History*. Columbus: Ohio State University Press, 1997.

Attie, Jeanie. *Patriotic Toil: Northern Women and the American Civil War*. Ithaca, NY: Cornell University Press, 1998.

Ayers, Edward L. *In the Presence of Mine Enemies: War in the Heart of America, 1859–1863*. New York: W. W. Norton, 2003.

Baumgartner, Kabria. *In Pursuit of Knowledge: Black Women and Educational Activism in Antebellum America*. New York: New York University Press, 2019.

Beier, Lucinda McCray. *Health Culture in the Heartland, 1880–1980: An Oral History*. Urbana: University of Illinois Press, 2009.

———. *A Matter of Life and Death: Health, Illness and Medicine in McLean County, 1830–1995*. Bloomington, IL: McLean County Historical Society, 1995.

Birk, Megan. *Fostering on the Farm: Child Placement in the Rural Midwest*. Urbana: University of Illinois Press, 2015.

Blight, David W. *Race and Reunion: The Civil War in American Memory*. Cambridge, MA: Harvard University Press, 2001.

Bloch, Marc. *The Historian's Craft*. New York: Vintage Books, 1953.

Bollet, Alfred Jay. *Civil War Medicine: Challenges and Triumphs*. Tucson, AZ: Galen Press, 2002.

Boris, Eileen. *Home to Work: Motherhood and the Politics of Industrial Homework in the United States*. Cambridge, UK: Cambridge University Press, 1994.

Boydston, Jeanne. *Home and Work: Housework, Wages, and the Ideology of Labor in the Early Republic*. New York: Oxford University Press, 1994.

Brimmer, Brandi C. *Claiming Union Widowhood: Race, Respectability, and Poverty in the Post-Emancipation South*. Durham, NC: Duke University Press, 2020.

Brooks, Jane, and Christine E. Hallett. *One Hundred Years of Wartime Nursing Practices, 1854–1953*. Manchester, UK: Manchester University Press, 2015.

Brown, Thomas J. *Dorthea Dix: New England Reformer*. Cambridge, MA: Harvard University Press, 1998.

Buhle, Mari Jo. *Women and American Socialism, 1870–1920*. Urbana: University of Illinois Press, 1983.

Buhler-Wilkerson, Karen. *No Place Like Home: A History of Nursing and Home Care in the United States.* Baltimore: Johns Hopkins University Press, 2001.
Carr, Edward Hallett. *What Is History?* New York: Vintage Books, 1961.
Cayton, Andrew R. L., and Susan E. Gray. "The Story of the Midwest: An Introduction." In *The American Midwest: Essays on Regional History*, edited by Andrew R. L. Cayton and Susan E. Gray. Bloomington: Indiana University Press, 2001.
Clement, Priscilla Ferguson. *Growing Pains: Children in the Industrial Age, 1860–1890.* New York: Trayne, 1997.
Cline, Patricia Cohen. *The Murder of Helen Jewett: The Life and Death of a Prostitute in Nineteenth-Century New York.* New York: Alfred A. Knopf, 1998.
Cmiel, Kenneth. *A Home of Another Kind: One Chicago Orphanage and the Tangle of Child Welfare.* Chicago: University of Chicago Press, 1995.
Cole, Sheila. *To Be Young in America: Growing Up with the Country, 1776–1940.* New York: Little, Brown, 2005.
Collins, Patricia Hill. *Black Feminist Thought: Knowledge, Consciousness, and the Politics of Empowerment.* New York: Routledge, 1990.
Cooling, Benjamin Franklin. *Fort Donelson's Legacy: War and Society in Kentucky and Tennessee, 1862–1863.* Knoxville: University of Tennessee Press, 1997.
Cox, Thomas C. "The Grasshopper Plague, 1874–1878, and Social Welfare: The Postbellum Prospects for Relief, Recovery, and Reform." In *The Struggle for Equality: Essays on Sectional Conflict, the Civil War, and the Long Reconstruction*, edited by Orville Vernon Burton, Jerald Podair, and Jennifer L. Weber. Charlottesville: University of Virginia Press, 2011.
Crane, Susan A. *Nothing Happened: A History.* Stanford, CA: Stanford University Press, 2020.
Crenson, Matthew A. *Building the Invisible Orphanage: A Prehistory of the American Welfare System.* Cambridge, MA: Harvard University Press, 1998.
Cutter, Barbara. *Domestic Devils, Battlefield Angels: The Radicalism of American Womanhood, 1830–1865.* DeKalb: Northern Illinois University Press, 2003.
D'Antonio, Patricia. *American Nursing: A History of Knowledge, Authority, and the Meaning of Work.* Baltimore: Johns Hopkins University Press, 2010.
Devine, Shauna L. *Learning from the Wounded: The Civil War and the Rise of American Medical Science.* Chapel Hill: University of North Carolina Press, 2014.
Downs, Jim. *Maladies of Empire: How Colonialism, Slavery, and War Transformed Medicine.* Cambridge, MA: Belknap Press, 2021.
———. *Sick from Freedom: African-American Illness and Suffering during the Civil War and Reconstruction.* Oxford, UK: Oxford University Press, 2012.
Doyle, Don Harrison. *The Social Order of a Frontier Community: Jacksonville, Illinois, 1825–1870.* Urbana: University of Illinois Press, 1978.
Doyle, Nora. *Maternal Bodies: Redefining Motherhood in Early America.* Chapel Hill: University of North Carolina Press, 2018.
Dublin, Thomas. *Women at Work: The Transformation of Work and Community in Lowell, Massachusetts, 1826–1860.* 2nd ed. New York: Columbia University Press, 1993.
Du Bois, W. E. B. *Black Reconstruction: An Essay Toward a History of the Part Which Black Folk Played in the Attempt to Reconstruct Democracy in America, 1860–1880.* New York: Harcourt, Brace and Company, 1935.

Edwards, Rebecca. *Angels in the Machinery: Gender in American Party Politics from the Civil War to the Progressive Era*. New York: Oxford University Press, 1997.

Edwards, Richard, and Jacob K. Friefeld. *The First Migrants: How Black Homesteaders' Quest for Land and Freedom Heralded America's Great Migration*. Lincoln: University of Nebraska Press, 2023.

Egge, Sara. *Woman Suffrage and Citizenship in the Midwest, 1870–1920*. 1st ed. Iowa City: University of Iowa Press, 2018.

Eleanore, Sister M. *On the King's Highway: A History of the Sisters of the Holy Cross of St. Mary of the Immaculate Conception at Notre Dame, Indiana*. New York: D. Appleton, 1931.

Epstein, Barbara Leslie. *The Politics of Domesticity: Women, Evangelism, and Temperance*. Middletown, CT: Wesleyan University Press, 1981.

Fahs, Alice, and Joan Waugh. *The Memory of the Civil War in American Culture*. Chapel Hill: University of North Carolina Press, 2004.

Fairman, Julie, and Joan E. Lynaugh. *Critical Care Nursing: A History*. Philadelphia: University of Pennsylvania Press, 1998.

Fass, Paula S. *The End of American Childhood: A History of Parenting from Life on the Frontier to the Managed Child*. Princeton, NJ: Princeton University Press, 2016.

Faust, Drew Gilpin. *Mothers of Invention: Women and the Slaveholding South in the American Civil War*. Chapel Hill: University of North Carolina Press, 1996.

———. *This Republic of Suffering: Death and the American Civil War*. Cambridge, MA: Harvard University Press, 2008.

Fea, John. *The Bible Cause: A History of the American Bible Association*. New York: Oxford University Press, 2016.

Fett, Sharla. *Working Cures: Healing, Health, and Power on Southern Slave Plantations*. Chapel Hill: University of North Carolina Press, 2002.

Field, Corinne T. *The Struggle for Equal Adulthood: Gender, Race, Age, and the Fight for Citizenship in Antebellum America*. Chapel Hill: University of North Carolina Press, 2014.

Fischer, Marilyn, Carol Nackenoff, and Wendy Chmielewski, eds. *Jane Addams and the Practice of Democracy*. Urbana: University of Illinois Press, 2008.

Foote, Lorien. *The Gentlemen and the Roughs: Violence, Honor, and Manhood in the Union Army*. New York: New York University Press, 2010.

Gallagher, Gary W., and Joan Waugh. *The American War: A History of the Civil War Era*. State College, PA: Flip Learning, 2015.

Gangel, Kenneth O., and Warren S. Benson. *Christian Education: Its History and Philosophy*. Eugene, Oregon: Wipf and Stock Publishers, 2002.

Giesberg, Judith. *Army at Home: Women and the Civil War on the Northern Home Front*. Chapel Hill: University of North Carolina Press, 2009.

———. *Civil War Sisterhood: The United States Sanitary Commission and Women's Politics in Transition*. Lebanon, NH: Northeastern University Press, 2000.

———. "Orphans and Indians: Pennsylvania's Soldiers' Orphan Schools and the Landscape of Postwar Childhood." In *Children and Youth during the Civil War Era*, edited by James Marten. New York: New York University Press, 2012.

Ginsberg, Carlo. "Microhistory: Two or Three Things That I Know about It." In *Threads and Traces: True False Fictive*, translated by Anne C. Tedeschi and John Tedeschi. Oakland: University of California Press, 2012.

Ginzberg, Lori D. *Elizabeth Cady Stanton: An American Life.* New York: Hill and Wang, 2009.
———. *Women and the Work of Benevolence: Morality, Politics, and Class in the Nineteenth-Century United States.* New Haven, CT: Yale University Press, 1992.
Glasson, William Henry. *Federal Military Pensions in the United States.* New York: Oxford University Press, 1918.
Glymph, Thavolia. *Out of the House of Bondage: The Transformation of the Plantation Household.* New York: Cambridge University Press, 2008.
———. *The Women's Fight: The Civil War's Battles for Home, Freedom, and Nation.* Chapel Hill: University of North Carolina Press, 2020.
Gordon, Linda. *Pitied but Not Entitled: Single Mothers and the History of Welfare, 1890–1935.* New York: The Free Press, 1994.
Gorn, Elliot J. *Mother Jones: The Most Dangerous Woman in America.* New York: Farrar, Straus and Giroux, 2015.
Greene, Daniel. "Nothing Daunts Chicago: Wartime Relief on the Home Front." In *Home Front: Daily Life in the Civil War North.* Chicago: University of Chicago Press, 2013.
Guelzo, Allen C. *Lincoln and Douglas: The Debates That Defined America.* New York: Simon & Schuster, 2008.
Hackemer, Kurt. "Civil War Veteran Colonies on the Western Frontier." In *The War Went On: Reconsidering the Lives of Civil War Veterans,* edited by Evan C. Rothera and Brian Matthew Jordan. Chapel Hill: University of North Carolina Press, 2020.
Hadley-Cousins, Sarah. *Bodies in Blue: Disability in the Civil War North.* Athens: University of Georgia Press, 2019.
Hall, Richard. *Women on the Civil War Battlefront.* Lawrence: University Press of Kansas, 2006.
Haller, John S. *Medical Protestants: The Eclectics in American Medicine, 1825–1939.* Carbondale: Southern Illinois University Press, 2013.
———. *The People's Doctors: Samuel Thomson and the American Botanical Movement, 1790–1860.* Carbondale: Southern Illinois University Press, 2001.
Halttunen, Karen. *Confidence Men and Painted Women: A Study of Middle-Class Culture in America, 1830–1870.* New Haven, CT: Yale University Press, 1982.
Harbour, Jennifer R. *Organizing Freedom: Black Emancipation Activism in the Civil War Midwest.* Carbondale: Southern Illinois University Press, 2020.
Harper, Judith E. *Women during the Civil War: An Encyclopedia.* Oxford, UK: Taylor & Francis, 2003.
Hewitt, Nancy. *Radical Friend: Amy Kirby Post and Her Activist Worlds.* University of North Carolina Press, 2018.
Hodes, Martha. *The Sea Captain's Wife: A True Story of Love, Race, and War in the Nineteenth Century.* New York: W. W. Norton, 2007.
Hoffman, Beatrix Rebecca. *Health Care for Some: Rights and Rationing in the United States Since 1930.* Chicago: University of Chicago Press, 2012.
Hoganson, Kristin. *The Heartland: An American History.* New York: Penguin Press, 2019.
Hogeland, Ronald W. "Coeducation of the Sexes at Oberlin College: A Study of Social Ideas in Mid-Nineteenth-Century America." In *Education,* edited by Nancy F. Cott. Boston: De Gruyter, 1993.

Holt, Marilyn Irvin. *Children of the Western Plains: The Nineteenth-Century Experience*. Chicago: Ivan R. Dee, 2003.
———. *The Orphan Trains: Placing Out in America*. Lincoln: University of Nebraska Press, 1992.
Hulbert, Anne. *Raising America: Experts, Parents, and a Century of Advice about Children*. New York: Alfred A. Knopf, 2003.
Humphreys, Margaret. *Intensely Human: The Health of the Black Soldier in the American Civil War*. Baltimore: Johns Hopkins University Press, 2008.
———. *Marrow of Tragedy: The Health Crisis of the American Civil War*. Baltimore: Johns Hopkins University Press, 2013.
Illick, Joseph. *American Childhoods*. Philadelphia: University of Pennsylvania Press, 2002.
Jackson, Robert. *Rethinking Religious Education and Plurality: Issues in Diversity and Pedagogy*. London: Routledge, 2013.
Jacoby, Carl. *The Strange Career of William Ellis: The Texas Slave Who Became a Mexican Millionaire*. New York: W. W. Norton, 2016.
Jalland, Patricia. *Death in the Victorian Family*. Oxford, UK: Oxford University Press, 1996.
Janney, Caroline E. *Remembering the Civil War: Reunion and the Limits of Reconciliation*. Chapel Hill: University of North Carolina Press, 2013.
Johnson, Joan Marie. *Funding Feminism: Monied Women, Philanthropy, and the Women's Movement, 1870–1967*. Chapel Hill: University of North Carolina Press, 2017.
Johnson, Paul E., and Sean Wilentz. *The Kingdom of Matthias: A Story of Sex and Salvation in 19th-Century America*. New York: Oxford University Press, 1995.
Jones, Marian Moser. *The American Red Cross from Clara Barton to the New Deal*. Baltimore: Johns Hopkins University Press, 2013.
Jones-Rogers, Stephanie. *They Were Her Property: White Women as Slave Owners in the American South*. New Haven, CT: Yale University Press, 2019.
Jordan, Brian Matthew, and Evan C. Rothera, eds. *The War Went On: Reconsidering the Lives of Civil War Veterans*. Baton Rouge: University of Louisiana Press, 2020.
Kellehear, Allan. *A Social History of Dying*. New York: Cambridge University Press, 2007.
Kelly, Patrick J. *Creating a National Home: Building the Veterans' Welfare State, 1860–1900*. Cambridge: Harvard University Press, 1997.
Kerber, Linda. *No Constitutional Right to Be Ladies*. New York: Hill and Wang, 1999.
Kerber, Linda K. "Separate Spheres, Female Worlds, Woman's Place: The Rhetoric of Women's History." In *Toward an Intellectual History of Women*. Chapel Hill: University of North Carolina Press, 1997.
Kirschmann, Anne Taylor. *A Vital Force: Women in American Homeopathy*. New Brunswick: Rutgers University Press, 2004.
Ladd-Taylor, Molly. *Mother-Work: Women, Child Welfare, and the State, 1890–1930*. Urbana: University of Illinois Press, 1994.
Lauck, Jon K. *The Good County: A History of the American Midwest, 1800–1900*. Norman: University of Oklahoma Press, 2022.
Levi, Giovanni. "On Microhistory." In *New Perspectives on Historical Writing*, edited by Peter Burke. University Park: Pennsylvania State University Press, 1991.

Lewis, Jan. "Mother's Love: The Construction of an Emotion in Nineteenth-Century America." In *Mothers & Motherhood: Readings in American History*, edited by Rima D. Apple and Janet Golden. Columbus: Ohio State University Press, 1997.

Limerick, Patricia Nelson. *The Legacy of Conquest: The Unbroken Past of the American West*. New York: W. W. Norton, 1987.

Linderman, Gerald. *Embattled Courage: The Experience of Combat in the American Civil War*. New York: The Free Press, 1987.

Litvin, Martin. *The Young Mary, 1817–1861: Early Years of Mother Bickerdyke, America's Florence Nightingale, and Patron Saint of Kansas*. Galesburg, IL: Log City Books, 1976.

Lüdtke, Alf. *The History of Everyday Life: Reconstructing Historical Experiences and Ways of Life*. Princeton, NJ: Princeton University Press, 1995.

Mahoney, Timothy R. *From Hometown to Battlefield in the Civil War Era: Middle Class Life in Midwest America*. Cambridge, UK: Cambridge University Press, 2016.

Marszalek, John F. *Sherman: A Soldier's Passion for Order*. New York: Free Press, 1993.

Marten, James. *Children for the Union: The War Spirit on the Northern Home Front*. New York: Ivan R. Dee, 2004.

———. *The Children's Civil War*. Chapel Hill: University of North Carolina Press, 1999.

Masarik, Elizabeth Garner. *The Sentimental State: How Women-Led Reform Built the American Welfare State*. Athens: University of Georgia Press, 2024.

Massey, Mary Elizabeth. *Bonnet Brigades*. New York: Alfred A. Knopf, 1966.

———. *Women in the Civil War*. Lincoln: University of Nebraska Press, 1994.

Masur, Louis P. *The Civil War: A Concise History*. New York: Oxford University Press, 2011.

McCarthy, Kathleen D. *Lady Bountiful Revisited: Women, Philanthropy, and Power*. New Brunswick, NJ: Rutgers University Press, 1990.

McClellan, B. Edward. *Moral Education in America: Schools and the Shaping of Character from Colonial Times to the Present*. New York: Teachers College Press, 1999.

McCurry, Stephanie. *Women's War: Fighting and Surviving the American Civil War*. Cambridge, MA: Harvard University Press, 2019.

McHenry, Elizabeth. *Forgotten Readers: Recovering the Lost History of African American Literary Societies*. Durham, NC: Duke University Press, 2002.

McKown, Robin. *Heroic Nurses*. New York: Putnam, 1966.

Meredith, Robert. *The Politics of the Universe: Edward Beecher, Abolition, and Orthodoxy*. Nashville, TN: Vanderbilt Press, 1968.

Michel, Sonya. "The Limits of Maternalism: Policies toward American Wage-Earning Mothers during the Progressive Era." In *Mothers of a New World: Maternalist Politics and the Origins of Welfare States*, edited by Sonya Michel and Seth Koven. New York: Rutledge, 1993.

Michel, Sonya, and Seth Koven, eds. *Mothers of a New World: Maternalist Politics and the Origins of Welfare States*. New York: Routledge, 1993.

Mink, Gwendolyn. *The Wages of Motherhood: Inequality in the Welfare State, 1917–1942*. Ithaca, NY: Cornell University Press, 1995.

Mintz, Steven. *Huck's Raft: A History of American Childhood*. Cambridge, MA: Harvard University Press, 2004.

Mintz, Steven, and Susan Kellogg. *Domestic Revolutions: A Social History of American Family Life*. New York: Free Press, 1988.

Morantz-Sanchez, Regina. *Sympathy and Science: Women Physicians in American Medicine.* Chapel Hill: University of North Carolina Press, 1985.
Moss, Hilary J. *Schooling Citizens: The Struggle for African American Education in Antebellum American.* Chicago: University of Chicago Press, 2009.
Neff, John R. *Honoring the Civil War Dead: Commemoration and the Problem of Reconciliation.* Lawrence: University of Kansas Press, 2005.
Nelson, Scott Reynolds. *Steel Driving Man: John Henry, the Untold Story of an American Legend.* New York: Oxford University Press, 2009.
Noll, Mark A. *The Scandal of the Evangelical Mind.* Grand Rapids, MI: William B. Erdman's Publishing, 1994.
Norton, Mary Beth. *Founding Mothers & Fathers: Gendered Power and the Forming of American Society.* New York: Vintage, 1997.
———. *Separated by Their Sex: Women in Public and Private in the Colonial Atlantic World.* Ithaca, NY: Cornell University Press, 2011.
Oates, Stephen B. *A Woman of Valor: Clara Barton and the Civil War.* New York: Free Press, 1994.
Painter, Nell Irvin. *Exodusters: Black Migration to Kansas after Reconstruction.* New York: W. W. Norton, 1977.
Pascoe, Peggy. *What Comes Naturally: Miscegenation Law and the Making of Race in America.* New York: Oxford University Press, 2009.
Pope, Clayne L. "Adult Mortality in America before 1900: A View from Family Histories." In *Strategic Factors in Nineteenth-Century American Economic History: A Volume to Honor Robert W. Fogel,* edited by Claudia Goldin and Hugh Rockoff. Chicago: University of Chicago Press, 1992.
Reverby, Susan M. *Ordered to Care: The Dilemma of American Nursing 1850–1945.* Cambridge, UK: Cambridge University Press, 1987.
Rockman, Seth. *Scraping By: Wage Labor, Slavery, and Survival in Early Baltimore.* Baltimore: Johns Hopkins University Press, 2009.
Rosenberg, Charles. *The Care of Strangers: The Rise of America's Hospital System.* New York: Basic Books, 1988.
Rothman, David J. *Strangers at the Bedside: A History of How Law and Bioethics Transformed Medical Decision Making.* New York: Basic Books, 1991.
Royster, Jacqueline Jones. *Traces of a Stream: Literacy and Social Change among African American Women.* Pittsburgh, PA: University of Pittsburgh, 2000.
Ryan, Mary P. *Cradle of the Middle Class: The Family in Oneida County, New York, 1790–1865.* New York: Cambridge University Press, 1981.
Schantz, Mark S. *Awaiting the Heavenly Country: The Civil War and America's Culture of Death.* Ithaca, NY: Cornell University Press, 2008.
Schmidt, James D. *Industrial Violence and the Legal Origins of Child Labor.* New York: Cambridge University Press, 2010.
Schultz, Jane E. *Women at the Front: Hospital Workers in Civil War America.* Chapel Hill: University of North Carolina Press, 2004.
Silber, Nina. *Daughters of the Union: Northern Women Fight the Civil War.* Cambridge, MA: Harvard University Press, 2005.

Silber, Nina, and Catherine Clinton. *Divided Houses: Gender and the Civil War*. New York: Oxford University Press, 1992.
Sizer, Lyde Cullen. *The Political Work of Northern Women Writers and the Civil War, 1850–1872*. Chapel Hill: University of North Carolina Press, 2003.
Sklar, Kathryn Kish. *Catharine Beecher: A Study in American Domesticity*. New Haven, CT: Yale University Press, 1973.
———. *Florence Kelley and the Nation's Work*. New Haven, CT: Yale University Press, 1995.
Skocpol, Theda. *Protecting Soldiers and Mothers: The Political Origins of Social Policy in the United States*. Cambridge, MA: Harvard University Press, 1995.
Smith, Katy Simpson. *We Have Raised All of You: Motherhood in the South, 1750–1835*. Baton Rouge: Louisiana State University Press, 2013.
Smith, Timothy B. *Rethinking Shiloh: Myth and Memory*. Knoxville: University of Tennessee Press, 2013.
Smith-Rosenberg, Carroll. *Religion and the Rise of the American City: The New York City Mission Movement, 1812–1870*. Ithaca, NY: Cornell University Press, 1971.
Starr, Paul. *The Social Transformation of American Medicine: The Rise of a Sovereign Profession and the Making of a Vast Industry*. New York: Basic Books, 1982.
Szijártó, Istvan M. *What Is Microhistory? Theory and Practice*. New York: Rutledge, 2013.
Taylor, Amy Murrell. *Embattled Freedom: Journeys through the Civil War's Slave Refugee Camps*. Chapel Hill: University of North Carolina Press, 2018.
Tetrault, Lisa. *The Myth of Seneca Falls: Memory and the Women's Suffrage Movement, 1848–1898*. Chapel Hill: University of North Carolina Press, 2014.
Trouillot, Michel-Rolph. *Silencing the Past: Power and the Production of History*. New York: Beacon Press, 1995.
Tsui, Bonnie. *She Went to the Field: Women Soldiers of the Civil War*. Guilford, CT: TwoDot, 2006.
Tucker, Spencer C. *Unconditional Surrender: The Capture of Forts Henry and Donelson*. Abilene, TX: McWhiney Foundation Press, 2001.
Ulrich, Laurel Thatcher. *A Midwife's Tale: The Life of Martha Ballard, Based on Her Diary, 1785–1812*. New York: Alfred A. Knopf, 1990.
Valenčius, Conevery Bolton. *The Health of the Country: How American Settlers Understood Themselves and Their Land*. New York: Basic Books, 2002.
Vandenberg-Daves, Jodi. *Modern Motherhood: An American History*. New Brunswick, NJ: Rutgers University Press, 2014.
Vanderpool, Harold Y. *Palliative Care: The 400-Year Quest for a Good Death*. Jefferson, NC: McFarland, 2015.
Vapnek, Lara. *Breadwinners: Working Women and Economic Independence, 1865–1920*. Urbana: University of Illinois Press, 2009.
Varon, Elizabeth R. *Armies of Deliverance: A New History of the Civil War*. New York: Oxford University Press, 2019.
Warner, John Harley. *Against the Spirit of System: The French Impulse in Nineteenth-Century American Medicine*. Princeton, NJ: Princeton University Press, 1998.
———. *The Therapeutic Perspective: Medical Practice, Knowledge, and Identity in America, 1820–1885*. Princeton, NJ: Princeton University Press, 1997.

Weiner, Lynn Y. *From Working Girl to Working Mother: The Female Labor Force in the United States, 1820–1980*. Chapel Hill: University of North Carolina Press, 1985.
West, Elliott. *Growing Up with the Country: Children on the Far Western Frontier*. Albuquerque: University of New Mexico Press, 1989.
Whelan, Jean C. *Nursing the Nation: Building the Nurse Labor Force*. New Brunswick, NJ: Rutgers University Press, 2021.
White, Barbara Anne. *The Beecher Sisters*. New Haven, CT: Yale University Press, 2003.
White, Deborah Gray. *Too Heavy a Load: Black Women in Defense of Themselves*. New York: W. W. Norton, 1999.
Wills, Brian Steel. *Inglorious Passages: Noncombat Deaths in the American Civil War*. Lawrence: University Press of Kansas, 2017.
Woodworth, Stephen E., ed. "Introduction." In *The Shiloh Campaign*. Carbondale: Southern Illinois University Press, 2009.
Wosh, Peter J. *Spreading the Word: The Bible Business in Nineteenth-Century America*. Ithaca, NY: Cornell University Press, 1994.
Yarbrough, Fay A. *Race and the Cherokee Nation: Sovereignty in the Nineteenth Century*. Philadelphia: University of Pennsylvania Press, 2008.
Young, Alfred F. *The Shoemaker and the Tea Party: Memory and the American Revolution*. Boston: Beacon Press, 2000.
Welter, Barbara. *Dimity Convictions: The American Woman in the Nineteenth Century*. Athens: Ohio University Press, 1976.

JOURNAL ARTICLES AND DISSERTATIONS

Abel, John H., and LaWanda Cox. "Andrew Johnson and His Ghost Writers: An Analysis of the Freedmen's Bureau and Civil Rights Veto Messages." *Mississippi Valley Historical Review* 48, no. 3 (1961): 460–79.
Albisetti, James C. "The Fight for Female Physicians in Imperial Germany." *Central European History* 15, no. 2 (1982): 99–123.
Barnhart, Terry A. "'A Common Feeling': Regional Identity and Historical Consciousness in the Old Northwest, 1820–1860." *Michigan Historical Review* (2003): 39–70.
Bell, Clark. "Medical Jurisprudence in America in the Nineteenth Century." *Texas Medical Journal* 16, no. 5 (1900): 201–9.
Bender, Robert Patrick. "Old Boss Devil: Sectionalism, Charity, and the Rivalry between the Western Sanitary Commission and the United States Sanitary Commission during the Civil War." PhD diss., University of Arkansas at Fayetteville, 2001.
Blake, Kellee. "'First in the Path of the Firemen': The Fate of the 1890 Population Census, Part 1." *Prologue: Quarterly of the National Archives and Records Administration* 28, no. 1 (Spring 1996). https://www.archives.gov/publications/prologue/1996/spring/1890-census.
Brace, Susan. "Consecrated by Sorrow: Mary Ann Bickerdyke, The War Years, 1861–1865." PhD diss., Institute of Contemporary Psychoanalysis, 1997.
Brevetti, Melissa. "Building Moral Bridges: The Childhood Experiences of Women Who Attended Parochial Schools in the 1950s and 1960s and the Role of the Theory of Care Which Shaped Families and Communities." *Journal of Thought* 54 (2020): 23–39.
Buchkoski, Courtney. "'Luke-Warm Abolitionists': Eli Thayer and the Contest for Civil War Memory, 1853–1899." *Journal of the Civil War Era* 9, no. 2 (2019): 249–74.

Campney, Brent M. S. "'Light Is Bursting upon the World!': White Supremacy and Racist Violence against Blacks in Reconstruction Kansas." *Western Historical Quarterly* 41, no. 2 (2010): 171–94.

Chappell, Marisa. "Protecting Soldiers and Mothers Twenty-Five Years Later: Theda Skocpol's Legacy and American Welfare State Historiography, 1992–2017." *Journal of the Gilded Age and Progressive Era* 17, no. 3 (2018): 546–73.

Cohn, Raymond L. "Nativism and the End of the Mass Migration of the 1840s and 1850s." *Journal of Economic History* 60, no. 2 (2000): 361–83.

Cronon, William. "A Place for Stories: Nature, History, and Narrative." *Journal of American History* 78, no. 4 (1992): 1347–76.

Culpepper, Marilyn Mayer, and Pauline Gordon Adams. "Nursing in the Civil War." *American Journal of Nursing* 88 (July 1988): 981–86.

Dinger, Steven C. "'The Doctors in This Region Don't Know Much': Medicine and Obstetrics in Mormon Nauvoo." *Journal of Mormon History* 42, no. 4 (2016): 51–68.

Eli, Shari, Laura Salisbury, and Allison Shertzer. "Ideology and Migration after the American Civil War." *Journal of Economic History* 78, no. 3 (September 2018): 822–61.

Erlandson, E. V. "The Story of Mother Bickerdyke." *American Journal of Nursing* 20, no. 8 (1920): 628–31.

Fairchild, James H. *Co-education of the Sexes as Pursued in Oberlin College*. College paper, 1868.

Fairman, Julie, and Patricia D'Antonio. "Reimagining Nursing's Place in the History of Clinical Practice." *Journal of the History of Medicine and Allied Sciences* 63, no. 4 (2008): 435–46.

Fischer, Leroy H. "Cairo's Civil War Angel, Mary Jane Safford." *Journal of the Illinois State Historical Society (1908–1984)* 54, no. 3 (1961): 229–45.

Flannery, Michael A. "The Early Botanical Medical Movement as a Reflection of Life, Liberty, and Literacy in Jacksonian America." *Journal of the Medical Library Association* 90, no. 4 (2002): 442–54.

Gardner, Sarah E. "When Service Is Not Enough: Charity's Purpose in the Immediate Aftermath of the Civil War." *Journal of the Civil War Era* 9, no. 1 (2019): 29–54.

Goggin, Jacqueline. "Challenging Sexual Discrimination in the Historical Profession: Women Historians and the American Historical Association, 1890–1940." *American Historical Review* 97, no. 3 (1992): 769–802.

Graff, Harvey J. "The Literacy Myth: Literacy, Education and Demography." *Vienna Yearbook of Population Research* 8 (2010): 17–23.

Green, Abigail. "Humanitarianism in Nineteenth-Century Context: Religious, Gendered, National." *Historical Journal* 57, no. 4 (2014): 1157–75.

Gregory, Brad S. "Is Small Beautiful? Microhistory and the History of Everyday Life." *History and Theory* 38, no. 1 (1999): 100–111.

Haines, Michael. "Fertility and Mortality in the United States." EH.Net Encyclopedia, edited by Robert Whaples. March 19, 2008.

Hamerow, Theodore S. "The Professionalization of Historical Learning." *Reviews in American History* 14, no. 3 (1986): 319–33.

Hilde, Libra Rose. "Worth a Dozen Men: Women, Nursing, and Medical Care during the American Civil War." PhD diss., Harvard University, 2003.

Hudson, Angela Pulley. "The Indian Doctress in the Nineteenth-Century United States: Race, Medicine, and Labor." *Journal of Social History* 54, no. 4 (2021): 1160–87.
Kastcher, Leopold. "Owen's Topolobampo Colony, Mexico." *American Journal of Sociology* 12, no. 2 (1906): 145–75.
LaPointe, Patricia M. "Military Hospitals in Memphis, 1861–1865." *Tennessee Historical Quarterly* 42, no. 4 (1983): 325–42.
Lepore, Jill. "Historians Who Love Too Much: Reflections on Microhistory and Biography." *Journal of American History* 88, no. 1 (2001): 129–44.
Lynaugh, Joan E. "Nursing the Great Society: The Impact of the Nurse Training Act of 1964." *Nursing Historical Review* (2008): 13–28.
Mahoney, Deirdre M. "'More Than an Accomplishment': Advice on Letter Writing for Nineteenth-Century American Women." *Huntington Library Quarterly* 66, nos. 3/4 (2003): 411–23.
Marten, James. "For the Good, the True, and the Beautiful: Northern Children's Magazines and the Civil War." *Civil War History* 41, no. 1 (1995): 57–75.
Matherly, Sarah Copenhaver. "'The Age of Associated Effort': Communitarian Reform at Topolobampo, Mexico, 1872–1896." PhD diss., Princeton University, 2019.
May, Ernest R. "Ghost Writing and History." *American Scholar* 22, no. 4 (1953): 459–65.
McCall, Laura. "'The Reign of Brute Force Is Now Over': A Content Analysis of 'Godey's Lady's Book,' 1830–1860." *Journal of the Early Republic* 9, no. 2 (1989): 217–36.
McClintock, Megan J. "Civil War Pensions and the Reconstruction of Union Families." *Journal of American History* 83, no. 2 (1996): 456–80.
McDonald, Jeanne Gillespie. "Edward Beecher and the Anti-Slavery Movement in Illinois." *Journal of the Illinois State Historical Society* 105, no. 1 (2012): 9–35.
Metheny, Hannah. "'For a Woman': The Fight for Pensions for Civil War Army Nurses." Undergraduate thesis, College of William & Mary, 2013.
Monahan, Thomas P. "Interracial Marriage and Divorce in Kansas and the Question of Instability of Mixed Marriages." *Journal of Comparative Family Studies* 2, no. 1 (1971): 107–20.
Monteiro, Lois A. "On Separate Roads: Florence Nightingale and Elizabeth Blackwell." *Signs* 9, no. 3 (1984): 520–33.
Muelder, Hermann R. "Galesburg: Hot-Bed of Abolitionism." *Journal of the Illinois State Historical Society (1908–1984)* 35, no. 3 (1942): 216–35.
Muhammad, Gholnecsar E. "The Literacy Development and Practices within African American Literary Societies." *Black History Bulletin* 75, no. 1 (2012): 6–13.
Nolen, Anita Lonnes. "The Feminine Presence: Women's Papers in the Manuscript Division." *Quarterly Journal of the Library of Congress* 32, no. 4 (1975): 348–65.
Norman, Matthew. "The Other Lincoln-Douglas Debate: The Race Issue in a Comparative Context." *Journal of the Abraham Lincoln Association* 31, no. 1 (2010): 1–21.
Novak, William J. "The Myth of the 'Weak' American State." *American Historical Review* 113, no. 3 (2008): 752–72.
Olney, James. "'I Was Born': Slave Narratives, Their Status as Autobiography and as Literature." *Callaloo*, no. 20 (1984): 46–73.
Pace, James, and Beverly Lunsford. "The Evolution of Palliative Care Nursing Education." *Journal of Hospice & Palliative Nursing* 13, no. 6 (November 2011): S8–S19.

Patterson, Jean A., Kathryn A. Mickelson, Jan L. Petersen, and Diane S. Gross. "Educating for Success: The Legacy of an All-Black School in Southeast Kansas." *Journal of Negro Education* 77, no. 4 (2008): 306–22.

Peterson, Lindsey R. "'Home-Builders': Free Labor Households and Settler Colonialism in Western Union Civil War Commemorations." *Journal of the Civil War Era* 15, no. 1 (2025): 33–54.

Randall, J. G. "Has the Lincoln Theme Been Exhausted?" *American Historical Review* 41, no. 2 (1936): 270–94.

Riley, Glenda. "Frederick Jackson Turner Overlooked the Ladies." *Journal of the Early Republic* 13, no. 2 (1993): 216–30.

Roberts, Richard. "Reversible Social Processes, Historical Memory, and the Production of History." *History in Africa* 17 (1990): 341–49.

Ross, Catherine J. "Families without Paradigms: Child Poverty and Out-of-Home Placement in Historical Perspective." *Ohio State Law Journal* 60 (Winter 1999): 1249–93.

Schultz, Jane E. "The Inhospitable Hospital: Gender and Professionalism in Civil War Medicine." *Signs* 17, no. 2 (1992): 363–92.

———. "Seldom Thanked, Never Praised, and Scarcely Recognized: Gender and Racism in Civil War Hospitals." *Civil War History* 48, no. 3 (2002): 220–36.

Senese, Gail. "Sarah Josepha Hale and Ladies' Magazine: A Reconstructed Image." PhD diss., University of Wyoming, 2003.

Silber, Nina. "Introductory Remarks: The Study of Gender and the Civil War." Society for Civil War Historians Conference, September 28, 2021.

Skocpol, Theda. "America's First Social Security System: The Expansion of Benefits for Civil War Veterans." *Political Science Quarterly* 108, no. 1 (1993): 85–116.

Small, Neil. "Social Work and Palliative Care." *British Journal of Social Work* 31, no. 6 (2001): 961–71.

Thomas, Richard Harlan. "Jenkin Lloyd Jones: Lincoln's Soldier of Civic Righteousness." PhD diss., Rutgers University, 1967.

Torreno, Evie. "The Art and Politics of Chicago's Sanitary Fairs." *Chicago History* (2015): 4–23.

Venet, Wendy Hamand. "The Emergence of a Suffragist: Mary Livermore, Civil War Activism, and the Moral Power of Women." *Civil War History* 48, no. 2 (2002): 143–64.

Ware, Susan. "The Book I Couldn't Write: Alice Paul and the Challenge of Feminist Biography." *Journal of Women's History* 24, no. 2 (2012): 13–36.

———. "Writing Women's Lives: One Historian's Perspective." *Journal of Interdisciplinary History* 40, no. 3 (2010): 413–35.

Welter, Barbara. "The Cult of True Womanhood: 1820–1860." *American Quarterly* 18 (Summer 1966): 151–74.

Whittelsey, Samuel, and William Williams. *The Mother's Magazine*. Edited by Abigail Goodrich Whittelsey. 1833–1849.

Wood, Ann Douglas. "The War within a War: Women Nurses in the Union Army." *Civil War History* 18, no. 3 (1972): 197–212.

Young, Alfred F. "George Roberts Twelves Hewes (1742–1840): A Boston Shoemaker and the Memory of the American Revolution." *William and Mary Quarterly* 38, no. 4 (October 1981): 561–623.

# Index

*Page numbers in italics refer to illustrations.*

Abbott, Amelia, 64–67
Abbott, Sherman, 64, *66*
abolitionism, 24–25, 81
Adams, Lemuel, 47
Allen, Sue, 166–67
amanuenses, 50, 116, 118, 162, 191n24, 204n29. *See also* Foster, Lydia
American Tract Society of Chicago, 106–7
Arapahoe people, 107
Army Nurses Pension Act (1892), 58, 139, 145
*As I Knew Her* (Kellogg), 179–181

Baker, Nina Brown, 27–28
Ball, Mary. *See* Bickerdyke, Mary Ann "Mother"
Battle of Belmont, 47
Battle of Fort Donelson, 47–48, 196n33; Bickerdyke's midnight rescue at, 50–53, 58–60, *61*; civilian response to, 53
Battle of Shiloh, 62
Beecher, Catharine, 14, 185
Beecher, Edward, 24
Beecher, Henry Ward, 24–25
Bellows, Henry, 82, 114, *115*
Bickerdyke, Hiram, *36*; adult life of, 125; early life of, 17, 34–36; education of, 79, 82–83; hieroglyphs by, *187*; and Mary Ann (mother), 83, 84–85, 177–78
Bickerdyke, James "J. R.", *35*; adult life of, 125, 132; death of, 177–78; early life of, 17, 34–36; education of, 79, 82–83; mother of, xiii, 83–85, 167–74, 177
Bickerdyke, Mary Ann "Mother", *2–3*, *45*; care-switching by, 31–38, 82–83, 112; Carleton's poetic ode to, 170–74; early life and family of, 14–17, 192n10, 200n45; early work life of, 20–23, 25–31; Foster and, 10, 12–13, 164–66, 180; funeral and burial of, 166–69; in Galesburg life Civil War, 23–25; historical remembrances of, 169–74, 179–82; independent postwar work of, 113–19; institutional care for children by, 91, 94–103; Kansas hotel and community aid work of, 103–11, 113; legacy of, 4, 166, 174–82; marriage and family life of, 17–20; maternal expediency of, 85–93; pension of and advocacy work by, 10, 135–54; postwar palliative care by, 97, 101, 112, 119–20, 129–32, 157, 172, 180–81; religion and, 19, 24, 33, 180, 193n62; socioeconomic conditions of, 78–84; statues of, xi, *xii*, *xiv*; USSC work by, xi, 28, 39, 70–71, 100–101, 197n70; wartime palliative care by, 3, 11, 12, 40–41, 50, 53, 63; working motherhood and maternal identity of, 5–10, 78–85
Bickerdyke, Mary "Mollie," *34*, 125–34, *133*
Bickerdyke, Robert, 17–19, 21, 166, 192n17
Bickerdyke Hotel, 105–11, 113
Black literacy rates, *160*. *See also* literacy
Black migration and families, 158–59. *See also* western migration
Black refugees, 69, 70–72, 84–85
Black women's marginalization, 10, 12–13, 164–66, 180. *See also* Black migration and families; Black refugees
Bolton, Thomas, 150–52
Boston Training School, 55
botanic remedies, 21–23, 63–67
*The Boys in Blue* (Hoge), 40, 54

British medical care model, 55–57
Brockett, L. P., 36, 74–75
Brown, Mahala, 159–60
Brown, Mary A., 159–60
Brown, Sarah, 159–60
*Bulletin of the Sanitary Commission* (pamphlet), 88
Burns, Ken, xiv–xv, 74. See also *The Civil War* (PBS series)
Burns, Robert, 170

Cairo, IL, 25–28, 42–47, 78–79
cancer, 125–26, 133
caregiving work, domestic, 16–17, 20, 29
care-switching, 31–38, 82–83, 112
Carleton, Will, 170–74
Chase, Julia, 174–76, 178, 180
Cheyenne people, 107
Chicago, Burlington, and Quincy Railroad, 104
Chicago Sanitary Commission, 39, 46, 52, 77, 82. See also US Sanitary Commission (USSC)
Chicago World's Fair, 155–56
children: age of innocence of, 37; guardianship of, 94, 96–97, 107–8, 146–53; institutional care for, 2, 91, 94–103
Christian Commission, 91
Cincinnati, OH, 14, 128, 129
*The Civil War* (television series), xiii–xv, 74. See also Burns, Ken
Clark, George Washington, 171
Connecticut Training School, 55
Cook, Eliza, 147–50
Cook, James H., 146–50
Cow and Hen Tour, 76–78
Crimean War, 56–57
cult of domesticity, 7–8
cult of true womanhood, 14
*Cyclone in Calico* (Baker), 27–29

Darley, F. O. C., 59
Davis, Caleb C., 141
death expectations, 4, 48–50

Dependent Pension Act (1890), 138, 153
diet and illness recovery, 76, 87–89
Dix, Dorothea, xi, 5, 57, 91, 117
Duffield, George, 116

Eastman family, 122
education, 79, 82–83

Foster, Eliza and Wesley, 158–159; interracial marriage of, 213n16
Foster, Lydia, 10, 12–13, 157–66, 180, 191n24, 214n31; family of, 158

Galesburg Academy of Music, 18, 19
Galesburg Congregational Church, 19, 24
Gayoso Hospital, 71–72, 76. See also Memphis, TN
gendered authority, 41–47
ghostwriters, 50, 116, 118, 162, 191n24, 204n29. See also Foster, Lydia
Goslin, A., 143
Grand Army of the Republic (GAR), 140–41, 156, 167
Grant, Ulysses S., 39, 47–48, 62, 70, 93
grasshopper plague, 107–10, 117
grief: of Bickerdyke, 20, 23, 132, 134, 167; social practices and, 49, 85, 94
guardianship of children, 94, 96–97, 107–8, 146–53. See also institutional care for children; maternal care; orphans

Hale, Sarah Josepha, 80, 185
Hayward, Laura A., 104
health campaign, 76
Henshaw, Sarah, 52–53, 62
historical remembrances, 156–57, 166, 169–82, 218n121
Hoge, Jane, 36, 39, 53, 54, 70, 81, 82
Home for the Friendless, 94, 95, 202n2. See also institutional care for children
hospitals: in Cairo, IL, 42, 43, 47; Gayoso Hospital, 71–72, 76; hospital ships, 51, 53–55, 197n67; modern East Coast, 17; wartime field, xiii, 2, 27, 31, 43

H.R. 700 (1886), 142
Hurlbut, Stephen A., 73, 75

Illinois Sanitary Commission, 76, 77
Illinois Soldiers' Orphans' Home, xiii, 95, 97–103, 111, 113, 204n32, 204nn31–32. *See also* institutional care for children; orphanages
Indigenous land dispossession, 107
insect plagues, 108–10, 117
institutional care for children, 2, 91, 94–103. *See also* Home for the Friendless; Illinois Soldiers' Orphans' Home
Irwin, Bernard J. D., 73
"I Would Not Live Alway" (hymn), 168–69

Janes, Theodore B., 122
Jones, Jenkin Lloyd, 9, 155–56, 180, 181–82

Kansas Constitution (1859), 158
Kansas State Historical Society, 175, 176, 178
Kellogg, Florence Shaw, 179–81
Kitson, Theo Alice Ruggles, xi
Knapp, Frederick N., 139–40, 141–42
Knox College, 116

"Lady with the Lamp" trope, 55, 57. *See also* Nightingale, Florence
laundry operations, 70–72
Leebrich, Elizabeth, 139
Liegenspeck, Emma, 95
Lincoln, Abraham, 23–24, 57
literacy, 80, 82, *160*
Livermore, Mary, xi; memoir by, 59–60, 180; reform work by, 108, 142; social service work by, 54, 70, 94; socioeconomic condition of, 29, 36, 81; wartime activism by, 81, 88–89
Long, Alice, 183–84
Longfellow, Henry Wadsworth, 56–57

Magee, Lottie, 123
Magee, William J., 123

male physicians' authority, 41–47, 80. *See also* medical care; physicians and medical care
marriage, 158, 214n16
Martin, George W., 176, 179
*Mary A. Bickerdyke, "Mother"* (Chase), 174–77
maternal care: authority and US military, 70–78; expediency of, vs. USSC, 85–93; at home and at war, 78–85; mother-guardian role, 94–111; mother-nurse role, 2, 112–34, 195n15; specialized, 63–67. *See also* Bickerdyke, Mary Ann "Mother"; motherhood, cultural meaning of; palliative care; wartime medicine
maternal guardianship. *See* guardianship of children
McCagg, E. B., 88, 90–91, 100–101
medical care: botanic remedies, 21–23, 63; financial compensation for, 78–80; on hospital ships, 54–55, 197n67; male vs. female authority in, 41–47, 80. *See also* maternal care; palliative care; wartime medicine
Medical College of Ohio, 30
medical education system, 4, 190n5
medical sovereignty, 119–24
memorial hymn card, *137*
Memphis, TN, 70–72, 78; Gayoso Hospital, 71–72, 76
"Midnight on the Battlefield" (illustration), 59, *61*
migration, 70–71, 84–85, 103–5, 158–59
milk, 76, 196n45. *See also* Cow and Hen Tour
monuments, xi, *xii, xiv*
Morris Husband, Mary, 138–39, 140
Mother Bickerdyke Home and Hospital, 183
Mother Bickerdyke Memorial Association, xi, xiii, 169
Mother Bickerdyke Memorial Cemetery, 184
mother-guardian role, 94–111. *See also* motherhood, cultural meaning of
motherhood, cultural meaning of, 1–2, 4, 5–6, 10, 13, 187–88. *See also* Bickerdyke, Mary Ann "Mother"; maternal care
"Mother knows best" (phrase), 1, 190n1

mother-nurse role, 112–34. *See also* motherhood, cultural meaning of; nurses

"Must Jesus Bear the Cross Alone?" (hymn), 136

*My Story of the War* (Livermore), 59–60, 180

*New Guide to Health; or Botanic Family Physician* (Thomson), 21, 22

New York Training School, 55

Nicholson, Harmon, 152–53

Nicholson, Lucy, 152–53

Nightingale, Florence, 9, 55–56, 61

nurses: Civil War, xi, *xii*, 52–53, 68, 92, 145, 183–84; nurse-mother role, 2, 112–34, 195n15; pensions for, 135, 138–39. *See also* Dix, Dorothea; Leebrich, Elizabeth; maternal care; Morris Husband, Mary; private nursing work; Richards, Augusta M.; Safford, Mary Jane; Stopes, Amanda; Tolam, Ellen S.

Oberlin College, 29, 193n61

orphanages, 20, 37, 54, 78; Illinois Soldiers' Orphans' Home, xiii, 95, 97–103, 111, 113, 204n32, 204nn31–32. *See also* institutional care for children; orphans

orphans, 91, 94–103, 203n11, 203n13, 203n17. *See also* guardianship of children

palliative care: medical establishment of, 122; by Bickerdyke after war, 97, 101, 112, 119–24, 129–32, 157, 172, 180–81; Bickerdyke during war, 3, 11, 12, 40–41, 50, 53, 63. *See also* maternal care; medical care; private nursing work; wartime medicine

"The Passing of the Mother" (poem), 172–73

patriotic domesticity, 31–34, 36–37

pension acquisition and advocacy work, 10, 135–54, 158, 209n6

physicians and medical care: botanicism, 21–23; education in, 4, 190n5; male authority in, 41–47, 80, 143. *See also* Mussey, Reuben D.; Woodward, Benjamin

plague, 108–10, 117

Porter, Eliza Chappell, 78–79, 81, 82, 87, 90

power of production, 156. *See also* Trouillot, Michel-Rolph

private nursing work, 119–24. *See also* palliative care

public motherhood, 39–41

railroads and western migration, 103–4

religious faith, 19, 24, 33, 180, 193n62

Republican Party, 23–24

Richards, William, 147–48, 211n52

Rogers, Henry, 48, 50

Safford, Mary Jane, 42–43, 44, 78–79

Salina, KS, 103–4; Bickerdyke's hotel in, 104, *106*, 107; development of, 105–7; "Indian raids" in 1868, 107, 108, 113, 175, 176, 177, 178

"Santa Filomena" (Longfellow), 56–57

Sherman, William T., 75, 85, 93, 100, 107

*Songs of Two Centuries* (Carleton), 171, 173

Stanton, Elizabeth Cady, 163

Starkweather family, 16

statues, xi, *xii*, *xiv*

Stopes, Amanda, 139

Swift's Specific (treatment), 126, 127

Temmen, Catharine E., *128*, 128–29

temperance hotel, 105–11, 113

Thomson, Samuel, 21, 22

Trouillot, Michel-Rolph, 156, 161–62

US Census, 82

US Pension Bureau, 149, 158

US Sanitary Commission (USSC), 115; Bickerdyke's work and, xi, 28, 39, 70–71, 100–101, 197n70; as organization, 41–42, 46; women's work in, 32, 56. *See also* Chicago Sanitary Commission

Vaughan, Mary, 36, 74–75

vegetable rations, 87–89

Vicksburg Memorial Park, xi

Wagstaff, Dan, 175, 176–77
wartime activism, 76–78, 80–81
wartime medicine: by Bickerdyke, 31–63, 91–93; Nightingale's model of, 55–58. *See also* maternal care; medical care; nurses; palliative care
Webb-Peck, Anna, 62
Weeks, George, 64
western migration, 103–5. *See also* Black migration and families
Western Sanitary Commission (WSC), 76–77, 143
White House Conference on the Care of Dependent Children (1909), 203n12

Wittenmyer, Annie, 203n17
*Woman's Work in the Civil War* (Brockett and Vaughn), 40, 74–75
*The Woman Who Battled for the Boys in Blue* (Burton), 58
Women's Relief Corps (WRC), 141, 157, 166–67, 169, 174–75, 183
*Women's War* (McCurry), 7
Woodward, Amanda, 26
Woodward, Benjamin, 25–29, 36–37, 195n12

Yates, Richard, xiii, 99–100
Yeatman, James, 77, 143

www.ingramcontent.com/pod-product-compliance
Lightning Source LLC
Chambersburg PA
CBHW021854230426
43671CB00006B/380